Respiratory Tract Infections: Advances in Diagnosis, Management and Prevention

Respiratory Tract Infections: Advances in Diagnosis, Management and Prevention

Edited by Richard Dempsey

AMERICAN
MEDICAL PUBLISHERS
www.americanmedicalpublishers.com

American Medical Publishers,
41 Flatbush Avenue,
1st Floor, New York,
NY 11217, USA

Visit us on the World Wide Web at:
www.americanmedicalpublishers.com

ISBN: 978-1-63927-467-3

Cataloging-in-Publication Data

Respiratory tract infections : advances in diagnosis, management and prevention / edited by Richard Dempsey.
p. cm.
Includes bibliographical references and index.
ISBN 978-1-63927-467-3
1. Respiratory infections. 2. Respiratory infections--Diagnosis. 3. Respiratory infections--Treatment.
4. Respiratory infections--Prevention. 5. Respiratory organs--Diseases. I. Dempsey, Richard.
RC740 .R47 2021
616.2--dc23

Table of Contents

Preface

The world is advancing at a fast pace like never before. Therefore, the need is to keep up with the latest developments. This book was an idea that came to fruition when the specialists in the area realized the need to coordinate together and document essential themes in the subject. That's when I was requested to be the editor. Editing this book has been an honour as it brings together diverse authors researching on different streams of the field. The book collates essential materials contributed by veterans in the area which can be utilized by students and researchers alike.

Respiratory tract infections are the infectious diseases that affect the respiratory tract, which is a part of the respiratory system and involved in respiration. These infections are classified into two groups - upper respiratory tract infections and lower respiratory tract infections. The upper respiratory tract is the airway above the glottis. It includes respiratory parts such as nose, pharynx, larynx, and sinuses. The infections of the upper respiratory tract include tonsillitis, sinusitis and otitis media and it causes symptoms such as sore throat, nasal congestion, headache and mild fever. The lower respiratory tract includes trachea, bronchioles, bronchial tubes and lungs. Its infections are more complicated than upper respiratory tract infections. Its most common examples include pneumonia and bronchitis. This book contains some path-breaking studies in the advancement of diagnosis, management and prevention of respiratory tract infections. Those in search of information to further their knowledge will be greatly assisted by this book. This book traces the progress of this field and highlights some of its key concepts and applications.

Each chapter is a sole-standing publication that reflects each author's interpretation. Thus, the book displays a multi-facetted picture of our current understanding of application, resources and aspects of the field. I would like to thank the contributors of this book and my family for their endless support.

Editor

1

Screening for genital tuberculosis in a limited resource country

Sadie Namani[1,3*], Emine Qehaja-Buçaj[1] and Diellëza Namani[2]

Abstract

Background: Screening for benign or malignant process of pelvis in young females is a challenge for a physician in a limited resource country. Tuberculosis should be always considered in the differential diagnosis of a pelvic mass in countries with high prevalence of tuberculosis. Negative results of analysis of peritoneal fluid for acid-fast staining, late cultures, and unavailability of new diagnostics methods such as polymerase chain reaction and adenosine deaminase of the aspirated fluid from peritoneal cavity can often result in invasive diagnostic procedures such as laparotomy.

Case presentation: We report a case of a 24 year old Albanian unemployed female living in urban place in Kosovo who presented with abdominal pain, loss of appetite, fever, headache, a weight loss, nonproductive cough and menstrual irregularity for three weeks. In this example case, the patient with cystic mass in tubo-ovarial complex and elevated serum cancer antigen 125 levels was diagnosed for genital tuberculosis after performing laparotomy. Caseose mass found in left tubo-ovarial complex and histopathological examination of biopsied tissue were the fastest diagnostic tools for confirming pelvis TB. The Lowenstein-Jensen cultures were positive after six weeks and her family history was positive for tuberculosis.

Conclusion: Young females with abdominopelvic mass, ascites, a positive family history for tuberculosis and high serum cancer antigen 125, should always raise suspicion of tuberculosis especially in a limited resource country. A laparoscopy combined with peritoneal biopsy should be performed to confirm the diagnosis as this could lead to a prevention of unnecessary laparotomies.

Keywords: Genital tuberculosis, CA-125, Developing countries, Kosovo

Background

The incidence of genital tuberculosis (TB) is low and often attacks middle-aged females. However, it is a frequent cause of chronic pelvic inflammatory disease (PID) and infertility in other parts of the world [1]. TB should be always considered in the differential diagnosis of a pelvic mass among immigrants from developing countries, especially those from Asia, the Middle East and Latin America, as well as the human immunodeficiency virus (HIV) positive patients [2]. The most common primary location of genital TB is in Fallopian tubes. The cancer antigen 125 (CA-125) marker is sensitive when used for monitoring the progress of an established tumor [3]. Elevated serum CA-125 is not specific to ovarian cancer, however, and a positive result can, at times, be misleading [2]. In this case report, the elevated serum CA-125, 40 times higher from normal value, was associated with the upper tract genital TB.

Case presentation

A 24-year-old female patient woman was admitted to our hospital complaining of abdominal pain, loss of appetite, fever, headache, a weight loss, nonproductive cough and menstrual irregularity. Her symptoms started three weeks earlier and she was treated with antibiotics and steroids for Erythema nodosa and Polyarthritis. She had a positive family history for tuberculosis since her father had died two years ago from Pulmonary TB.

At admission, the patient was febrile, intoxicated, hypotensive, anemic, no palpable lymph nodes were

* Correspondence: sadie_namani@yahoo.com
[1]Clinic of Infectious Diseases, University Clinical Center of Kosovo, Prishtinë, Kosovo
[3]Medical Faculty, University of Prishtina, Kongresi i Manastirit 3A, Prishtinë, Kosovo
Full list of author information is available at the end of the article

noted, normal heart sounds, lungs with rales bilaterally, blood pressure was 90/60 mmHg, respirations 24/min, Pulse 80 beats/min, enlarged liver and spleen, with dolente tenderness in lower left abdominal quadrant, meningeal sings were negative and the rest of physical examinations were normal.

From laboratory analysis revealed elevated ESR = 40/, HB = 8.7 g/dl, leucocytes = 5.2×10^9/L, CRP = 48, liver enzymes, urea, glucose and kreatinin in normal levels, total proteins = 64 g/L, albumins = 36 g/L, LDH = 492 U/L, Fe = 8.6 mmol/L, blood cultures sterile, Wright negative, Widal negative. Chest x rays bilateral adenitis as shown in Fig.1, Mantoux probe 15 mm, HIV negative, serum CA 125 = 1430...1455, CA 19-9, AFP, CEA and CA 15-3 in normal levels. Ultrasound and MRI of abdomen revealed cystic formation on left tubo-ovarial complex and ascites as shown in Figs. 2 and 3.

Abdominal paracentesis was performed and revealed clear exudative fluid with benign cells. In consultation with gynecologist, the patient underwent operation, suprapubic transversal laparotomy. During operation, in the left tubo-ovarial complex was found caseose mass which was sent together with samples from omentum, peritoneum and ascites for histopathology and microbiological examination. On histopathological examination were seen epiteloidal granulomas with gigantic multinuclear cells, lymphocyte infiltrations and caseous necrosis. On Lowenstein-Jensen cultures was isolated Mycobacterium tuberculosis sensitive to Rifampicin (RIF), Izoniazid (INH), Ethambutol (ETH) and Streptomycin (STM). The patient was treated with a 4-drug TB treatment regimen consisting of RIF, INZ, Pyrazinamide, and ETH for the first two months and with two antituberculotics (RIF and INH) for another 7 months and recovered completely. Her serum cancer antigen 125 level was elevated for three months.

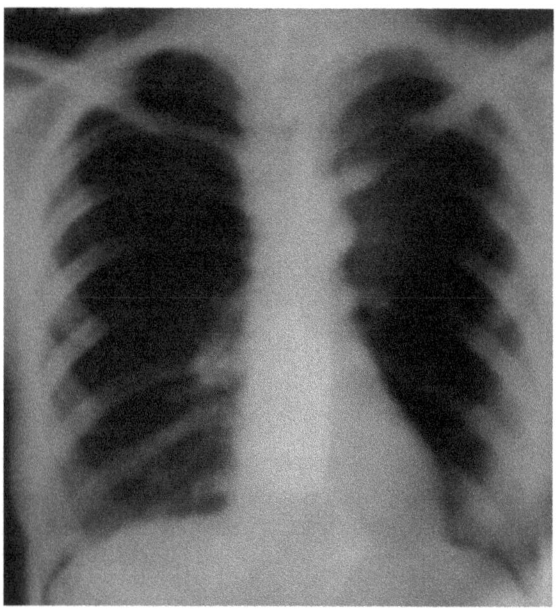

Fig. 1 Chest X ray Adenitis hilly bill

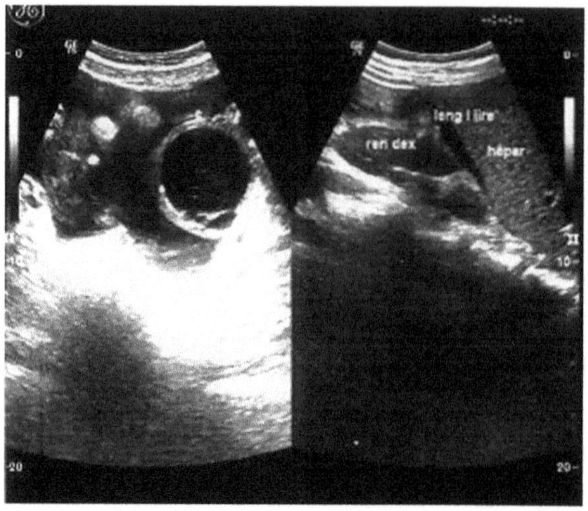

Fig. 2 Abdominal ultrasound: cystic formation in left tubo-ovarial complex and ascites

Discussion

Extrapulmonary tuberculosis is rarely seen at our Infectious Diseases Clinic in Prishtina, with less than 1% (20 cases or 0.6%) of the total 3156 patients hospitalized during 2014. Of the 20 cases treated for extrapulmonary tuberculosis 17 patients were treated for TB Meningitis, and single cases of TB lymphadenitis, TB peritonitis and TB of genital tract.

Abdominal TB, which may involve the genitourinary or gastrointestinal tract, peritoneum, lymph nodes or solid viscera, constitutes up to 12% of extrapulmonary TB and 1–3% of the total, and its nonspecific signs and symptoms may be similar to gastrointestinal (GI) or ovarian cancers [4]. Signs and symptoms of our patients were similar to those observed from previous reports [5–7]. Fever was the main symptom of our patient and it was the most common finding (73%) in the series reported by Muneef et al. [6]. Also, weight loss, menstrual irregularity, ascites, pelvic mass and a positive family history of TB, young age and geographic location in developing countries with high incidence of TB should direct the clinician to the diagnosis of upper genital tract TB. Helpful can be a positive TB skin test which is reported in about a quarter of patients in most reports [7]. Presence of TB at other sites and a positive family history of TB may be helpful in suggesting the diagnosis, but this was reported to occur in somewhat less than 30% of patients [5].

Pelvic TB can be caused by reactivation of the organism (spread via blood stream, lymphatic system or direct from

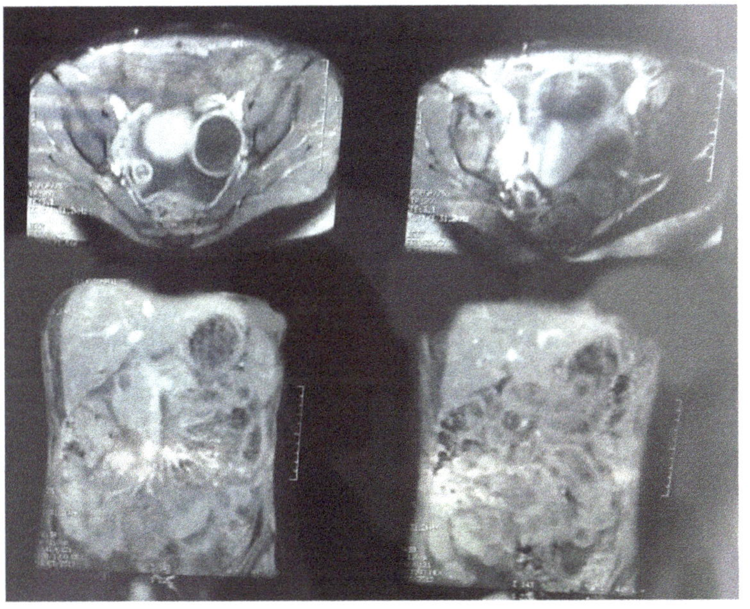

Fig. 3 Abdominal MRI: Cystic formation in left tubo-ovarial complex

the involved abdominal organs such as intestines) or rarely by venereal transmission [1]. Abdominal ultrasound and MRI of the pelvis was helpful for finding a cystic formation and directing us to suspect of a non-malignant disorder of the genital tract. Non-invasive methods such as tuberculin skin test, chest radiographs or acid-fast staining and culture of the aspirated fluid from peritoneal cavity are usually insufficient to provide the diagnosis of peritoneal or pelvic TB [8, 9]. Abdominal paracentesis revealing clear exudative fluid with benign cells was not helpful, while polymerase chain reaction (PCR) of the aspirated fluid can't be done in developing countries such as ours. Some recently published studies argue that a positive PCR assay or high adenosine deaminase (ADA) level in aspirated fluid is diagnostic for TB [10, 11]. None of them can be done in our country.

Serum CA-125 is a specific marker for ovarian cancer but can be elevated in various conditions including peritoneal and pelvic TB, endometriosis, pelvic inflammatory disease, liver cirrhosis, chronic renal failure, pleural effusion and pancreas [1, 11–13]. A value of 35 U/mL for CA-125 is considered the upper limit of normal [14]. In this case example, the level of serum CA-125 was 40 times higher from normal value. Cystic formation found by imaging, a positive TB skin test, a positive family history of tuberculosis, abdominal paracentesis were not helpful considering the high level of serum CA-125 found in this case which influenced the decision of the consultant gynecologist for laparotomy instead of laparoscopy. Caseose mass found in left tubo-ovarial complex by suprapubic transversal laparotomy and histopathological examination of biopsied tissue were the fastest diagnostic tools for confirming pelvis TB. The Lowenstein-Jensen cultures of the taken samples confirmed the suspected genital TB although 6 weeks later. For any suspicious mass of the upper genital tract, laparoscopy and histopathological examination of biopsied tissue should be the first intervention to prevent unnecessary surgery and starting appropriate and timely therapy.

Conclusion

Young females with abdominopelvic mass, ascites, and high serum cancer antigen 125, should always raise suspicion of tuberculosis especially in a limited resource country. A laparoscopy combined with peritoneal biopsy should be performed to confirm the diagnosis as this could lead to a prevention of unnecessary laparotomies.

Abbreviations

ADA: Adenosine deaminase; AFP: Alpha Fetoprotein; CA-125: Cancer antigen 125; CEA: Carcinoembryonic Antigen; CRP: C reactive protein; ESR: Erythrocyte sedimentation rate; ETH: Ethambutol; GI: Gastrointestinal; HB: Hemoglobin; HIV: human immunodeficiency virus; INH: Izoniazid; LDH: Lactat dehydrogenase; MRI: Magnetic resonance imaging; PCR: Polymerase chain reaction; PID: Pelvic inflammatory disease; RIF: Rifampicin; STM: Streptomycin; TB: Tuberculosis

Acknowledgements

Staff of the Institute of Radiology of the University Clinical Center of Kosovo for their help in processing abdominal ultrasound and MRI images for publication.

Funding

The authors declare that they have no funding source.

Authors' contributions

All authors have read and approved the final manuscript. SN made primary contributions to the design of the study, data collecting, comparing the results with other publications and drafted manuscript. EQ-B contributed to the data collection and participated in additional correction and design. DN scientific writer.

Authors information

Not applicable.

Competing interests

The authors declare that they have no competing interests.

Consent for publication

Written informed consent was obtained from the patient for publication of this case report and any accompanying images. Also, a statement for ethical approval was obtained from ethical committee of Medical Faculty, University of Prishtina. A copy of the written consent from the patient and a statement for ethical approval is available for review by the Editor of this journal.

Author details

[1]Clinic of Infectious Diseases, University Clinical Center of Kosovo, Prishtinë, Kosovo. [2]Smart Center, Prishtinë, Kosovo. [3]Medical Faculty, University of Prishtina, Kongresi i Manastirit 3A, Prishtinë, Kosovo.

References

1. Hasanzadeh M, Naderi HR, Hoshyar AH, Shabane S, Shahidsales S. Female genital tract tuberculosis presenting as ovarian cancer. J Res Med Sci. 2014;19(2):184–9.
2. Rock J, Jones HW. Te Linde's operative gynecology, vol. 30. 10th ed. Philadelphia: Lippincott Williams and Wilkins; 2008. p. 677–8.
3. Carlson KJ, Skates SJ, Singer D. Screening for ovarian cancer. Ann Intern Med. 1994;121:124–32.
4. Sheer TA, Coyle WJ. Gastrointestinal tuberculosis. Curr Gastroenterol Rep. 2003;5:273–8.
5. Uzunkoy A, Harma M, Harma M. Diagnosis of abdominal tuberculosis: experience from 11 cases and review of the literature. World J Gastroenterol. 2004;10:3647–9.
6. Muneef MA, Memish Z, Mahmoud SA, Sadoon SA, Bannatyne R, Khan Y. Tuberculosis in the belly: a review of forty-six cases involving the gastrointestinal tract and peritoneum. Scand J Gastroenterol. 2001;36:528–32.
7. Demir K, Okten A, Kaymakoglu S, Dincer D, Besisik F, Cevikbas U, et al. Tuberculous peritonitis-reports of 26 cases, detailing diagnostic and therapeutic problems. Eur J Gastroenterol Hepatol. 2001;13:581–5.
8. Adali E, Dulger C, Kolusari A, Kurdoglu M, Yildizhan R. Pelvic-peritoneal tuberculosis simulating peritoneal carcinomatosis: high clinical suspicion and a minimally invasive procedure. Arch Gynecol Obstet. 2009;280:867–8.
9. Tinelli A, Malvasi A, Vergara D, Martignago R, Nicolardi G, Tinelli R, et al. Abdominopelvic tuberculosis in gynaecology: laparoscopical and new laboratory findings. Aust N Z J Obstet Gynaecol. 2008;48:90–5.
10. Tewari M, Sahoo SP, Shukla HS. Tuberculosis. In: Abdominal tuberculosis. 2nd ed. India: Jaypee Brothers Medical Publishers; 2009. p. 288.
11. Simsek H, Savas MC, Kadayifci A, Tatar G. Elevated serum CA 125 concentration in patients with tuberculosis peritonitis: a case-control study. Am J Gastroenterol. 1997;92:1174–6.
12. Thakur V, Mukherjee U, Kumar K. Elevated serum cancer antigen 125 levels in advanced abdominal tuberculosis. Med Oncol. 2001;18:289–91.
13. Bilgin T, Karabay A, Dolar E, Develioglu OH. Peritoneal tuberculosis with pelvic abdominal mass, ascites and elevated CA 125 mimicking ovarian carcinoma: a series of 10 cases. Int J Gynecol Cancer. 2001;11:290–4.
14. Finkler NJ. Clinical utility of CA 125 in preoperative diagnosis of patients with pelvic masses. Obstet Gynecol Reprod Biol. 1993;49(1–2):105–7.

2

Health seeking behaviour and delayed management of tuberculosis patients in rural Bangladesh

K. A. T. M. Ehsanul Huq[1*], Michiko Moriyama[1], Khalequ Zaman[2], Mohammod Jobayer Chisti[2], Julie Long[3], Akramul Islam[4], Shahed Hossain[2], Habiba Shirin[2], Mohammad Jyoti Raihan[2], Sajeda Chowdhury[5] and Md Moshiur Rahman[1]

Abstract

Background: Early diagnosis of tuberculosis (TB) and involvement of the public-private partnership are critical to eradicate TB. Patients need to receive proper treatment through the National Tuberculosis Control Programme (NTP). This study describes various predictors for health seeking behaviour of TB patients and health system delay made by the different health care providers.

Methods: A cross-sectional study was conducted in a public health facility of a rural area in Bangladesh. Newly diagnosed smear positive pulmonary TB (PTB) patients who were ≥ 15 years of age were sequentially enrolled in this study. The socio-demographic characteristics and proportion of health care utilization by the patients, and health system delay made by the health care providers were calculated. Multivariate analysis was conducted to determine the independent association of the risk factors with the time to seek medical care.

Results: Two hundred and eighty patients were enrolled in this study. Among them, 73.6% were male and 26.4% were female. A hundred percent of patients primarily sought treatment for their cough, 170 (60.7%) first consulted a non-qualified practitioner while 110 patients (39.3%) first consulted with qualified practitioners about their symptoms. Pharmacy contact was the highest (27.9%) among the non-qualified practitioners, and 58.9% non-qualified practitioners prescribed treatment without any laboratory investigation. The average health system delay was 68.5 days. Multiple logistic regressions revealed a significant difference between uneducated and educated patients (OR 2.33; CI 1.39–3.92), and qualified and non-qualified practitioners (OR 2.34; CI 1.38–3.96) to be independent predictors of health system delay.

Conclusions: Compared to men, fewer women sought TB treatment. Uneducated patients and questionably qualified practitioners made for a longer delay in detecting TB. Increasing public health awareness and improving health seeking behavior of females and uneducated patients, and greater participation of the qualified practitioners in the NTP are highly recommended.

Keywords: Tuberculosis, Health seeking, Delay, Health care provider, Bangladesh

* Correspondence: d163965@hiroshima-u.ac.jp
[1]Graduate School of Biomedical & Health Sciences, Hiroshima University, Kasumi 1-2-3 Minami-ku, Hiroshima 734-8553, Japan
Full list of author information is available at the end of the article

Background

Tuberculosis (TB) is a major public health problem and is, globally, the ninth leading cause of death. In 2016, of the 10.4 million new cases worldwide, 1.3 million resulted in death [1]. This infectious disease is most commonly spread by coughing [2] and is most prevalent among productive-age adults between 15 and 59 years [3]. According to 'The End TB Strategy' in the Sustainable Development Goals (SDGs), early diagnosis of TB and engagement of public and private health care providers is essential [1, 4]. To reduce the case fatality rate from 16 to 10% between 2015 and 2020, it is necessary to diagnose and treat patients without any delay [1]. Patients who are not diagnosed and treated early, act as reservoirs for spreading the disease [5]. Access to TB services for diagnosis, treatment and prevention is necessary to promote and protect human rights and gender equalities [6]. Currently, the world is experiencing a pulmonary TB epidemic. The increased incidence of multi-drug resistant tuberculosis has contributed to the increased global burden of TB [7].

The chance of catching the infection depends on the close contact, frequency and duration of exposure with TB patients [8]. Delayed diagnosis and close contact with a TB patient significantly increase the risk of transmission of infection [9]. Moreover, delays in TB diagnosis may cause a significant adverse outcome, which may increase fatality rates [10]. A systematic review found that the average health system delay for treating TB was nearly the same in developing and developed countries (28.5 and 21.5 days respectively) [11]. The public health response to the increased threat of TB in the community is to prevent the transmission of TB [10, 12]. This is achievable by treating active TB patients and screening and using chemoprophylaxis for those who come in contact with active cases [10]. However, a systematic review found that in many countries, more than half of the TB cases remain undiagnosed in the community despite active surveillance [12].

Universal access to quality treatment for all TB patients is necessary to achieve the goal of a TB free world [1]. Most countries now provide free treatment facilities through the National Tuberculosis Control Programme (NTP). NTP is normally implemented by the government health services of a country's national health system. However, many private health care providers and non-government organizations (NGOs) are also involved in the NTP delivery system [13, 14].

In many settings, patients with symptoms like persistent cough, have an equal opportunity to utilize both public health care providers within the NTP as well as private providers, such as drug sellers and traditional healers, who are not under the NTP [13]. Because of the weak health infrastructure in some countries, patients seek care outside the NTP. Moreover, some public central hospitals that provide health services for prisoners, police and army personnel are also not covered by the NTP [13]. While still, some countries based their official reports only on information about patients within NTP facilities, resulting in a risk of under-reporting patients who attend facilities outside the NTP. Despite the availability of standard NTP treatment, patients may utilize private providers and receive inadequate treatment, which contributes to the development of multi-drug resistance TB [13]. In many developing countries, like Bangladesh, most TB patients' first contact with a private physician is at the primary health care facility of their choice, which is not directly linked with the NTP [15]. Pharmacists and drug sellers who specifically treat poor patients may not be aware of the standard guidelines for proper TB management and the referral system. They are not the part of NTP and have no specific training on TB management [15].

With the public facilities, TB patients also practiced self-medication, and went to private practitioners and traditional healers for their primary consultation. Patient's lack of awareness about TB symptoms and lack of free treatment facilities in the public health care facilities and dissatisfaction with the public health care systems resulted in more delays [16]. It is noteworthy that public-private partnership could improve TB case notifications, treatment success rates, decreased defaulter patients, service accessibility and increase referral system of TB patients to the NTP [17]. In the End TB Strategy of WHO, all care providers are included in the NTP [1]. In underprivileged countries, the TB control programme is often more effective than other health services due to its highly-trained staff, uninterrupted drug supply, proper diagnostic and treatment facilities, a good reporting system and, most importantly, all services are free of charge [13]. Most of the countries with a high TB burden allocate a large portion of the national health budget to the TB control program. Additional funds are provided from the Global Fund according to the single stream funding policy for the sustainability of the TB project [1, 18]. Despite an adequately financed and effective TB management programme that exist in Bangladesh, the morbidity and mortality from TB are still high [1]. The incidence rate was almost static between 2000 and 2016; moreover, the notifications of new and relapse cases increased significantly over that period of time [1]. Compared to massively growing urban areas, NTP is more effective in the rural areas. Overcrowded and high density residences, inadequate and packed public transportation make for easy transmission of TB. Poor people, particularly those moving from rural areas to urban areas, live in extremely overcrowded slums and they move from one slum to another with shorter intervals, which impacts adversely on their access to health facilities and proper treatment. Consequently, the prevalence of TB is significantly higher in urban areas [19].

Understanding of TB patients' health care seeking patterns is helpful for improving the organization of the National Tuberculosis Program (NTP), which in turn improves early detection of TB and helps patients receive proper treatment without delay. The primary aim of this study was to explore the patterns of health care utilization by TB patients before starting treatment at a government health care facility in rural Bangladesh. As a secondary objective, the study attempted to shed light on the relationship between different factors such as demographic and socio-economic characteristics and treatment delays within the health system.

Methods

Study design and study population

This was a cross-sectional study. The study was conducted in a rural area called Matlab Upazila in Bangladesh about 55 km from the capital, Dhaka. The population of this community was 227,853, with 46% being male and 54% female and 68% of the population was aged ≥15 years in 2013. Thirty percent had no formal education, and 86% were Muslim. Male and female literacy was 75 and 67%, respectively. The primary sources of income were from agriculture, other daily labour, and small business. The coverage of the Bacillus Calmette-Guerin (BCG) vaccine for the prevention of tuberculosis was 97.9% or more [20, 21]. All the TB patients were prospectively enrolled from the Upazila (Sub-district) Health Complex (UHC) between April 2005 and May 2009 to minimize biases. Patients, who had smear positive pulmonary tuberculosis, were interviewed after diagnosis. We evaluated the health care seeking patterns of the TB patients before commencing treatment at the Upazila Health Complex, in order to assess the delay for the diagnosis of TB.

Data collection

After the diagnosis of TB (smear positive TB case) at the UHC, patients were invited to participate in the study. A Field Research Assistant (FRA) usually contacted the patient at home on the day following the diagnosis, and a voluntary informed consent form (ICF) was signed. The FRA also administered a structured questionnaire to collect required study information. Both the ICF and the questionnaire were translated into Bengali from English. Study procedures took 30–40 min to complete per participant. The questionnaire contained questions regarding the type of health seeking and utilization patterns, referral attitude and action of the health care providers, use of health care providers, reasons for changing provider, time taken to receive treatment at the UHC, knowledge about the free treatment facilities, and socio-demographic characteristics of the patients. The time taken to receive treatment (health system delay) was calculated using data about type and number of health care providers the patient visited before the diagnosis of TB at UHC.

Diagnosis and treatment

In Bangladesh, each Upazila Health Complex has around 30 to 50 beds, including both indoor and outdoor facilities. In the Matlab Upazila Health Complex (UHC) all suspected TB cases with a history of cough for more than 3 weeks were seen by a study physician. The physician performed a physical examination and gave advice regarding laboratory testing. UHC has facilities to examine sputum for acid-fast bacilli (AFB), perform chest X-rays and other routine examinations. Three sputum spot samples (overnight, morning, and following day) were collected (about 5 ml per sample) for microscopic examination for the AFB test. Sputum samples were collected and examined by the UHC laboratory technician. Standard guidelines were followed for the diagnosis and treatment in accordance with the National Tuberculosis Control Programme algorithm [22].

Sample size calculation

We assumed the proportion of smear positive TB patients seeking care from qualified and non-qualified health care providers was 25 and 75%, respectively [23]. The calculated sample size was 288 with a 95% confidence interval and 5% error [24]. It took 4 years to complete the study. All sputum smear positive patients who attended the Matlab Upazila Health Complex were enrolled. According to UHC records, approximately 75 TB patients were diagnosed each year for a total of nearly 300 smear positive cases during the study period.

Operational definitions

A systematic review, analyzing 52 studies, found that the delay in treatment could be stratified by patients' delay, health system delay and total delay [11]. Health system delay was considered as a delay between the first consultation with a formal or informal provider and the diagnosis of TB. This delay ranged from 2 to 87 days. The length of health system delays differed depending on whether patients sought treatment from formal or informal health care providers [11]. For the purpose of our study, we defined health system delay as the time between first consultation with any health care professional (both qualified and non-qualified practitioner) and the initiation of proper TB treatment. Based on the previous study in Bangladesh, we calculated the mean health system delay to be ≥45.6 days [25]. Considering the health system delay, we have recognized "considerable delay" to be 45.6 days and above and "acceptable delay" to be less than 45.6 days for our study. Moreover, in our analyses, proper 'action taken' is defined as referral to UHC. Whereas, 'qualified practitioner' is defined as a medical doctor or a special government-training certificate for TB management who worked at the UHC.

Data analysis

All questionnaires were checked for validity, consistency, and completeness. After tabulating the data, frequency distributions were checked for each variable to identify any abnormalities or extreme values. With respect to 'delay' in using health care system by the TB patients, we estimated the odds ratios with 95% CIs. All key variables used are mentioned in Tables 1 and 2. Finally, using the significant predictors of considerable delay, multivariate analyses in the form of a logistic regression were performed to reflect on the relationship between individuals' background characteristics, and considerable delay with adjustment for other variables. Data analyses were performed using software package SPSS version 17.0 (SPSS Inc., Chicago, USA). One US dollar (USD) was considered equivalent to 76 Bangladeshi Taka (BDT).

Results

In accordance with the sample size estimation, 280 patients were diagnosed with pulmonary TB-they all consented and were successfully interviewed. Two hundred and six patients (73.6%) were male and 74 (26.4%) were female. Most (66.5%) of the male patients were older than 45 years of age, but most (62.2%) of the female patients were between 15 and 45 years of age. The basic demographic characteristics of the patients suggest that their average household size was 5.4 ± 2.3 with a median (range) of 5.0 (4.0–6.7). The average monthly household income was 4312.5 BDT and 198 out of the 280 (70.7%) patients lived below the poverty line. The maximum monthly income was BDT 20,000, and minimum was BDT 1000, reflecting a disparity in the community (Table 1).

Among the patients, 86.1% were Muslims and 13.9% were Hindus; 43.6% had no formal education, 33.2% had 1-5 years, 20.4% had 6-10 years, and only 2.9% had more than 10 years of formal education. In terms of occupation, 33.2% were unemployed; and among the employed most (21.1%) were involved in the agriculture. The data indicated that 83.2% had not received the BCG vaccine, 68.9% were smokers (with 71.5% of smokers smoking for more than 10 years) and 41.8% of the patients had a history of TB in the family (Table 2).

All (100%) patients were seeking treatment for their cough. Among the patients, 170 (60.7%) patients had first consulted a non-qualified practitioner while 110 (39.3%) had consulted a qualified practitioner about their symptoms. The patients received a different quality of care during consultations from the non-qualified and qualified practitioners before attending the UHC (Fig. 1). Among all those who consulted non-qualified practitioners (170),

Table 1 Distribution of age, family size and monthly income

Items	Male	Female
	n (%)	*n* (%)
Age:		
15–45 years	69 (33.5)	46 (62.2)
> 45 years	137 (66.5)	28 (37.8)
Total	206 (73.6)	74 (26.4)
Family size and monthly income		
	Mean (SD)	Median (IQR)
Family size mean (SD)	5.37 (2.3)	5.0 (4.0–6.7)
Average monthly income (BDT)	4312.5 (2281.6)	4000 (3000–5000)

SD Standard deviation, *IQR* Interquartile range, *BDT* Bangladesh Taka

Table 2 Basic demographic characteristics of this study

Items	*n*	%
Religion		
Muslim	241	86.1
Hindu	39	13.9
Occupation		
Agriculture	59	21.1
Day Laborer	22	7.9
Fisherman	8	2.9
Boatman	2	0.7
Service	12	4.3
Teacher	2	0.7
Rickshaw puller	11	3.9
Business	41	14.6
Student	5	1.8
Doctor/Engineer/Lawyer	1	0.4
Unemployed	93	33.2
Driver	1	0.4
Garment/Factory worker	2	0.7
Others	21	7.5
Received BCG vaccine		
No	233	83.2
Yes	47	16.8
Smoking habits		
No	87	31.1
Yes	193	68.9
Duration of Smoking		
≤ 10 Years	55	28.5
> 10 Years	138	71.5
History of TB in Family		
Yes	117	41.8%
No	163	58.2%

BCG Bacillus Calmette-Guerin, *TB* Tuberculosis

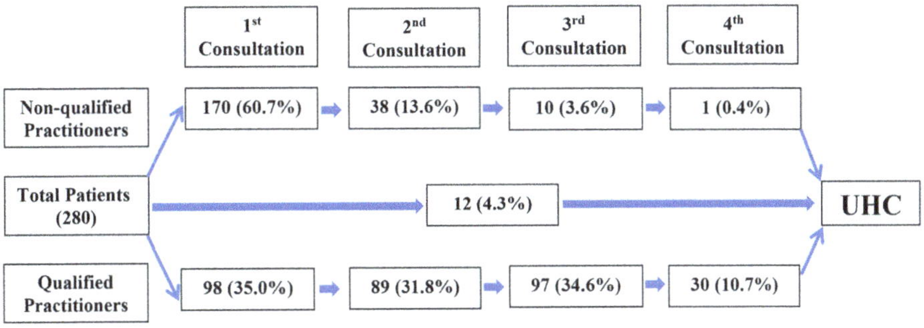

Fig. 1 Flow chart of patients' consultation for non-qualified and qualified practitioners. *Note*: the dropout patients directly consulted at Upazila Health Complex (UHC)

pharmacy contact was the most common, (78 or 45.9% of all patients who sought care from non-qualified practitioners). The remaining patients had sought treatment from other diverse types of non-qualified practitioners such as licentiate of medical faculty (LMF), village doctors, medical assistants, sub-assistant community medical officers (SACMOs) who are designated helping hands of qualified physicians, and traditional and faith healers. Moreover, of the patients who took advice from non-qualified practitioners, only 31 (18.2%) were referred to the UHC (i.e. proper action taken) (Table 3).

Among all patients, 165 (58.9%) were prescribed with drugs at the first consultation without performing any laboratory investigation. Seventy-five (26.8%) patients were advised to undergo laboratory investigations, 5 (1.8%) were referred to a TB clinic elsewhere and 2 (0.7%) received advice on cough management only and 1 (0.4%) patient was referred to doctors who were a chest or pulmonary specialist (not shown in table).

Table 3 Distribution of health care providers at first consultation

Items	*n*	(%)
First Consultation		
Non-qualified Practitioner	170	60.7
Pharmacy	78	27.9
Others	72	25.7
NGO Paramedics	18	6.4
Homeopath	1	0.4
Ayurvedic	1	0.4
Qualified Practitioner	110	39.3
Private Practitioner	64	22.9
icddr,b	33	11.8
UHC	12	4.3
DOTS Centre	1	0.4

NGO Non-governmental organization, *UHC* Upazila Health Complex, *icddr,b* International Centre for Diarrhoeal Disease Research, Bangladesh, *DOTS* Directly-observed treatment short-course

Most of the patients (90%) had knowledge/awareness of the free treatment facilities provided by the government and NGOs (BRAC, a private for profit). Moreover, 76.1% patients knew the signs and symptoms of TB. Patients who sought treatment from other health care providers had an average delay of 68.5 days till proper initiation of TB treatment at the UHC (Table 4). Health system delay according to the patients' demographic characteristics in respect to non-qualified and qualified practitioners is shown in Table 4.

The results of the bivariate analyses suggest that education, BCG vaccination and types of health care providers during the first consultation were significantly associated with the duration of the delay. The results suggest that an acceptable delay was 2.17 times more likely if the patient was educated in comparison to being uneducated. Participants who received the BCG vaccination were 2.13 times likely to have an acceptable delay in comparison with those who were not vaccinated. However, our result shows that patients who consulted qualified personnel were 2.08 times less likely to make an acceptable delay (Table 5).

Finally, the binary logistic regression model, using the significant predictors of acceptable delay as a dependent variable, patients' lack of education and first consultation with a qualified service provider were independently associated with the delay in the initiation of proper TB treatment. The result suggests that primarily the odds of an acceptable delay was 2.33 times higher for educated patients and 2.34 times greater if the patient sought care from a non-qualified person (Table 6). Age, sex and income did not confound the size of the effect of the statistically significant variables, as they remained similar when adjusted for age, sex and income level.

Discussion

These findings indicate that patients' education, BCG vaccination status and first consultation with qualified persons were significant predictors for delay initiation of proper TB treatment. Educated patients who primarily sought care

Table 4 Health system delay in the initiation of TB treatment among patients first receiving advice from non-qualified or from qualified practitioners

Characteristics	Non-qualified Practitioner Days Mean	SD	Qualified Practitioner Days Mean	SD	Overall delay Days Mean	SD
All	66.52	80.24	70.90	207.66	68.50	151.61
Age						
≤ 44	67.66	85.58	70.84	97.09	69.07	90.47
> 44	65.70	76.65	70.93	257.22	68.11	182.80
Sex						
Male	61.01	78.13	72.95	234.65	66.57	169.70
Female	80.60	84.70	64.55	81.84	73.88	83.33
Religion						
Muslim	69.36	83.79	78.43	225.94	73.35	162.10
Hindu	45.22	40.93	32.86	42.84	38.56	41.89
Education						
Uneducated	78.72	85.34	74.05	81.92	76.38	84.13
Educated	61.25	57.23	71.81	64.51	66.53	62.87
Income						
≤ 3500	70.07	91.03	71.56	273.58	70.75	173.91
> 3500	58.26	46.13	69.22	100.46	63.07	74.65
BCG vaccination						
No	76.46	89.71	78.81	80.38	77.63	87.10
Yes	64.79	68.34	71.23	74.51	68.01	78.42

SD Standard deviation, *BCG* Bacillus Calmette-Guerin

from health care personnel were more likely to have an acceptable delay in starting proper TB treatment in comparison to uneducated patients. Moreover, qualified personnel had longer delays before initiation of TB management. A lower proportion of women were diagnosed with TB at the facility, and they had a higher rate of considerable delay before initiating treatment. For this study, being educated reduces the odds of considerable delay in getting proper treatment of TB. In fact, despite proper diagnosis or guidance during the first consultation, uneducated patients may suffer a considerable delay in the initiation of proper TB treatment. Reasons include time wasted to seek a second or even third opinion due to psychological factors of denial among the patients diagnosed with this stigmatized disease [26–28].

Whereas, in terms of a considerable delay made before initiation of proper TB treatment after the first consultation with qualified personnel, it could be explained that some of the private practitioners with less awareness about TB may not want to acknowledge failure in diagnosing; therefore, they do not refer patients to UHC. This may justify the longer delay made in this sample who first sought care from private practitioners, and similar findings are evident also in another study in Bangladesh [29] and elsewhere [12]. This is often observed, as private practitioners repeatedly prescribe different diagnosis procedures and treatments for cough before referring the patients to UHC, or did not refer patients at all. In this case, the patients sought treatment from other places causing a further delay in the initiation of proper TB treatment (Fig. 1).

The tendency for patients to seek care from private practitioners in this rural setting, was much lower than that observed in another study that covered populations from all over Bangladesh in which 43.8% first sought care from the private practitioners before reporting to public health facilities [29]. Two other studies in Indonesia and India have shown that 27.3 and 48.7% respectively visited private facilities [30, 31].

A study in rural Tanzania [32] observed a somewhat lesser health system delay in the initiation of treatment (57 days) than our study, while the average delay was 151 days in Afghanistan [33] and 16 days in China [34].

Furthermore, the knowledge and awareness of TB in this study population was higher (76.1%) than in the neighboring country of India, where 56% of the people knew about TB and only 20% knew about the cause and mode of TB transmission [35]. Most of our study population did not receive BCG vaccine during their childhood, which indicates that vaccination coverage in this area has increased [20, 21].

Table 5 Relationship of demographic and socio-economic factors with time delayed

Variable		Accepted delay (< 45.6 days)	Considerable Delay (≥ 45.6 days)	OR (95% CI)
Age	≤ 44	66 (62.3%)	40 (37.7%)	Ref.
	> 44	124 (71.3%)	50 (28.7%)	0.66 (0.34–1.11)
Sex	Male	145 (70.4%)	61 (29.6%)	Ref.
	Female	45 (60.8%)	29 (39.2%)	1.53 (0.88–2.66)
Religion	Muslim	159 (66.0%)	82 (34.0%)	Ref.
	Hindu	31 (79.5%)	8 (20.5%)	0.51 (0.22–1.14)
Patient's Occupation	Unemployed	21 (80.8%)	5 (19.2%)	Ref.
	Employed	169 (66.5%)	85 (33.5%)	2.11 (0.77–5.80)
Patient's Education Status	Uneducated	94 (77.0%)	28 (23.0%)	Ref.
	Educated	96 (60.8%)	62 (39.2%)	2.17 (1.27–3.68)
Average monthly income	≤ 3500	82 (69.5%)	36 (30.5%)	Ref.
	> 3500	108 (66.7%)	54 (33.3%)	1.14 (0.68–1.90)
Receiving BCG vaccine	No	165 (70.8%)	68 (29.2%)	Ref.
	Yes	25 (53.2%)	22 (46.8%)	2.13 (1.13–4.04)
Smoking	No	60 (69.0%)	27 (31.0%)	Ref.
	Yes	130 (67.4%)	63 (32.6%)	1.08 (0.62–1.86)
Smoking duration	≤ 15 years	115 (69.7%)	50 (30.3%)	Ref.
	> 15 years	40 (34.8%)	35 (21.2%)	1.23 (0.74–2.04)
Family member who have TB	No	144 (66.7%)	72 (33.3%)	Ref.
	Yes	46 (71.9%)	18 (28.1%)	0.78 (0.42–1.45)
Family member who had TB	No	106 (65.0%)	57 (35.0%)	Ref.
	Yes	84 (71.8%)	33 (28.2%)	0.73 (0.43–1.22)
First Consultation	Non- qualified person	90 (52.9%)	80 (47.1%)	Ref.
	Qualified person	77 (70.0%)	33 (30.0%)	0.48 (0.30–0.80)
Having knowledge and awareness about TB and free TB treatment	No	19 (67.9%)	9 (32.1%)	Ref.
	Yes	171 (67.9%)	81 (32.1%)	1.00 (0.43–2.30)
Who referred at MUHC	Self/Relative	29 (59.2%)	20 (40.8%)	Ref.
	Other	161 (69.7%)	70 (30.3%)	0.63 (0.33–1.19)

OR Odds ratio, *CI* Confidence interval, *Ref.* Reference, *BCG* Bacillus Calmette-Guerin, *TB* Tuberculosis, *MUHC* Matlab Upazila Health Complex

Table 6 Multivariable analysis showed the associations between independent (x) background factors and dependent (y) variables as acceptable delay

Variable	Categories	OR (95% CI)
Education	Uneducated	Ref.
	Educated	2.33 (1.39–3.92)
BCG Vaccine	Not received	Ref.
	Received	1.41 (0.73–2.71)
First Consultation	Qualified person	Ref.
	Non-qualified person	2.34 (1.38–3.96)

OR Odds ratio, *CI* Confidence interval, *Ref*, Reference, *BCG* Bacillus Calmette-Guerin

Our study found that less women sought treatment than men, though the gender distribution in the catchment was the same, which is in concordance with the national prevalence of TB in Bangladesh (male and female ratio more than 3:1, [1] 1.45:0.48 [25] and findings from other middle and low-income countries [36]. The reasoning for less female attendance may be attributed to the social stigma associated with TB [25, 28]. Women prefer to visit traditional healers and seek alternative medicine rather than mainstream medical health professionals [28]. Even though fewer women consult with qualified health care providers, clinicians are not able to aggressively investigate for the diagnosis of TB [20, 37, 38]. As a result, further evaluation of the low rates of female hospital attendance and TB among women is needed.

It is likely that access to health care was limited due to poor socio-economic conditions of this study population. This might have made the patients choose non-qualified practitioners, especially pharmacists, due to easy access and low-price of drugs. This finding is similar to a WHO report on the National Tuberculosis Control Programme of Bangladesh [15].

This paper suggests that all medical service providers, both qualified and non-qualified, should be integrated into the National Tuberculosis Control Programme (NTP). This integration could improve the proper referral system, increase awareness and reduce the stigma surrounding TB. It may also help to increase the utilization of free and complete treatment facilities for TB provided by the government.

In order to achieve the Sustainable Development Goals (SDGs), TB needs to be further highlighted in the National Health Policy of Bangladesh and incorporated into various public health programmes to increase knowledge, awareness, reduce gender differences and stigma in the National Tuberculosis Programme (NTP).

Limitations

The limitations of this study were that we excluded all the patients who were less than 15 years, as well as extra-pulmonary TB patients, because it was very difficult to diagnose this age group due to nonspecific clinical symptoms. We also did not enroll those patients who did not visit the Upazila Health Complex, but sought treatment from private health care providers. The study was carried out in a single health facility; therefore, the findings are not representative of the whole of rural Bangladesh. The study delay data relied on patients recall and was thus prone to recall bias. This is a cross-sectional study, and thus no causal inferences could be made. Because of the above-mentioned limitations, the results may not be extrapolated to depict the TB situation in Bangladesh.

Conclusions

In conclusion, though most patients knew about the signs and symptoms of TB and the existence of free TB treatment facilities, the majority of the patients primarily consulted a non-qualified practitioner for their symptoms. Educated patients and non-qualified practitioners experienced less delay for proper TB treatment. Also, females were less likely to seek treatment. This study has identified a critical knowledge gap regarding patients and their health seeking behavior. This study's findings suggest that less-educated and female patients need to increase their awareness and more qualified practitioners need to be integrated into the NTP. These discoveries may help assist further the implementation of future health intervention for proper diagnosis and treatment of TB patients.

Abbreviations

AFB: Acid-fast bacilli; BCG: Bacillus Calmette-Guerin; BDT: Bangladesh Taka; CI: Confidence interval; DOTS: Directly-observed treatment short-course; FRA: Field research assistant; icddr,b: International Centre for Diarrhoeal Disease Research, Bangladesh; ICF: Informed consent form; IQR: Interquartile range; LMF: Licentiate of medical faculty; MUHC: Matlab Upazila Health Complex; NGOs: Non-government organizations; NTP: National Tuberculosis Control Programme; OR: Odds ratio; PTB: Pulmonary tuberculosis; SACMO: Sub-assistant community medical officer; SD: Standard deviation; SDGs: Sustainable Development Goals; SPSS: Statistical package for social sciences; TB: Tuberculosis; UHC: Upazila Health Complex; USD: United State Dollar; WHO: World Health Organization

Acknowledgements

We acknowledge all the tuberculosis patients who participated in this study. We thank the study staff for their valuable efforts. We also especially give thanks to Professor Lars Åke Persson, Department of Women's and Children's Health, Uppsala University, Sweden for his supportive supervision. We thank the donors who provide unrestricted support to icddr,b for operations and research. Current donors include: Australian Agency for International Development (AusAID), Government of the People's Republic of Bangladesh, Canadian International Development Agency (CIDA), Swedish International Development Cooperation Agency (SIDA), and the Department for International Development, UK (DFID).

Funding

This work was funded by the United States Agency for International Development (USAID) and The Global Fund (GFATM) Grant number GR-00230. The funding agencies had no role in the design of the study, data collection, analysis, interpretation, manuscript writing, approval of the manuscript and submission for publication.

Authors' contributions

KATMEH and KZ conceptualized the study. AI, SH, HS and SC involved in project administration. KATMEH, KZ and MJR conducted the data analysis. KZ, MM and KATMEH supervised the research activities. KZ, KATMEH and MJR wrote the original draft. MM, MJC, JL and MMR reviewed and edited the manuscript. Finally, all authors read and approved the manuscript.

Ethics approval and consent to participate

The study was approved by the Research Review Committee (RRC) and Ethical Review Committee (ERC) of the International Centre for Diarrhoeal Disease Research, Bangladesh (icddr,b) (PR-2006-011). A written informed consent was taken from all the study participants individually before enrollment. A parental written informed consent including ascent from the participants was also obtained for those patients who were less than 18 years of age. Data were handled confidentially and processed and presented anonymously. Patients could withdraw from the study at any point in the study period without giving any reason and without suffering any negative effect on their further treatment.

Consent for publication

Not applicable.

Competing interests

The authors declare that they have no competing interests.

Author details
[1]Graduate School of Biomedical & Health Sciences, Hiroshima University, Kasumi 1-2-3 Minami-ku, Hiroshima 734-8553, Japan. [2]International Centre for Diarrhoeal Disease Research, Dhaka, Bangladesh. [3]University of Colorado, Denver, USA. [4]Health Programme, BRAC, Dhaka, Bangladesh. [5]Institute of Biomedical & Health Sciences, Hiroshima University, Hiroshima, Japan.

References

1. World Health Organization. Global tuberculosis report 2017. Geneva. p. 2017. http://www.who.int/tb/publications/global_report/en/
2. Turner RD, Bothamley GH. Cough and the transmission of tuberculosis. J Infect Dis. 2015;211(9):1367–72.
3. Uchimura K, Ngamvithayapong-Yanai J, Kawatsu L, Ohkado A, Yoshiyama T, Ito K, Ishikawa N. Permanent employment or public assistance may increase tuberculosis survival among working-age patients in Japan. Int J Tuberc Lung Dis. 2015;19(3):312–8.
4. Surya A, Setyaningsih B, Nasution HS, Parwati CG, Yuzwar YE, Osberg M, et al. Quality tuberculosis Care in Indonesia: using patient pathway analysis to optimize public–private collaboration. J Infect Dis. 2017;216(Suppl 7):S724–32.
5. Wang L, Zhang H, Ruan Y, Chin DP, Xia Y, Cheng S, et al. Tuberculosis prevalence in China, 1990-2010; a longitudinal analysis of national survey data. Lancet. 2014;383(9934):2057–64.
6. The Global Fund. Investing to end epidemics: The Global Fund strategy 2017–2022. https://www.theglobalfund.org/media/2531/core_globalfundstrategy2017-2022_strategy_en.pdf?u=636486807150000000
7. Falzon D, Mirzayev F, Wares F, Baena IG, Zignol M, Linh N, et al. Multidrug-resistant tuberculosis around the world: what progress has been made? Eur Respir J. 2015;45(1):150–60.
8. Centers for Disease Control and Prevention. Introduction to the core curriculum on tuberculosis: what the clinician should know. 6th. 2013. https://www.cdc.gov/tb/education/corecurr/pdf/corecurr_all.pdf
9. Rahayu SR, Katsuyama H, Demura M, Katsuyama M, Ota Y, Tanii H, et al. Factors associated with tuberculosis cases in Semarang District, Indonesia: case–control study performed in the area where case detection rate was extremely low. Environ Health Prev Med. 2015;20(4):253–61.
10. Lee CH, Wang JY, Lin HC, Lin PY, Chang JH, Suk CW, et al. Treatment delay and fatal outcomes of pulmonary tuberculosis in advanced age: a retrospective nationwide cohort study. BMC Infect Dis. 2017;17(1):449.
11. Sreeramareddy CT, Panduru KV, Menten J, Van den Ende J. Time delays in diagnosis of pulmonary tuberculosis: a systematic review of literature. BMC Infect Dis. 2009;9:91.
12. Kranzer K, Afnan-Holmes H, Tomlin K, Golub JE, Shapiro AE, Schaap A, et al. The benefits to communities and individuals of screening for active tuberculosis disease: a systematic review. Int J Tuberc Lung Dis. 2013;17(4):432–46.
13. World Health Organization. Framework for conducting reviews of tuberculosis programmes. 2014. http://apps.who.int/iris/bitstream/handle/10665/127943/9789241507103_eng.pdf?sequence=1
14. Ministry of Foreign Affairs of Japan, Ministry of Health, Labour and Welfare of Japan, Japan International Cooperation Agency, Japan Anti-Tuberculosis Association, Stop TB Partnership Japan. Stop TB Japan Action Plan: Public-private partnership for international cooperation towards the elimination of tuberculosis. 2008. http://www.mofa.go.jp/policy/health_c/action0807.pdf
15. World Health Organization. Fifth Joint Monitoring mission of the Bangladesh National Tuberculosis Control Programme 2010; BAN TUB 45.
16. Samal J. Health seeking behaviour among tuberculosis patients in India: a systematic review 2016. J Clin Diagn Res. 2016;10(10):LE01–6.
17. Lei X, Liu Q, Escobar E, Philogene J, Zhu H, Wang Y, et al. Public–private mix for tuberculosis care and control: a systematic review. Int J Infect Dis. 2015:34:20–32.
18. The Global Fund to fight AIDS, Tuberculosis and Malaria. Update on the Implementation of the new grant architecture. Third replenishment 2011–2013. file:///Users/mdmoshiurrahman/Downloads/Replenishment_2010HagueNewGrantArchitecture_Update_en.pdf.
19. Goldberg ML. Fighting urban TB in Bangladesh. UN Dispatch, United Nations News & Commentary Global News – Forum. 2011. https://www.undispatch.com/fighting-urban-tb-in-bangladesh/
20. International Centre for Diarrhoeal Disease Research, Bangladesh (icddr,b). Health and Demographic Surveillance System–Matlab. 2015;47: Scientific Report No. 126. http://dspace.icddrb.org:8080/jspui/bitstream/123456789/6325/1/icddrbScientificReport-126.pdf
21. International Centre for Diarrhoeal Disease Research, Bangladesh (icddr,b). Matlab Demographic workbook: Matlab HDSS annual reports 1983–2013. http://www.icddrb.org/activity/index.jsp?activityObjectID=2878
22. National Tuberculosis Control Programme. National guidelines and operational manual for tuberculosis control (Fourth edition). NTP/DGHS. 2015.
23. Rifat M, Rusen ID, Islam MA, Enarson DA, Ahmed F, Ahmed SM, et al. Why are tuberculosis patients not treated earlier? A study of informal health practitioners in Bangladesh. Int J Tuberc Lung Dis. 2011;15(5):647–51.
24. Charan J, Biswas T. How to calculate sample size for different study designs in medical research? Indian J Psychol Med. 2013;35(2):121–6.
25. Weiss MG, Auer C, Somma DB, Abouihia A, Kemp J, Jawahar MS, et al. Gender and tuberculosis: cross-site analysis and implications of a multi-country study in Bangladesh, India, Malawi, and Colombia. Social, economic and Behavioural research, report series no.3: World Health Organization on behalf of the special Programme for research and training in tropical diseases; 2006. http://www.who.int/tdr/publications/documents/sebrep3.pdf?ua=1
26. Nogueira BMF, Rolla VC, Akrami KM, Kiene SM. Factors associated with tuberculosis treatment delay in patients co-infected with HIV in a high prevalence area in Brazil. PLoS One. 2018;13(4):e0195409.
27. Bonadonna LV, Saunders MJ, Guio H, Zegarra R, Evans CA. Socioeconomic and behavioral factors associated with tuberculosis diagnostic delay in Lima, Peru. Am J Trop Med Hyg. 2018;98(6):1614–23.
28. Krishnan L, Akande T, Shankar AV, McIntire KN, Gounder CR, Gupta A, et al. Gender-related barriers and delays in accessing tuberculosis diagnostic and treatment services: a systematic review of qualitative studies. Tuberc Res Treat. 2014;2014:215059.
29. Rifat M, Hall J, Oldmeadow C, Husain A, Milton AH. Health system delay in treatment of multidrug resistant tuberculosis patients in Bangladesh. BMC Infect Dis. 2015;15:526.
30. Mahendradhata Y, Syahrizal BM, Utarini A. Delayed treatment of tuberculosis patients in rural areas of Yogyakarta province, Indonesia. BMC Public Health. 2008;8:393.
31. Dhanvij P, Joshi R, Kalantri SP. Delay in diagnosis of tuberculosis in patients presenting to a tertiary care hospital in rural Central India. J MGIMS. 2009; 14(ii):56–63.
32. Verhagen LM, Kapinga R, van Rosmalen-Nooijens KA. Factors underlying diagnostic delay in tuberculosis patients in a rural area in Tanzania: a qualitative approach. Infection. 2010;38(6):433–46.
33. Sabawoon W, Sato H, Kobayashi Y. Delay in the treatment of pulmonary tuberculosis: a report from Afghanistan. Environ Health Prev Med. 2012; 17(1):53–61.
34. Zhou C, Tobe RG, Chu J, Gen H, Wang X, Xu L. Detection delay of pulmonary tuberculosis patients among migrants in China: a cross-sectional study. Int J Tuberc Lung Dis. 2012;16(12):1630–6.
35. Jurcev-Savicevic A, Kardum G. Health-care seeking behaviour for tuberculosis symptoms in Croatia. Eur J Pub Health. 2012;22(4):573–7.
36. Horton KC, MacPherson P, Houben RM, White RG, Corbett EL. Sex differences in tuberculosis burden and notifications in low- and middle-income countries: a systematic review and meta-analysis. PLoS Med. 2016; 13(9):e1002119.
37. Uplekar M, Rangan S, Ogden J. Gender and tuberculosis control: towards a strategy for research and action. Geneva: World Health Organization (WHO/CDS/TB/2000.280); 1999. http://www.who.int/tb/publications/gender-strategy/en/
38. Sendagire I, Loeff MSVL, Mubiru M, Konde-Lule J, Cobelens F. Long delays and missed opportunities in diagnosing smear-positive pulmonary tuberculosis in Kampala, Uganda: a cross-sectional study. PLoS One. 2010; 5(12):e14459.

3

Clinical management of respiratory syndrome in patients hospitalized for suspected Middle East respiratory syndrome coronavirus infection in the Paris area from 2013 to 2016

A. Bleibtreu[1,2,6,7*], S. Jaureguiberry[2], N. Houhou[3], D. Boutolleau[4], H. Guillot[2], D. Vallois[1], J. C. Lucet[5,6,7], J. Robert[8,9], B. Mourvillier[6,7,10], J. Delemazure[11], M. Jaspard[2], F. X. Lescure[1,6,7], C. Rioux[1], E. Caumes[2†] and Y. Yazdanapanah[1,6,7†]

Abstract

Background: Patients with suspected Middle East respiratory syndrome coronavirus (MERS-CoV) infection should be hospitalized in isolation wards to avoid transmission. This suspicion can also lead to medical confusion and inappropriate management of acute respiratory syndrome due to causes other than MERS-CoV.

Methods: We studied the characteristics and outcome of patients hospitalized for suspected MERS-CoV infection in the isolation wards of two referral infectious disease departments in the Paris area between January 2013 and December 2016.

Results: Of 93 adult patients (49 male (52.6%), median age 63.4 years) hospitalized, 82 out of 93 adult patients had returned from Saudi Arabia, and 74 of them were pilgrims (Hajj). Chest X-ray findings were abnormal in 72 (77%) patients. The 93 patients were negative for MERS-CoV RT-PCR, and 70 (75.2%) patients had documented infection, 47 (50.5%) viral, 22 (23.6%) bacterial and one *Plasmodium falciparum* malaria. Microbiological analysis identified *Rhinovirus* (27.9%), *Influenza* virus (26.8%), *Legionella pneumophila* (7.5%), *Streptococcus pneumoniae* (7.5%), and non-MERS-coronavirus (6.4%). Antibiotics were initiated in 81 (87%) cases, with two antibiotics in 63 patients (67.7%). The median duration of hospitalization and isolation was 3 days (1–33) and 24 h (8–92), respectively. Time of isolation decreased over time ($P < 0.01$). Two patients (2%) died.

Conclusion: The management of patients with possible MERS-CoV infection requires medical facilities with trained personnel, and rapid access to virological results. Empirical treatment with neuraminidase inhibitors and an association of antibiotics effective against *S. pneumoniae* and *L. pneumophila* are the cornerstones of the management of patients hospitalized for suspected MERS-CoV infection.

Keywords: Middle East respiratory syndrome coronavirus (MERS-CoV), Pilgrims, Saudi Arabia, Isolation ward, Respiratory tract infection, Legionella

* Correspondence: alexandre.bleibtreu@aphp.fr
†E. Caumes and Y. Yazdanapanah contributed equally to this work.
[1]APHP, Hôpital Bichat Claude Bernard, Service des Maladies Infectieuses et Tropicales, Paris Diderot University, Paris, France
[2]APHP, Hôpitaux Universitaires Pitié Salpêtrière-Charles Foix, Service des Maladies Infectieuses et Tropicales, Paris, France
Full list of author information is available at the end of the article

Summary
During the 2013–2016 period, 93 patients were managed in two Parisian referral centers for possible MERS-CoV infection. None of them were confirmed as MERS-CoV positive. Seasonal and influenza viruses were the most common pathogens but bacterial pneumonia was also diagnosed.

Background
Middle East respiratory syndrome coronavirus (MERS-CoV) is a single-stranded positive-sense RNA virus firstly isolated in 2012 in the Kingdom of Saudi Arabia (KSA) [1]. In December 2016, the World Health Organization (WHO) reported 1917 laboratory-confirmed cases of MERS-CoV, and 684 deaths in 27 different countries [2]. MERS-CoV is a zoonotic virus of incompletely elucidated origin. Dromedary camels are suspected of being the reservoir, with bats as a possible origin because they harbor related viral sequences [3–8]. Human-to-human transmission requires close contact with infected people [9]. To date, all reported MERS-CoV cases have occurred in individuals from Arabian Peninsula countries, in travelers returning from this area or traced to an ill traveler.

Each year, during the Muslim Hajj and Umrah pilgrimage, millions of people travel to the Middle East. During this period there is a high risk among pilgrims of acquisition of respiratory tract infections, including MERS-CoV [10]. Although the risk of MERS-CoV acquisition is extremely low in pilgrims and travelers, the consequences of such acquisitions can be dreadful, as illustrated by a South Korean outbreak in which one index case led to 186 secondary and tertiary cases, including 36 deaths [11–13]. Nosocomial epidemic events have also been described in the KSA, where new cases in residents are still reported monthly [13–15]. These reports show that MERS-CoV is mostly characterized by nosocomial transmission and family clusters [13]. Interestingly, it has been shown that cross-transmission can be contained at home as well as in hospital settings when suspected cases are put under contact restriction and enhanced hygiene procedures are applied in combination with rapid testing for MERS-CoV [16].

In France, a national plan was set up in 2012/13 in which reference wards were identified in each region for rapid isolation of suspected cases, with prompt case ascertainment based on epidemiological and clinical characteristics with the help of the national institute of health [17]. Despite this framework, one case of MERS-CoV infection identified in 2013 in a traveler from the Middle East region led to a secondary case after nosocomial acquisition [18]. The clinical symptoms of MERS-CoV infection have low specificity [19]. Therefore the "true" etiology of an acute respiratory syndrome can be overlooked when focusing only on MERS-CoV infection in a suspected case and this may result in a lost opportunity [20]. This is particularly true during the period when people return from the Hajj, where the number of suspected cases increases greatly during a short time.

Here we report our four-year experience in the Paris area on the management and outcome of patients hospitalized in two isolation wards for suspected MERS-CoV infection. We performed a descriptive analysis to better define viruses or bacteria causing infections in this MERS-CoV negative population.

Methods
This retrospective analysis was carried out in the infectious diseases departments of two university hospitals (Bichat Claude Bernard and Pitié-Salpêtrière) in Paris, France. Both departments are part of the Paris/Ile de France regional plan for the management of contagious emerging infectious diseases in adults. They serve as referral centers for emerging infectious diseases in the Paris area and have isolation wards and dedicated rooms with anterooms and negative pressure. We enrolled patients who had been admitted to these two wards after being classified as possible cases of MERS-CoV infection, as defined by the WHO epidemiological bulletins [21].

In hospitalized patients, epidemiological data were collected: demographic characteristics, travel history, purpose of the travel, contact with animals or sick people and inpatient or outpatient visits during the travel. Also recorded were the nature of the initial symptoms, and the lag time between symptom onset and both the date of departure from the at-risk region, and hospitalization in an isolation ward.

Upon admission to the isolation wards, clinical symptoms and comorbidities were studied, the initial laboratory findings were assessed, and chest X-ray was defined as normal or showing alveolar and interstitial infiltrates.

Clinical management was evaluated in terms of the place of hospitalization, antibiotic treatment, antiviral use and oxygen administration. Microbiological parameters recorded included all bacteriological and virological tests performed during the hospital stay of the patient. Nasopharyngeal specimens were collected for real-time RT-PCR analysis. Respiratory specimens were obtained as soon as possible during the course of the illness (within 21 days after symptom onset). Laboratory confirmation of MERS-CoV infection has been performed on site since 2013, during the opening hours of the local laboratories and in the Pasteur Institute reference laboratory at night and weekends. Confirmation was performed by specific real-time RT-PCR assay, using two different MERS-CoV genomic target sites, the region upstream of the envelope gene and the site of *ORF1* [22]. Film Array Rapid multiplex PCR was performed for simultaneous qualitative detection and identification of multiple respiratory viral and bacterial nucleic acids in nasopharyngeal swabs (FilmArray® Respiratory Panel

Biomérieux Lyon France): adenovirus, coronaviruses, human metapneumovirus, influenza A and B viruses, parainfluenza viruses, respiratory A and B viruses, *Bordetella pertussis*, *Chlamydophila pneumoniae*, and *Mycoplasma pneumoniae*. Bacteria were documented using diverse methods including blood cultures, serology, urinary antigens, sputum and pulmonary samples, respectively. Blood smear for malaria was performed in at-risk travelers. Isolation was maintained until a negative result was obtained for MERS-CoV if the symptoms were more than 4 days old (otherwise a second sample was needed). Duration of isolation and total duration of hospitalization were recorded.

Comparisons were performed using Kruskal-Wallis tests for continuous variables and Pearson's χ^2 or Fisher's exact test for categorical variables. Statistical analysis was performed using R (v3.2.0, Vienna, Austria); significance was set at a p-value < 0.05.

According to the French Health Public Law (CSP Art L1121–1.1), such an investigation does not require specific informed consent or ethics committee approval because it is a retrospective study without medical intervention.

Results

Clinical characteristics

From January 2013 to December 2016, 93 adult patients, classified as possible MERS-CoV cases, were hospitalized in the two participating isolation wards. The male: female ratio was 1.1 and the median age was 63.4 years (interquartile range; IQR, 56–71.5). Of 82 (88.2%) patients who were returning from the KSA, 74 (90.2%) had travelled for the pilgrimage, two (2.1%) for professional reasons, and four (4.9%) for tourism; two (2.4%) were KSA residents (Fig. 1). There was an obvious seasonal trend with a major annual increase in the number of admitted patients during the annual Hajj period (Fig. 2). The median travel duration was 23 days (IQR = 17–27). The median lag time between the first symptoms and admission to the isolation ward was 8.2 days (IQR, 0–28). The median lag time between arrival in France and admission to the isolation ward was 2 days (IQR, 1–5 days), and only 19 (20.4%) patients had the first symptoms after their arrival in France.

The first symptoms described by the patients were cough (n = 62, 67%), influenza-like symptoms (n = 18, 19%), and dyspnea (n = 6, 6%). Other symptoms were diarrhea (n = 2, 2%), fever (n = 2, 2%), vomiting (n = 1, 1%), general illness (n = 1, 1%) and headache 1(1%). Thirty-four (36.5%) patients had consulted a physician in the at-risk countries and nine (9.7%) had prior hospitalization in these countries.

Close contact with ill travelers with respiratory symptoms during travel was found in 43 (46.7%) patients. Exposure to dromedary camels or contaminated camel milk or meat was found in five (5.4%) patients.

Initial clinical findings of patients admitted to isolation wards are reported in Tables 1 and 2. The most common signs were cough (95.7%), with 63 (70.7%) patients having sputum production, and 26 (29.3%) dry cough. Pulmonary auscultation revealed crackles in 61 (65.5%) patients, bilateral in 25 (26.9%). Ten (11%) patients required oxygen therapy at initial evaluation. Other clinical symptoms are listed in Table 2. Ten patients (11%) were admitted to intensive care directly (n = 6) or after evaluation in isolation wards (n = 5).

Seventy-five (80.6%) patients had underlying medical conditions with a median of 2 (1–3) different comorbidities

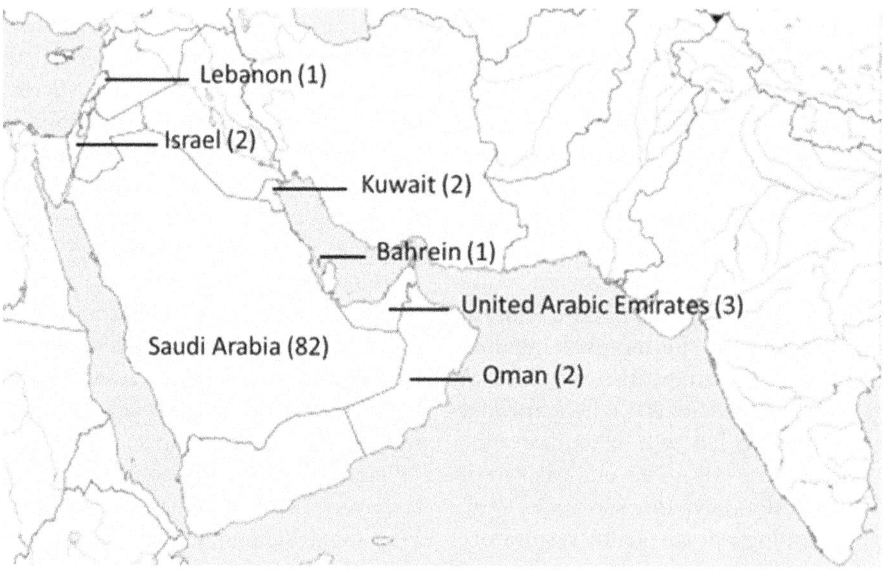

Fig. 1 Geographic distribution of the 93 patients prior to their hospitalization in an isolation ward for suspected MERS-COV infection. Adapted from Виктор В https://fr.wikipedia.org/wiki/Fichier:Outline_map_of_Middle_East.svg

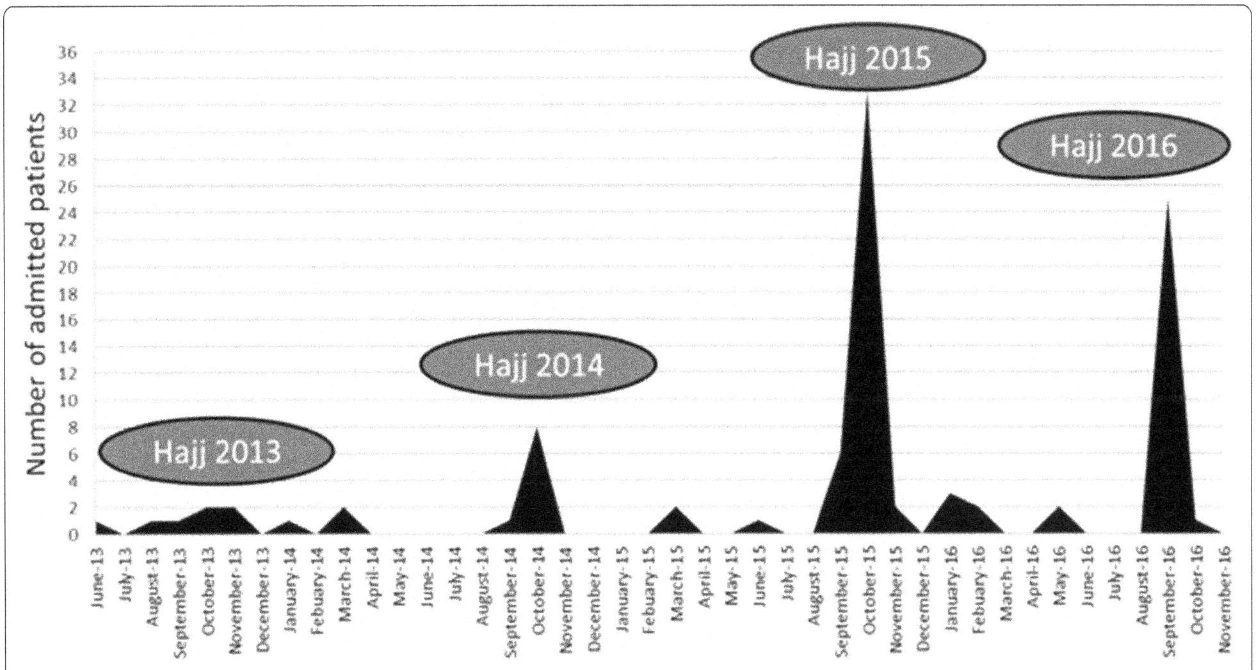

Fig. 2 Total number of admissions for suspected MERS-CoV infection according to the time of year, with special reference to the Hajj pilgrimage. The vertical axis represents the number of patients admitted per month. The horizontal axis represents dates. Boxes inside the diagram indicate the annual Hajj pilgrimage

Table 1 Clinical and travel characteristics of 93 patients with possible MERS-CoV infection hospitalized during 2013–2016

Characteristics		
Sex ratio M/F		49/44
		Median (IQR)
Age (year)		63.4 (56–71.6)
Temperature (°C)		38.4 (37.2–39)
Systolic blood pressure (mm Hg)		133 (120–148.5)
Diastolic blood pressure (mm Hg)		77 (66.5–83.5)
Heart rate (beats/min)		91 (81.5–108-5)
Respiratory frequency/min		20 (18–24)
Oxygen saturation		96 (93–98)
NYHA score		2 (1–3)
Duration of travel (days)		6.5 (4–12)
Time of illness (days) median (IQR) 6.5 (4–12)		
Reason for travel	N	%
Pilgrimage	74	79.6
Business	4	4.3
Tourism	11	11.8
Resident	4	4.3
Duration of travel (days) 23 (17–27)		

New York Heart Association (*NYHA*) Functional *Classification*, *KSA* Kingdom of Saudi Arabia, *UAE* United Arab Emirates

Table 2 Presenting symptoms and laboratory findings on admission in 93 patients with possible MERS-CoV infection hospitalized during 2013–2016

Symptoms	N	%
Cough	89	95.7
Fever (> 38 °C)	61	65.6
Lung crackles	61	65.6
Rhinorrhea	42	45.2
Myalgia	30	32.3
Headhache	26	28.0
Thoracic pain	22	23.7
Diarrhea	20	21.5
Abdominal pain	13	14.0
Vomiting	12	12.9
Nausea	11	11.8
Hemoptysis	9	9.7
Laboratory tests (n)	Median	IQR
CRP mg/dL (81)	122	41–247
WBC G/L (90)	9.295	6.45–12.325
Neutrophils G/L (75)	8.285	4.61–10.26
Lymphocytes G/L (63)	1.300	0.93–2.02
Platelets G/L (89)	268.	179–320
Serum creatinine μmol/L (89)	78.3	57–87

CRP C-reactive protein, *WBC* white blood cell count

such as hypertension ($n = 57$, 61.3%), chronic respiratory diseases ($n = 22$, 23.6%), chronic cardiac disease ($n = 21$, 22.6%), or obesity ($n = 19$, 20.4%). Nine patients (9.7%) had a history of neoplastic or hematological disease, six (6.4%) were receiving corticosteroids, and six (6.4%) immunosuppressive drugs.

Chest X-ray evaluation and laboratory results

Initial chest X-ray was available for 90 patients (96.7%), and findings were abnormal in 72 (80%). Thirty-nine of these 72 (54.1%) exhibited alveolar opacities with 4 (10.4%) bilateral localization, 20 (27.7%) interstitial syndrome, including 12 (60%) with bilateral localization, and 13 (18%) alveolar and interstitial syndrome, with bilateral localization in 9 (69.2%) (Additional file 1: Figure S1).

Laboratory findings are reported in Table 2. On admission, the median C-reactive protein was 122 mg/dL (21–247) and above 50 mg/dL in 57 (70.3%) patients. Neutrophil count was increased in 15 patients. Median neutrophil count was 8.285 G/L (4.61–10.26).

Therapeutic management

Among the 93 patients, 81 (87.1%) initially received antibiotic therapy: 63 (69.3%) antibiotic combinations (AC), and 18 (19.4%) a single antibiotic. AC were administered for a median duration of 48 h (IQR, 24–116), and were secondarily switched in 48 (76.2%) cases and discontinued in 15 (23.8%). AC were third-generation cephalosporin and macrolides in 55 patients (87.3%), aminopenicillin and macrolides in three patients and third-generation cephalosporin and fluoroquinolone in four patients. An AC was maintained in 10 (19.2%) cases, with aminopenicillin–spiramycin in six and quinolones plus spyramicin or rifampicin in four. Thirty-eight (60.3%) patients were switched to a single antibiotic as amoxicillin-clavulanate in 12 (31.5%), third-generation cephalosporin in eight, amoxicillin in seven, spiramycin in six, levofloxacin in three, and piperacillin-tazobactam and doxycycline each in one.

Single antibiotics initially prescribed were amoxicillin-clavulanate in nine patients (50%), amoxicillin in five, or third-generation cephalosporin in four. This antibiotic was maintained throughout treatment in 14 cases and switched to oral amoxicillin-clavulanate in four cases, with no discontinuation in the 48 first hours of treatment.

Empirical antiviral treatment with neuraminidase inhibitors

Oseltamivir was given to 35 patients (37.6%) for a median duration of 120 h (24–120). It was discontinued after 48 h in 12/35 (34.3%) patients, between 48 h and 5 days in 4 (11%) patients and kept for the entire treatment duration in 19 (54.3%) patients.

Oxygen therapy was required for 42 patients (45.6%), with a median maximal flow of 3 L/min (IQR = 2–4). Five (5.4%) patients had an oxygen flow of more than 6 L/min and were transferred to intensive care.

Microbiological documentation

None of the patients hospitalized for suspected MERS-CoV inhibition was found to be positive on MERS-CoV PCR. A microbiological etiology was identified in 70 (75.4%) patients (Table 3).

A viral infection was documented in 47 patients (50.3%), including 26 (37%) with human rhinovirus (HRV) and 25 (35.6%) influenza virus. For the latter, each type of virus was identified in approximately half of the cases.

A bacterial infection was documented in 22 patients (23.6%), the most common etiologies being *Legionella pneumophila* and *Streptococcus pneumoniae* in 10 patients (31.8%) each. Patients with Legionnaires' disease (LD) had more chronic cardiac disease and were more immunosuppressed than other patients (data not shown). Finally, those with LD had a longer duration of hospital management (11 days vs. 4 days, $p = 0.001$). *Plasmodium falciparum* malaria was diagnosed once.

A mixed infection was documented in 16 (17.4%) patients, 43% being mixed viral infections and 56% mixed virus-bacterial infections.

Empirical antibiotic therapy was prescribed to 21/22 patients with a documented bacterial infection, and was effective in 21 against the bacterial strains secondarily documented during the course of the disease. Among the 47 patients with a documented viral infection, 39 had received empirical antibiotic therapy. Lastly, of 23 patients without any documentation 21 had received empirical antibiotic therapy. Of the 25 patients with documented influenza virus, 13 (52%) had received neuraminidase inhibitors (oseltamivir).

Isolation precautions

The duration of isolation was calculated from the initial confinement triggered by the suspicion of MERS-CoV infection, upon the removal order by the physician following receipt of the negative result of the MERS-CoV analysis. The median duration of isolation precautions was 24 h (IQR, 24–32.5) and ranged from 8 to 144 h. The duration of isolation decreased significantly over the years from a median of 36 h in 2013 to 24 h in 2016 ($p < 0.01$) (Fig. 3). Patients were hospitalized in the isolation ward for a median of three days (IQR 2–5.22), and the total management duration from alert to hospital discharge was four days (IQR 3–8).

Mortality

Two of the 93 (2.1%) patients died of malignant flu and with a *Staphylococcus aureus* related prosthetic heart valve infective endocarditis, respectively.

Table 3 Pathogens in the 70 patients with microbiological data

	Monomicrobial infection	Mixed Infection							
	No other microorganism	Human Coronarovirus	*Influenza* A	*Influenza* B	*K. pneumoniae*	*S. pneumoniae*	*S. mitis*	*S. aureus*	Total
Non MERS Coronavirus_	3		1						4
Influenza A	13			1		2	1		17
H. influenzae	1		1						2
L. pneumophilia	6		1						7
Rhinovirus	16	2	3		1	2		1	25
S. paratyphi	1								1
Streptococcus A	1								1
Coxiella burnetti	1								1
HSV-1	1								1
Metapneumovirus	2								2
Infleunza B	2								2
P. falciparum	1								1
Parainfluenza	2								2
S. pneumoniae	3								3
Negative	23								23
Total	76	2	6	1	1	4	1	1	92

Discussion

During a four-year period including four Hajj and Umrah pilgrimages, our two centers managed 93 patients for possible MERS-CoV infection. None of the patients returning from endemic countries and classified as possible cases were confirmed as MERS-CoV positive.

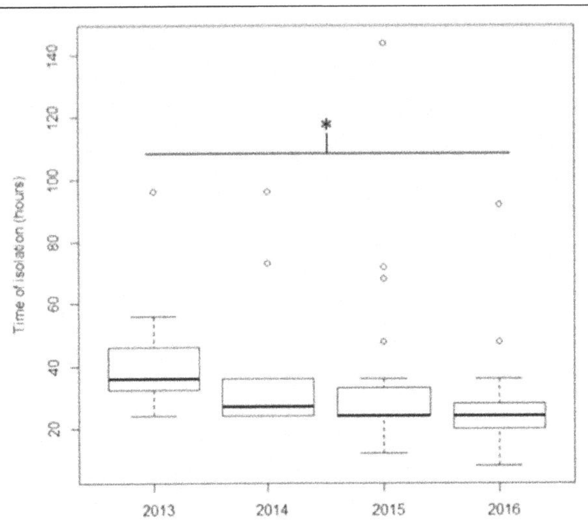

Fig. 3 Duration of isolation precautions in the isolation ward from 2013 to 2016. Each boxplot represents the duration of isolation for patients hospitalized per year, horizontal bars in the boxes represent the median, horizontal bars outside the boxes represent interquartile range (IQR), and circles represent outliers. The asterisk and the black bar represent *p*-valued under 0.05 using the Kruskal-Wallis test

Seasonal viruses and influenza viruses were the most common pathogens identified, but life-threatening bacterial pneumonia was also diagnosed.

Influenza viruses were found in 35% of the microbiologically documented patients, which is consistent with other results showing prevalence ranging from 13 to 64% for patients with suspected MERS-CoV infection [23–25]. In an Iranian study, influenza prevalence was around 10% in pilgrims with upper respiratory tract infections [26]. These results suggest that empirical oseltamivir therapy should be initiated in patients admitted to the isolation ward for suspected MERS-CoV infection. This antiviral treatment should be discontinued when PCR results prove negative for influenza. Moreover, these results illustrate the importance of preventive flu vaccine prior to pilgrimage and in all travelers to areas such as those where MERS-CoV is endemic [27].

In our study, 31.4% of the patients were positive for HRV, compared with 10 and 23% in two other studies [10, 28]. This is also in agreement with a study in French pilgrims that demonstrated acquisition of HRV during the trip using a pre- and post-travel routine screening [10]. HRV involvement in acute respiratory infection remains controversial, and further studies on phylogenetic and epidemiological characteristics are necessary to clarify the clinical impact of this virus [29].

Altogether, about one-quarter of our patients had species infections associated or not with viral infection. The two most frequently documented bacteria were *S.*

pneumoniae and *L. pneumophila*. Pneumococcal disease was diagnosed in seven patients; all had received empirical antibiotics effective against *S. pneumoniae*. It has been showed that *S. pneumoniae* carriage increases in French pilgrims during the Hajj [10], whereas vaccine coverage was low (7%) in 300 French Hajj pilgrims [30]. Therefore, pneumococcal vaccination should be proposed to at-risk persons before the Hajj pilgrimage.

Seven patients presented *L. pneumophila* infection. They all had previous underlying conditions with greater chronic cardiac disease and more immunosuppressed status. At initial evaluation, they presented with more headache, increased respiratory frequency, more intense dyspnea and a more prolonged duration of hospitalization. None of them died, but two patients required admission to intensive care units. LD has already been reported as an alternate diagnosis of MERS-CoV infection in a series of 77 suspected patients where 22 had positive results for alternative respiratory pathogens including two LD [23].

Pilgrims during the Hajj frequently stayed in accommodation opened only during the pilgrimage. *Legionella spp.*, the causative bacterium, is found naturally in fresh water and can contaminate hot tubs and cooling towers of air conditioners. The conditions of accommodation could partly explain LD acquisition during travel, as recently reported by the European Centre for Disease Prevention and Control, with more than 30 laboratory-confirmed cases of LD diagnosed in travelers from the European Union to Dubai since October 2016 [31], representing a significant increase over the average incidence. The probability of LD in patients with possible MERS-CoV infection highlights the need for an initial antibiotic combination with anti-Legionella efficacy, and local surveillance in pilgrim facilities.

One patient had a *P. falciparum* infection. This patient had made a stopover in Mali without antimalarial chemoprophylaxis during his return trip to France. Antimalarial treatment should be proposed to every patient with suspected MERS-CoV infection when they come back from a malarial endemic region.

A few sporadic travel-associated MERS-CoV cases have been reported outside the Arabian Peninsula, with 26 different countries involved, including Republic of South Korea (RSK). Regarding the very high number of travelers who stay in at-risk countries, especially during the Hajj, MERS-CoV transmission remains rare. In a recent MERS-CoV surveillance study conducted in the KSA during the annual Hajj pilgrimage, of 888 people screened during September 2015, none tested positive for MERS-CoV [32]. This is also supported by the absence of person-to-person MERS-CoV transmission during the mass gatherings at the Hajj in 2013–15 [33].

Nosocomial transmission of MERS-CoV, as in the KSA and RSK could be contained if every suspected case is managed with strict isolation precautions. This organization is implemented in France, with an alert system and referral departments trained and organized to receive possibly infected patients. This organization requires transfer of patients from the first care facility, where the suspicion arises, to the referral isolation ward. This might delay appropriate management of patients with acute respiratory infection and result in a lost opportunity as already detailed in one of our two case [20]. During our study period, patients with possible MERS-CoV infection were mostly (78.5%) admitted during short time periods linked to pilgrimage periods (Fig. 2). Moreover, the low specificity of the clinical symptoms [19] could lead to medical mistakes, and life-threatening diseases not fully covered by empirical antimicrobial treatment. Laboratory tests are limited in this setting excluding blood cultures. In our study, four diagnoses were likely delayed and not covered by the empirical treatment prescribed: Q fever, malaria, *S. aureus* endocarditis and HSV-1 stomatitis.

Our study had some limitations: it was retrospective and some data could not be obtained from all patients. There were only two MERS-CoV documented cases in the North of France [18]. Since these two cases, no new cases were described, but every year thousands of pilgrims and travelers return from endemic countries with respiratory syndrome, which engages the MERS-CoV procedure and leads to the transfer of these patients to isolation wards for diagnosis exclusion. Taking a control group with French non-traveler patients hospitalized for Respiratory infection seemed inappropriate. In a similar way, using travelers hospitalized for Respiratory tract infection did not seemed relevant because the only difference would be the travel destination as shown in travelers during the H1N1 pandemic [34]. Our Knowledge of MERS-CoV has grown over the years, and during this time management of possible cases has improved in terms of empirical treatment, which could have influenced our results. MERS-CoV RT-PCR was made available locally in 2013, thus reducing the time of diagnosis, which was also influenced by the time and day of the patient's arrival linked to the local laboratories opening hours.

Conclusions

Empirical antiviral treatment with neuraminidase inhibitors as well as antibiotic treatment effective against infection due to *L. pneumophila* and *S. pneumoniae* should be considered in any patients with suspected MERS-CoV infection. Altogether, our results argue for specific infectious disease units dedicated to emerging infectious disease management, but also for the development of new tools to simplify and expedite the diagnostic process in patients with suspected MERS-CoV infection in order to interrupt isolation procedures earlier.

Abbreviations

HSV-1: Herpes simplex virus1; IQR: Interquartile range; KSA: Kingdom of Saudi Arabia; LD: Legionnaires' disease; MERS-CoV: Middle East respiratory syndrome coronavirus; RSK: Republic of South Korea; RSV: Rhinovirus; RT-PCR: Real Time Polymerase Chain Reaction; UAE: United Arab Emirates; WHO: World Health Organization

Acknowledgments

Thanks to David Marsh and Guia Carrara for English copyediting.

Authors' contributions

AB collected and analyzed the data and performed illustrations. EC and YY contribute equally to the work. AB, SJ, YY, EC were major contributors in writing the manuscript. NH, DB performed virological analysis. JCL and JR supervised infection control. BM and JD were in charge with ICU patients. AB, SJ, HG, DV, MJ, FXL, CR, EC and YY were in charge with patients hospitalized in isolation wards. All authors read and approved the final manuscript.

Consent for publication

Not available.

All data generated or analyzed during this study are included in this published article and its supplementary information files.

Competing interests

The authors declare that they have no competing interests.

Author details

[1]APHP, Hôpital Bichat Claude Bernard, Service des Maladies Infectieuses et Tropicales, Paris Diderot University, Paris, France. [2]APHP, Hôpitaux Universitaires Pitié Salpêtrière-Charles Foix, Service des Maladies Infectieuses et Tropicales, Paris, France. [3]Virology Department, APHP-Bichat-Claude Bernard Hospital, Paris, France. [4]AP-HP, Hôpitaux Universitaires Pitié Salpêtrière-Charles Foix, Service de Virologie, et Sorbonne Universités, UPMC Univ Paris 06, CR7, CIMI, INSERM U1135, Paris, France. [5]APHP, Infection control unit, Bichat Claude Bernard hospital, Paris Diderot University, Paris, France. [6]INSERM, IAME, UMR 1137, Paris, France. [7]Univ Paris Diderot, IAME, UMR 1137, Sorbonne Paris Cité, Paris, France. [8]AP-HP, Hôpitaux Universitaires Pitié Salpêtrière-Charles Foix, Bactériologie-Hygiène Hospitalière, Paris, France. [9]Faculté de Médecine P. & M. Curie Paris-6 - Site Pitié, Centre d'Immunologie et des Maladies Infectieuses (CIMI) - E13, Paris, France. [10]APHP- Hôpital Bichat Claude Bernard, Service de Réanimation médicale et Infectieuse, Paris, France. [11]Service de pneumologie et réanimation Département R3S, AP-HP, Hôpitaux Universitaires Pitié Salpêtrière-Charles Foix, unité de Soin de Réadaptation Post Réanimation (SRPR), Paris, France.

References

1. Zaki AM, van Boheemen S, Bestebroer TM, Osterhaus ADME, Fouchier RAM. Isolation of a novel coronavirus from a man with pneumonia in Saudi Arabia. N Engl J Med. 2012;367:1814–20.
2. Who. http://www.who.int/emergencies/mers-cov/en/.
3. de Groot RJ, Baker SC, Baric RS, Brown CS, Drosten C, Enjuanes L, et al. Middle East respiratory syndrome coronavirus (MERS-CoV): announcement of the coronavirus study group. J Virol. 2013;87:7790–2.
4. Azhar EI, El-Kafrawy SA, Farraj SA, Hassan AM, Al-Saeed MS, Hashem AM, et al. Evidence for camel-to-human transmission of MERS coronavirus. N Engl J Med. 2014;370:2499–505.
5. Ali MA, Shehata MM, Gomaa MR, Kandeil A, El-Shesheny R, Kayed AS, et al. Systematic, active surveillance for Middle East respiratory syndrome coronavirus in camels in Egypt. Emerg Microbes Infect. 2017;6:e1.
6. Wernery U, Lau SKP, Woo PCY. Middle East respiratory syndrome (MERS) coronavirus and dromedaries. Vet J Lond Engl 1997. 2017;220:75–9.
7. Memish ZA, Mishra N, Olival KJ, Fagbo SF, Kapoor V, Epstein JH, et al. Middle East respiratory syndrome coronavirus in bats, Saudi Arabia. Emerg Infect Dis. 2013;19:1819–23.
8. Su S, Wong G, Shi W, Liu J, Lai ACK, Zhou J, et al. Epidemiology, Genetic Recombination, and Pathogenesis of Coronaviruses. Trends Microbiol. 2016; 24:490–502.
9. Hui DS, Azhar EI, Kim YJ, Memish ZA, Oh MD, Zumla A. Middle East respiratory syndrome coronavirus: risk factors and determinants of primary, household, and nosocomial transmission. Lancet Infect Dis. 2018;3099(18): 30127–0. [Epub ahead of print] Review. PubMed PMID: 29680581. https://doi.org/10.1016/S1473-3099(18)30127-0.
10. Benkouiten S, Charrel R, Belhouchat K, Drali T, Nougairede A, Salez N, et al. Respiratory viruses and bacteria among pilgrims during the 2013 Hajj. Emerg Infect Dis. 2014;20:1821–7.
11. Lim PL. Middle East respiratory syndrome (MERS) in Asia: lessons gleaned from the South Korean outbreak. Trans R Soc Trop Med Hyg. 2015;109:541–2.
12. Ki M. 2015 MERS outbreak in Korea: hospital-to-hospital transmission. Epidemiol Health. 2015;37:e2015033.
13. Alhamlan FS, Majumder MS, Brownstein JS, Hawkins J, Al-Abdely HM, Alzahrani A, et al. Case characteristics among Middle East respiratory syndrome coronavirus outbreak and non-outbreak cases in Saudi Arabia from 2012 to 2015. BMJ Open. 2017;7:e011865.
14. ProMED-mail [Internet]. [cited 2017 Feb 20]. Available from: http://www.promedmail.org/.
15. Hijawi B, Abdallat M, Sayaydeh A, Alqasrawi S, Haddadin A, Jaarour N, et al. Novel coronavirus infections in Jordan, April 2012: epidemiological findings from a retrospective investigation. East Mediterr Health J Rev Sante Mediterr Orient Al-Majallah Al-Sihhiyah Li-Sharq Al-Mutawassit. 2013;19(Suppl 1):S12–8.
16. Kim KH, Tandi TE, Choi JW, Moon JM, Kim MS. Middle East respiratory syndrome coronavirus (MERS-CoV) outbreak in South Korea, 2015: epidemiology, characteristics and public health implications. J Hosp Infect. 2017;95:207–13.
17. Avis du Haut conseil de la santé publique relatif à la définition et au classement des cas possibles et confirmés d'infection à MERS- CoV ainsi qu'aux précautions à mettre en œuvre lors de la prise en charge de ces patient. HCSP; 2015. https://www.hcsp.fr/explore.cgi/avisrapportsdomaine?clefr=506.
18. Guery B, Poissy J, el Mansouf L, Séjourné C, Ettahar N, Lemaire X, et al. Clinical features and viral diagnosis of two cases of infection with Middle East respiratory syndrome coronavirus: a report of nosocomial transmission. Lancet Lond Engl. 2013;381:2265–72.
19. Mohd HA, Memish ZA, Alfaraj SH, McClish D, Altuwaijri T, Alanazi MS, et al. Predictors of MERS-CoV infection: a large case control study of patients presenting with ILI at a MERS-CoV referral hospital in Saudi Arabia. Travel Med Infect Dis. 2016;14:464–70.
20. Bleibtreu A, Arias P, Vallois D, Debit A, Lermuzeaux M, Rioux C, et al. Delayed management of Staphyloccocus aureus infective endocarditis in a Middle East respiratory syndrome coronavirus possible case hospitalized in 2015 in Paris, France. Clin Microbiol Infect Off Publ Eur Soc Clin Microbiol Infect Dis. 2017;23:416–7.
21. mers_cov_interim_case_definition_Jul2015.pdf [Internet]. [cited 2017 Apr 10]. Available from: http://www.who.int/csr/disease/coronavirus_infections/mers_cov_interim_case_definition_Jul2015.pdf?ua=1.
22. Corman VM, Eckerle I, Bleicker T, Zaki A, Landt O, Eschbach-Bludau M, van Boheemen S, Gopal R, Ballhause M, Bestebroer TM, Muth D, Müller MA, Drexler JF, Zambon M, Osterhaus AD, Fouchier RM, Drosten C. Detection of a novel human coronavirus by real-time reverse-transcription polymerase chain reaction. Euro Surveill. 2012;17(39).
23. Thomas HL, Zhao H, Green HK, Boddington NL, Carvalho CFA, Osman HK, et al. Enhanced MERS coronavirus surveillance of travelers from the Middle East to England. Emerg Infect Dis. 2014;20:1562–4.
24. Gautret P, Charrel R, Benkouiten S, Belhouchat K, Nougairede A, Drali T, et al. Lack of MERS coronavirus but prevalence of influenza virus in French pilgrims after 2013 Hajj. Emerg Infect Dis. 2014;20:728–30.
25. Shahkarami M, Yen C, Glaser C, Xia D, Watt J, Wadford DA. Laboratory testing for Middle East respiratory syndrome coronavirus, California, USA, 2013-2014. Emerg Infect Dis. 2015;21:1664–6.
26. Moattari A, Emami A, Moghadami M, Honarvar B. Influenza viral infections among the Iranian Hajj pilgrims returning to Shiraz, Fars province, Iran. Influenza Other Respir Viruses. 2012;6:e77–9.
27. BEH-hors-serie-Recommandations-sanitaires-pour-les-voyageurs-2016) [Internet]. Available from: http://invs.santepubliquefrance.fr.

28. Annan A, Owusu M, Marfo KS, Larbi R, Sarpong FN, Adu-Sarkodie Y, et al. High prevalence of common respiratory viruses and no evidence of Middle East respiratory syndrome coronavirus in Hajj pilgrims returning to Ghana, 2013. Trop Med Int Health TM IH. 2015;20:807–12.
29. Greenberg SB. Update on human rhinovirus and coronavirus infections. Semin Respir Crit Care Med. 2016;37:555–71.
30. Sridhar S, Belhouchat K, Drali T, Benkouiten S, Parola P, Brouqui P, et al. French Hajj pilgrims' experience with pneumococcal infection and vaccination: a knowledge, attitudes and practice (KAP) evaluation. Travel Med Infect Dis. 2015;13:251–5.
31. European Centre for Disease Prevention and Control. Increase of cases of Legionnaires' disease in EU travellers returning from Dubai, October-December 2016. 22 Dec 2016 [Internet]. Available from: http://ecdc.europa.eu/en/publications/Publications/20-Dec-2016-RRA-Legionella-United%20Arab%20Emirates.pdf.
32. Saeed AAB, Abedi GR, Alzahrani AG, Salameh I, Abdirizak F, Alhakeem R, et al. Surveillance and testing for Middle East respiratory syndrome coronavirus, Saudi Arabia, April 2015-February 2016. Emerg Infect Dis. 2017; 23:682–5.
33. Mackay IM, Arden KE. MERS coronavirus: diagnostics, epidemiology and transmission. Virol J. 2015;12:222.
34. Jauréguiberry S, Boutolleau D, Grandsire E, Kofman T, Deback C, Aït-Arkoub Z, et al. Clinical and microbiological evaluation of travel-associated respiratory tract infections in travelers returning from countries affected by pandemic A(H1N1) 2009 influenza. J Travel Med. 2012;19:22–7.

4

Modeling tuberculosis dynamics with the presence of hyper-susceptible individuals for Ho Chi Minh City from 1996 to 2015

Dao Nguyen Vinh[1*], Dang Thi Minh Ha[1,2], Nguyen Thi Hanh[1], Guy Thwaites[1,3], Maciej F. Boni[3,4], Hannah E. Clapham[1,3] and Nguyen Thuy Thuong Thuong[1,3]

Abstract

Background: The depletion of CD4 cell is the underlying reason for TB hyper-susceptibility among people with HIV. Consequently, the trend of TB dynamics is usually hidden by the HIV outbreak.

Methods: Here, we aim to evaluate the trend of TB dynamics quantitatively by a simple mathematical model using the known prevalence of hyper-susceptible individuals in the population. In order to estimate the parameters governing transmission we fit this model in a maximum likelihood framework to both reported TB cases and data from samples tested with Interferon Gamma Assay from Ho Chi Minh City - a city with high TB transmission and strong synchronization between HIV/AIDS and TB dynamics.

Results: Our results show that TB transmission in HCMC has been declining among people without HIV; we estimate a 18% (95% CI: 9–25%) decline in the transmission parameter between 1996 and 2015. Furthermore, we show that co-infected patients have limited contribution to the transmission process. For hyper-susceptible individuals, our model suggests that the risk of a new active TB infection occurring is significantly higher than the risk of relapsed active TB, while this is not the case for people without hyper-susceptibility.

Conclusions: The increase of TB notifications in Ho Chi Minh City from 1996 to 2008 is evitable when, as occurred, the number of hyper-susceptible individuals increased faster than the decrease of TB transmission rate. The sharp decrease in TB notifications observed in this city from 2008 to 2015 is the combined result of the decrease of TB transmission rate and the decrease of hyper-susceptible individuals in the population. For hyper-susceptible individuals, we propose that the reason for the reduced relapsed active TB risk is HIV treatment delay. According to HIV treatment guidelines issued by Vietnam's Ministry of Health, hyper-susceptible individuals usually have to wait until their CD4 cell count falls under 350 cells/μl to start ART. Once patients begin ART, they will remain on ART for the rest of their life and thus have greater protection against relapses of TB. We therefore hypothesize that the delay in using ART imposes considerable TB burden on HCMC despite the declining transmission process.

Keywords: Tuberculosis, AIDS, Hyper-susceptible, Maximum likelihood estimation

* Correspondence: vinhdn@oucru.org
[1]Wellcome Trust Major Overseas Programme, Hospital for Tropical Diseases, Oxford University Clinical Research Unit, 764 Vo Van Kiet Street, District 5, Ho Chi Minh City, Vietnam
Full list of author information is available at the end of the article

Background

Among infectious diseases, tuberculosis (TB) is a leading cause of mortality worldwide with 1.5 million deaths annually, mainly occuring in low and middle income countries [1]. In Vietnam, TB is still one of the top ten leading causes of death among all ages [2] despite substantial attempts to reduce its burden. The Direct Observed Treatment, Short Course (DOTS), the heart of the TB elimination strategy recommended by the World Health Organization (WHO) [3, 4], was implemented in Vietnam in 1994. By 1998 it covered about 96% of the Vietnamese population [5, 6]. After DOTS was adopted, a large amount of National Tuberculosis Control Program's (NTP) funding was spent on public engagement to educate people about how to prevent transmission of TB in the population. However, annual TB notifications in Vietnam increased from around 75 per 100,000 in 1996 to over 100 per 100,000 in 1998, and remained stable at about 110 per 100,000 until 2014 [6, 7]. In Ho Chi Minh City (HCMC), the biggest city in Vietnam and a high TB transmission setting, an advanced monitoring program for TB relapses in which individuals with active TB are monitored more carefully was implemented by the NTP in 2003. In this program, patients who receive successful treatment are asked to come back to district tuberculosis units (DTUs) for a TB examination two to four months after treatment. However, the number of TB notifications in HCMC increased from about 10,000 in 1996 to about 13,000 in 2008. Subsequently, the number of notifications declined until 2015 – the last year that the TB data used in this paper are available.

It is important to emphasize that when DOTs was implemented, HIV had started to spread widely in the Vietnamese population. The first HIV case in Vietnam was detected in 1990 in HCMC. Two years later, only 11 HIV cases had been reported [8], and in 1993, the first cases of AIDS in Vietnam were reported. The reported number of new AIDS cases per year has increased sharply since then, peaking in 2008 at around 17,000. After that, like TB, this number also appeared to decline until 2015 – the last year that the HIV/AIDS data used in this paper are available. In HCMC, the Vietnam HIV program estimates the numbers of people with HIV and AIDS in 2015 were about 50,000 and 20,000 respectively [9]. Hence, the total number of people living with HIV in HCMC in 2015 was about 70,000, approximately 0.8% to 1% of the HCMC population.

The emergence of HIV/AIDS to human population enhanced the tuberculosis dynamics by creating a massive number of TB hyper-susceptible individuals in the human population. Consequently, high HIV prevalence settings such as Africa becomes target of many modelling HIV/TB studies such as [10–15]. The studies [11, 15] offers an overview about HIV/TB about nine different African countries. There was a strong synchronization between HIV and TB dynamics in these countries. When the HIV prevalence peaks at 10–25%, the number of TB notifications are about five times higher (at about 800 notifications/year). These studies also shows that ART wide use in the population benefits the TB dynamics. The study [10] only focused on the HIV/TB in a South Afican township indicates that HIV positive may account for 75% of TB notifications in a high HIV prevalence area. In the low HIV prevalence settings (≤ 1% HIV prevalence), HIV positives also accounts for a substantial part of TB patients. From October 2003 to Febuary 2005, 40% of TB patients were diagnosed with HIV positive in a small non-modelling study conducted in Cambodia – a developing country with only 0.5% HIV prevalence [16]. In Thailand – a high TB burden country with low HIV prevalence, strong correlation between HIV/AIDS and TB dynamics was observed for past 20 years [7].

Unlike the HIV/TB modeling works cited in this paper which focuses on the effect of various measures, the main aim of this paper is quantitatively investigating the trend of TB transmission in HCMC from 1996 to 2015 – period that HIV/AIDS emerged to HCMC's population. In order to archive this aim, we need to identify the impact of HIV/AIDS to TB dynamic in HCMC's population. Because we use multiple data sources for analyzing HCMC's TB dynamics, we do need a mathematical model to combine all of these sources into a simple framework for interpretation. There has been a considerable amount of modeling research on TB dynamics not including HIV/AIDS [17–22]. After HIV/AIDS was recognized as a crucial factor for TB, many modeling papers focused on the effect of HIV/AIDS on TB epidemiology at the population scale [10–12, 23–28]. However, none of the models cited in this paper includes all three aspects: HIV status (HIV+/HIV-), form of TB (pulmonary TB /extra pulmonary TB), and history of previous TB treatment (new/relapsed TB cases). As a result, it is difficult to apply these models for quantitatively analyzing our data sets. Thus, we modified the model presented by [20] to describe TB transmission in the presence of hyper-susceptible individuals in the population. Unlike the other HIV/TB modeling studies, the model developed in this study ignores the HIV transmission and HIV progression process. Furthermore, we used the AIDS prevalence to depict the dynamics of hyper-susceptible individuals in the population because [29, 30] indicates that about 90% of co-infected patients have CD4 cell count per μl less than 350–400 and the risk of TB increases exponentially with the decline of CD4 cell count. After that, we estimate parameters of the model by fitting this model to TB data collected from the NTP.

Methods

Tuberculosis transmission model (TTM)

For an uninfected individual, TB exposure results in either active TB (approximately 10% of the time) or latent TB (approximately 90% of the time); latent TB is defined as the state in which persistent immune response to Mycobacterium tuberculosis antigens but not clinical evidence of active TB exists. It is also possible for a patient with latent TB to develop active TB due to a new infection. This process is called *exogenous reinfection*. Note that TB exposure may cause the phenomenon in which mycobacteria remains in lungs and is not transmissible. The term *endogenous reactivation* describes the process in which these mycobacteria are activated, leading to active TB in an individual with a previously latent infection. Individuals who are experiencing active TB for the first time are classified as new cases. For every subsequent time they experience an active TB infection, individuals are classified as relapsed cases. Successful TB treatment eliminates all TB and its clinical symptoms, and stops transmission. However, there is no microbiological testing available to confirm that all mycobacteria are completely killed in the body of TB patients after successful TB treatment. Therefore, it is possible for individuals who have recovered from active TB to be infectious with TB again in the future due to both exogenous reinfection and endogenous reactivation.

We modified the model presented by [20] to describe TB transmission in HCMC. The model used in our study is shown in Fig. 1. Hyper-susceptibility is taken into account in our model by dividing the whole population into two groups: the *not hyper-susceptible* (G1) group and the *hyper-susceptible* (G2) group. In this model, we assumed that infectivity of extra-pulmonary TB cases is negligible, so transmission occurs due to effective contact with pulmonary TB cases only. For the G1 group, people stay in uninfected class (*U*) from the time they were born. In this class they are subject to the force of infection $\lambda(t)$. When individuals acquire a new infection, they have probability Φ to develop active TB, and probability $1-\Phi$ to stay in the latent state (*L*). People in the latent class (*L*) can develop active TB through both exogenous reinfection or endogenous reactivation. An active TB case has probability δ_p to develop pulmonary TB (*PTBn*), and $1-\delta_p$ to develop extra-pulmonary TB (*ExPTBn*). After recovery, individuals move to the recovered class (*R*). In the recovered class (*R*), similar to people in the latent class (*L*), people can become infectious through exogenous reinfection or endogenous reactivation. Relapsed pulmonary and extra-pulmonary TB cases go to the *PTBr* and *ExPTBr* states respectively. For G2 group, a similar diagram is used. We assume that there are no protection due to previous TB infection among people in G2. Individuals who had active TB while they were HIV-uninfected are

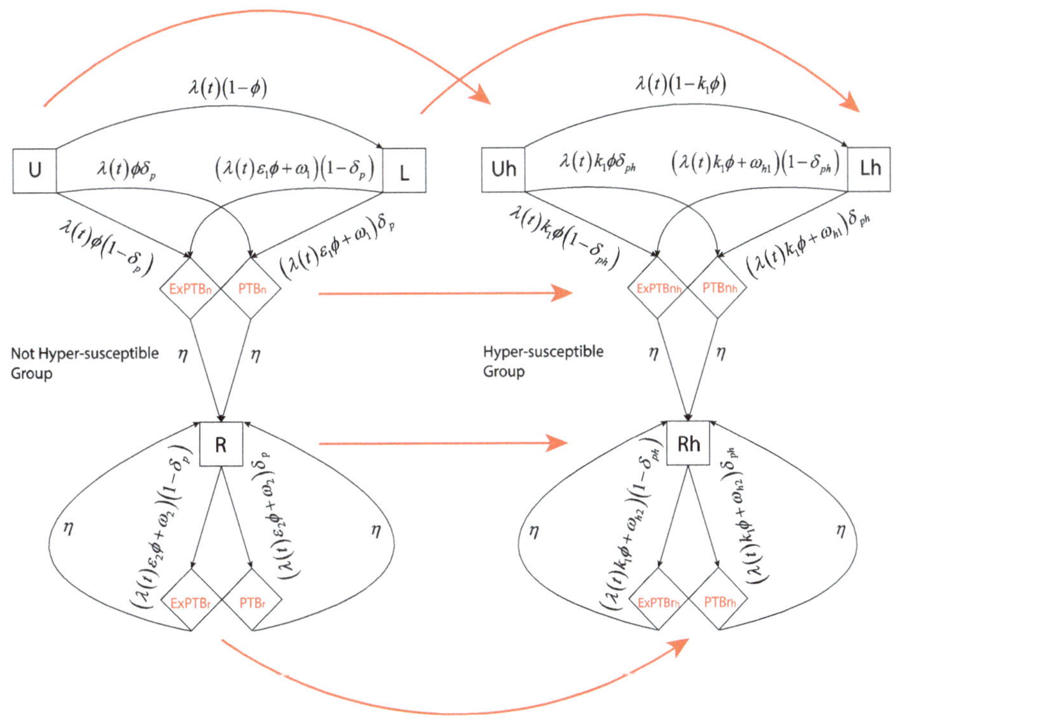

Fig. 1 Tuberculosis transmission model. The capital letters *U*, *L*, and *R* stands for uninfected, latent, and recovered. The notations *PTB* and *ExPTB* correspond to active pulmonary TB and extra-pulmonary TB respectively. In order to distinguish new and relapsed cases, the subscripts *n* and *r* are used. The subscript *h* is used for hyper-susceptible individuals. The red arrows show the hyper-susceptibility progression process by which individuals move from group G1 to group G2

Table 1 Parameter summary

Prms	Meaning	Fixed	Reference	Infer	Note
$\lambda(t)$	TB force of infection function			NA	See Fig. 2
β_1	Transmission rate of the year 1996			Yes	
β_2	Transmission rate of the year 2015			Yes	
Φ	Probability that a new infection results in an active TB.	10%	[18, 20, 21]	No	
ε_1	Relative rate that a new infection results in an active TB between people in *L* and *U*.	0.21	[53]		
ε_2	Relative rate that a new infection results in an active TB between people in *R* and *U*.			Yes	
ω_1	TB reactivation rate of people in *L*.	0.00098 p-yrs	[54]		The life-time risk: 5–10%
ω_2	TB reactivation rate people in *R*.			Yes	
k_1	Relative rate that a new infection results in an active TB case between hyper-susceptible individuals (*Ua*, *La*, and *Ra*) and uninfected people (*U*).			Yes	
ω_{h1}	TB reactivation rate of hyper-susceptible individuals with latent TB (*La*).			Yes	
ω_{h2}	TB reactivation rate of hyper-susceptible individuals with recovered TB (*Ra*).			Yes	
δ_p	Probability of an active TB in G1 develop into pulmonary TB.	78%	HCMC Report	No	
δ_{ph}	Probability of an active TB in G2 develop into pulmonary TB.	57%	HCMC Report	No	
d_{ptb}	Death probability of PTB case.	1%	HCMC Report	No	
d_{Exptb}	Death probability of ExPTB case.	10%	HCMC Report	No	
s_{ptb}	Probability of successful treatment for PTB	95%	HCMC Report	No	
s_{Exptb}	Probability of successful treatment for ExPTB	80%	HCMC Report	No	
η	Recovery rate	2		No	Average infectious time: 6 months.
γ	Infectivity of co-infected pulmonary cases			Yes	
$r_{new\text{-}tb}(t)$	Reporting rate of new TB cases at year$t$			NA	
$r_{relapsed\text{-}tb}(t)$	Reporting rate of relapsed TB cases at year t			NA	
r_1	Parameter of $r_{new\text{-}tb}(t)$ and $r_{relapsed\text{-}tb}(t)$			Yes	See Fig. 2
r_2	Parameter of $r_{relapsed\text{-}tb}(t)$			Yes	
Breaking-year	Parameter of $r_{relapsed\text{-}tb}(t)$ - breaking year.			Yes	
b	Birth rate			No	Parameter *b* is adjusted to sustain the HCMC population size GSO's report.
N	Population Size		[32]	No	
μ	Natural death rate	0.0054	[32]	No	
sc	Scaling parameter	1.9508		No	See Section 1.1 of supplement
est	Expected survival time of hyper-susceptible individuals.	1 yr		No	

classified as relapsed TB if it occurs after HIV infection. Furthermore, we assume that the process that people move from G1 to G2 happens to be uniform across TB states. The difference in exogenous reinfection and endogenous reactivation between G1 and G2 groups can be seen from the meaning of hyper-susceptibility- related parameters which are listed in Table 1. Because the TB dynamics is very slow [17, 31], data collected for couple decades are not enough for distingquish between infection and reactivation processes. Therefore, in order to to improve the identifiability of our analysis, we fix ε_1 and ω_1 in advance. For reporting purpose, we fix the expected survival time of people (*est*) in G2 group at one year. Analyses with different values of *est* are shown in supplement.

On top of birth, death, and hyper-susceptibility progression processes, we used deterministic model that is depicted by Fig. 1 to describe the transmission process of TB:

$$
\begin{aligned}
\dot{U} &= -\lambda(t)U \\
\dot{L} &= \lambda(t)(1-\phi)U-(\lambda(t)\varepsilon_1\phi+\omega_1)L \\
Ex\dot{PTB}n &= [\lambda(t)\phi U+(\lambda(t)\varepsilon_1\phi+\omega_1)L](1-\delta_p)-\eta s_{\text{Exptb}}ExPTBn-\eta d_{\text{Exptb}}ExPTBn \\
P\dot{T}Bn &= [\lambda(t)\phi U+(\lambda(t)\varepsilon_1\phi+\omega_1)L]\delta_p-\eta s_{\text{ptb}}PTBn-\eta d_{\text{ptb}}PTBn \\
\dot{R} &= \eta s_{\text{ptb}}PTBn+\eta s_{\text{Exptb}}ExPTBn+\eta s_{\text{Exptb}}ExPTBr+\eta s_{\text{ptb}}PTBr-[\lambda(t)\varepsilon_2\phi+\omega_2]R \\
Ex\dot{PTB}r &= [\lambda(t)\varepsilon_2\phi+\omega_2]R(1-\delta_p)-\eta s_{\text{Exptb}}ExPTBr-\eta d_{\text{Exptb}}ExPTBr \\
P\dot{T}Br &= [\lambda(t)\varepsilon_2\phi+\omega_2]R\delta_p-\eta s_{\text{ptb}}PTBr-\eta d_{\text{ptb}}PTBr \\
\dot{U}_h &= -\lambda(t)(1-k_1\phi)U_h-\lambda(t)\phi k_1U_h \\
\dot{L}_h &= \lambda(t)(1-k_1\phi)U_h-(\lambda(t)k_1\phi+\omega_{h1})L_h \\
Ex\dot{PTB}n_h &= [\lambda(t)\phi k_1U_h+(\lambda(t)k_1\phi+\omega_{h1})L_h](1-\delta_{ph})-\eta s_{\text{Exptb}}ExPTBn_h-\eta d_{\text{Exptb}}ExPTBn_h \\
P\dot{T}Bn_h &= [\lambda(t)\phi k_1U_h+(\lambda(t)k_1\phi+\omega_{h1})L_h]\delta_{ph}-\eta s_{\text{ptb}}PTBn_h-\eta d_{\text{ptb}}PTBn_h \\
\dot{R}_h &= \eta s_{\text{ptb}}PTBn_h+\eta s_{\text{Exptb}}ExPTBn_h+\eta s_{\text{Exptb}}ExPTBr_h+\eta s_{\text{ptb}}PTBr_h-[\lambda(t)k_1\phi+\omega_{h2}]R_h \\
Ex\dot{PTB}r_h &= [\lambda(t)k_1\phi+\omega_{h2}]R_h(1-\delta_{ph})-\eta s_{\text{Exptb}}ExPTBr_h-\eta d_{\text{Exptb}}ExPTBr_h \\
P\dot{T}Br_h &= [\lambda(t)k_1\phi+\omega_{h2}]R_h\delta_{ph}-\eta s_{\text{ptb}}PTBr_h-\eta d_{\text{ptb}}PTBr_h
\end{aligned}
\tag{1}
$$

Where the force of infection is defined by:

$$
\lambda(t)=\beta(t)\frac{PTBn(t)+PTBr(t)+\gamma PTBn_h(t)+\gamma PTBr_h(t)}{\text{Total Population Size at year } t} \tag{2}
$$

Demographic and hyper-susceptible individual data

In order to build and simulate the TB transmission model, the population size of G1 and G2 groups each year in HCMC are required in advance. Firstly, information about the population size of HCMC from 1993 to 2015 is derived from the General Statistics Office of Vietnam (GSO) [32]. The natural death rate of the population in HCMC is fixed at 0.0054 – the average death rate reported by GSO. The birth rate was adapted to maintain the population size as GSO reports. Second, because we assume the number of AIDS is representative for the number of individuals in G2 group, the reported number of new AIDS cases of Vietnam from 1993 to 2015 is collected from the Vietnam Ministry of Health [9, 33]. Note that due to lack of data for the year 2014, the reported number from the year 2014 is interpolated by averaging this number of the year 2013 and 2015. Then, the number of individuals in G2 group in a given year is reconstructed using the four following assumptions:

1. The number of AIDS cases is representative of the number of individuals in G2 group.
2. The number of annual newly AIDS cases in HCMC is proportional to that number in Vietnam.
3. The expected survival time of people in G2 group is constant over time.
4. The population size of G2 group in HCMC in 2015 is 19,973 as estimated by Vietnam's HIV program [9].

Only three first assumptions are needed to identify the shape of G2's population size curve. Then, we employ scaling parameter (*sc*) to adjust this curve to satisfy the fourth assumption. The number of individuals in G2 group in any given year follows after that. Further details of how these four assumptions are implemented is shown in Section 1 of supplement.

Tuberculosis data

We fit the model to three sources of data. Firstly, annual TB notification data from HCMC are collected from the Annual Tuberculosis Report from 1996 to 2015. This report is the combination of quarterly reports from all 24 DTUs in HCMC and Pham Ngoc Thach hospital, a national referral hospital for lung diseases and tuberculosis. Location of collecting sites are shown in Additional file 1: Figure S7. In summary, each annual report includes the number of new and relapsed pulmonary TB and total extra-pulmonary TB cases treated at the DTUs in the corresponding years. From 2009, extra-pulmonary TB cases were also classified into new and relapsed. Because pediatric TB is under-reported in Vietnam [34], more than 95% of reported cases of this data set are from adult. We call this data D1.

Secondly, blood samples are collected from 78 Vietnamese healthy subjects working at Oxford University Clinical Research Unit in HCMC and Interferon-Gamma Release Assays (IGRAs) are used to examine the history of TB exposure. These subjects have never been diagnosed as having active TB. IGRAs measure Interferon-Gamma produced by T lymphocytes in response to TB antigens. The assays are employed to identify latent TB in healthy volunteers who are in working age. In total, 46/78 (59%) of these subjects is tested positive and we adopt this as an estimate of the proportion of latent TB in HCMC in this work. Since the sensitivity and specificity of this test are over 96% [35], we do not consider the type 1 and type 2 error of the test. We call this data D2.

Thirdly, in order to investigate the prevalence of hyper-susceptible individuals among TB patients, we collect the HIV status of 1000 random TB patients in HCMC each year from 1996 to 2014 from patient records of all districts. Further information about those patients are anonymous. We call this data D3.

Simulation and maximum likelihood estimation

The model fitting method that is employed in this paper is maximum likelihood estimation. In order to compute the likelihood of a parameter set, we simulate the system depicted by eq. (1). After that, we compute the likelihood value of this parameter set. We use standard simplex method [36] in GSL library of C++ for the maximum likelihood estimation. The detail of simulation and maximum likelihood method is shown in Section 1.2 and 1.3 of supplement.

Hypothesis testing

In order to exloring the TB epidmiology scenario of HCMC, we investigate two additional hypotheses about the pattern of TB transmission and reporting of relapsed TB over the past 20 years by fitting the model described by eqs. (1) to HCMC's TB data. These two hypotheses are shown in Fig. 2. We have four different scenarios of TB transmission and reporting rate of relapsed TB:

1. Both contact parameter and reporting rate of relapsed TB are constant over time.
2. The contact parameter is time-varying and relapsed TB reporting rate is constant.
3. The contact parameter is constant and relapsed TB reporting rate is time-varying.
4. Both contact parameter and relapsed TB reporting rate are time-varying.

Hereinafter, we use the word *hypothesis* to refer to one of these four scenarios (enumerated from *H1 to H4*). The Akaike information criterion (AIC) is used for comparing different epidemiological scenarios [37].

Results

Epidemiological hypothesis selection

The summary of epidemiological hypothesis selection is shown in Table 2. The hypothesis H4 are more likely than the others by AIC. This hypothesis assumes that contact parameter declines linearly from 1996 to 2015 and the reporting rate of relapsed cases is time-varying (Table 2). According to this hypothesis, the estimate of contact parameter dropped from 37.8 in 1996 to 31.1 in 2015 (about 18% reduction) and the reporting rate of relapsed cases reached over 95% after 2003 (Table 3). Other hypotheses tend to fail in explaining either the DTU's reporting data or IGRA data (Additional file 1: Figure S2 –S4). The AIC difference between H4 and others is at least 385 units (Table 2). Therefore, we use H4 for presenting goodness of fit in Fig. 3. Goodness of fit for other hypotheses can be seen from Additional file 1: Figure S2 to S5.

Goodness of fit

Because there are only seven years (from 2009 to 2015) in which extra-pulmonary TB cases were classified as

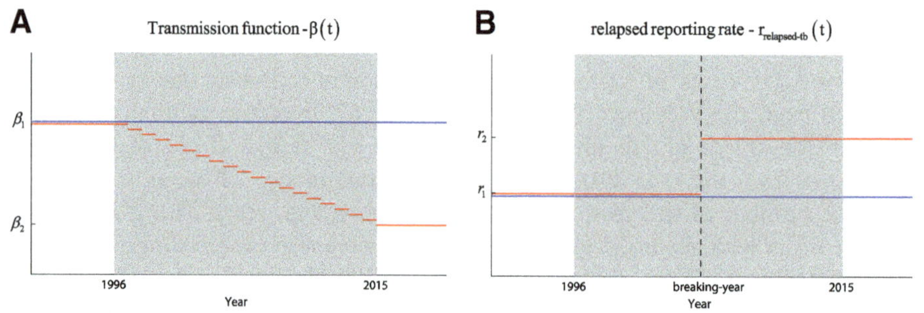

Fig. 2 Hypothesis of contact parameter and relapsed reporting rate. The grey area shows the period TB data were collected. In panel (**a**), the blue line and red line represent two different scenarios on transmission rate function *ß(t)*. While the blue line stands for the case in which transmission function is constant over time, the red line shows the case where this function is assumed to be piece-wise and linearly decreasing (or increasing) from 1996 to 2015. In total, two parameters at most (β_1 *and* β_2) are employed to parameterize for the transmission function. In panel (**b**), the blue and the red line represent two different hypotheses of relapsed reporting rate $r_{relapsed\text{-}tb}(t)$. The blue line corresponds to the case in which reporting rate of relapsed cases is constant over time. The red line corresponds to the case that the relapsed reporting rate changed over time. Note that the incidence reporting rate $r_{new\text{-}tb}(t)$ is always assumed to be constant over time, and equal r_1. Therefore, in total, three unknowns at most (r_1, r_2, and *breaking-year*) are used to describe both $r_{new\text{-}tb}(t)$ and $r_{relapsed\text{-}tb}(t)$. The *breaking-year* just takes discrete value from 1996 to 2015

Table 2 Summary of AIC comparison of different epidemiological hypotheses

Hypothesis	Assumption		#optimized parameters	AIC – min(AIC)
	ß(t)	*$r_{relapsed\text{-}tb}(t)$*		
H1	*Constant*	Constant	8	1886.96
H2	Time-varying	Constant	9	385.16
H3	Constant	Time-varying	10	1787.5
H4	Time-Varying	Time-Varying	11	**0.0**

The quantity AIC - min(AIC) of the best hypothesis is zero (in bold)

new or relapsed, we merge new extra-pulmonary and relapsed extra-pulmonary groups as Ex-Ptb for reporting the goodness of fit. As can be seen from Fig. 3, as the model relies on the annual counts of new hyper-susceptible individuals, the reconstructed TB dynamics is not smooth. However, it can capture qualitatively the pattern of collected TB data as both reconstructed dynamics and data peaked in 2007–2008. The panel B shows that the model captures the large increase of reported cases that was observed in 2003. In panel C, we see that the reconstructed dynamics of extra-pulmonary TB fit the data less well. The underlying reason is that we fixed the probabilities of developing extra-pulmonary and pulmonary TB in both G1 and G2 groups (δ_p and δ_{ph}) while these numbers were reported to be year-varying. This phenomenon likely comes from variation in skill of lab technician and sensitivity of mycobacteria detection overtime in DTUs rather than any relation to TB epidemiology change. In panel D, the un-infected group (without active TB history) is estimated to be about 40% of the population which is consistent with the IGRA data. The dynamics of co-infected patients are captured neatly by the model as shown in panel E. Panel F shows the goodness of fit by plotting data and reconstructed dynamics in per 100,000 form. The number of active TB cases per 100,000 among people in G1 group decreased from 1996 to 2005. In contrast, the number of active TB cases per 100,000 for the whole population follows a different trend. After 2002, this number increased, and peaked in 2008. It suggests that despite the increase of TB in the population, the risk of active TB among people in group G1 decreases in time.

Table 3 Estimate and 95% confidence intervals of parameters in H4. Because *breaking-year* takes discrete values, the confidence interval of this parameter is skipped

Prms	MLE	95% CI
$ß_1$	37.8	[36–40.1]
$ß_2$	31.1	[29.7–32.7]
ε_2	0.37	[0.29–0.45]
ω_2	0.0017	[0.0014–0.0022]
k_1	0.42	[0–10]
ω_{h1}	0.152	[0.09–0.163]
ω_{h2}	0.06	[0.01–0.09]
γ	0.15	[0.06–0.25]
r_1	0.57	[0.54–0.61]
r_2	0.99	[0.96–1]
breaking-year	2003	NA

Hyper-susceptibility and risk of active TB

As can be seen from Table 3, the confidence intervals (CIs) of k_1, the parameter used to describe the relative rate of developing active TB due to exogenous infection process between uninfected class (U) and G2 group (U_h, L_h, and R_h), are wide. The lowerbound of these CIs are zero. It indicates that the decrease in (re-)infection can be compensened by increase in reactivation. In other words, these two processes among individuals in G2 are not distinguishable from each other.

Another striking point shown in Table 3 is the risk of developing TB among people in G2. The reactivation rate of class Rh (ω_{h2}) is estimated to be lower than that of class Lh (ω_{h1}). Remember that we assume that the infection process is identical for individuals in Uh, Lh, and Rh. Therefore, our model suggests that people in Rh is more protected (in term of active TB) than in Lh. However, this is not the case for people in G1 group. The reactivation rate (ω_2) of people in R is estimated to be stable, at about 0.0017 person-years, and is estimated to be consistently higher than reactivation rate (ω_1) of people in L. Furthermore, because the relative rate of class R (ε_2) is estimated higher than that of class L (ε_1), the exogeneous (re-)infection process appears to have more impact on R class rather than L class. In total, it indicates that for people in group G1, the risk of relapsed active TB is higher than the risk of new active TB.

Infectivity of hyper-susceptible TB patients

It is important to notice that the estimate of co-infected pulmonary case's infectivity (γ) is low. It reveals that the contribution of co-infected patients to TB transmission in G1 is limited.

Discussion

We have constructed a simple mathematical model to describe the TB dynamics in a population containing hyper-susceptible individuals. We consider four different epidemiological hypotheses with different assumptions about the trends in the contact parameter and reporting rate. Under these hypotheses, we fitted the model to TB data collected from HCMC. We employed AIC to identify the most likely epidemiological hypothesis occuring in HCMC from 1996 to 2015.

In summary, based on the AIC, the analysis presented in this work shows that the contact parameter of TB in

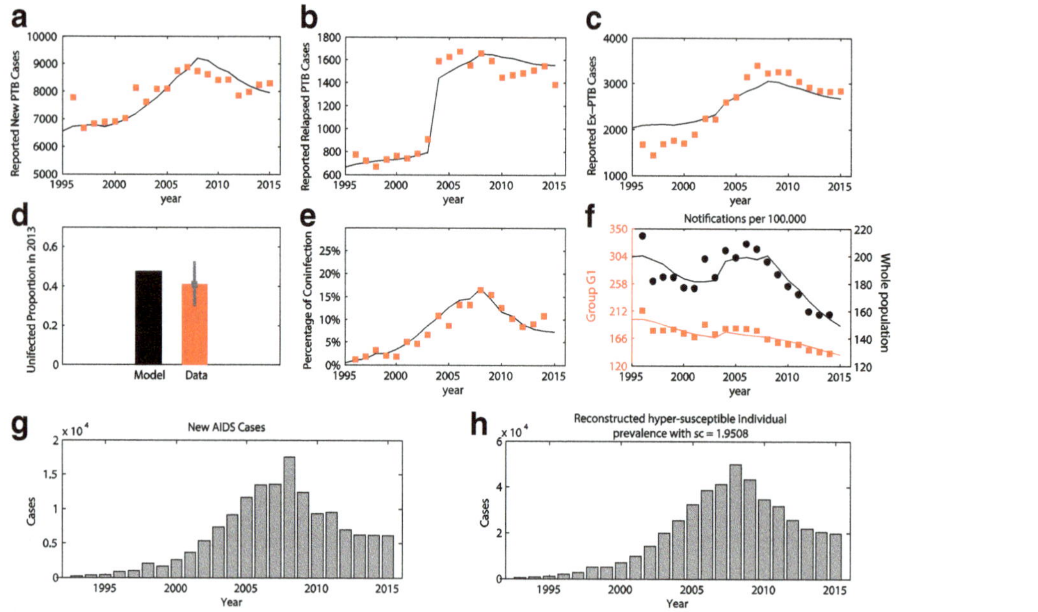

Fig. 3 Model fit under hypothesis H4. In panels (**a**, **b**, **c**, **e**, and **f**), he dots (red and black) are the data. The continuous lines (red and black) show the reconstructed dynamics using parameters estimated by Maximum Likelihood Estimation (MLE). In panel (**d**), the black and red bar shows the uninfected proportion inferred from our model and IGRA data respectively. The gray bar shows the confidence interval of uninfected proportion computed from our IGRA data with assumption of binomial distribution. In panel (**f**), the red and black graphs (correspond to left and right y-axis) show the TB notifications of G1 group and the total population respectively. The TB notifications of G1 group are inferred by combining data set D1 and D3. Panel (**g** and **h**) shows the AIDS data and reconstructed hyper-susceptible individual curve

HCMC reduced by around 18% from 1996 to 2015. This analysis also indicates that the reporting rate of relapsed TB patients to National Tuberculosis Control Program changed significantly to more than 95% after 2003, under the policy in which TB patients with successful treatment are asked to return for TB examination. The overall reporting rate ranges from 58 to 66%. The annual incidence is estimated at about 230 cases per 100,000. Furthermore, our estimate shows that the infectivity (γ) of an active TB cases with hyper-susceptibility is consistently low.

This study illustrates how HIV/AIDS drives TB dynamics in HCMC. Firstly, the wide spread of HIV/AIDS from the beginning of 1990s resulted in the increase of hyper-susceptible hosts in HCMC's population. Consequently, the annual TB notifications in HCMC increased sharply from 1996 to 2008. This number peaked in 2008 – the year that co-infected patients accounted for about 15% of annual TB notifications. After this year, the number of TB notifications followed a decline as HIV/AIDS dynamics started to go down. Co-infected patients accounted for about 7% of TB notifications in 2015. However, after removing the impact of HIV/AIDS on TB, the Panel F Fig. 3 indicates that the annual TB notifications among people in group G1 declined from 1996 to 2015 consistently. Especially, during the growth phase of HIV/AIDS epidemics (from 1996 to 2008), the risk of active TB for people in group G1 went down despite the fact that there were more TB cases in the population (because of HIV/AIDS). Note that exogeneous (re-)infection is the main pathway in which active TB develops in G1 group. It indicates that the TB transmission (of G1) decreased in time which is consistent with hypothesis H4 – the most likely epidemiological hypothesis. Furthermore, it also implies that co-infected patients appears to have small impact on individuals in G1 group. As a result, estimate of the infectivity (γ) of co-infected patients is low (Table 3). In other words, the role of co-infected patients to TB transmission process in HCMC is quite limited. At this point, it is unclear that low infectivity γ is due to the hyper-susceptibility or the contact pattern between individuals in G1 and G2. However, it suggests that the increase in annual TB notifications per year observed from 1996 to 2008 in HCMC is inevitable when, as occurred, the number of hyper-susceptible individuals increased faster than the decrease of TB transmission rate. The sharp decrease in TB notifications observed in HCMC from 2008 to 2015 is the combined result of the decrease of TB tranmission rate and the decrease of G2's population size.

The limited effect of HIV/AIDS to the trend of TB in people in G1 is quite consistent with [11]. However, the difference in underlying mechanism should be mentioned. The [11] suggests that limited interaction between HIV/AIDS comes from the difference between slow and fast dynamics of TB and HIV/AIDS respectively. Our model suggests that the underlying mechanism is low infectivity of co-infected patients. This indicates that how we model TB in group G2 has almost no impact on the trend of TB among people in G1. The low infectivity may be the result of contact pattern of the population. If this is a cases, there is a small sub-population (such as low income people) in which both HIV/AIDS and TB more co-circulate, and this sub-population is quite isolated from the whole population (in term of active TB). It is not necessary for these two populations to have the identical forces of infection as we model (in term of TB). It indicates that modelling for co-circulation of HIV-TB is problematic as there are many unknowns about contact pattern of this sub-population.

One important papers that is related to this work is [38]. This paper showed that latent TB is likely independent of HIV status in HIV high-risk group in Mexico. Therefore, the MTB prevalence among HIV positives is likely determined by the contact pattern of high-risk groups rather than HIV infection. Although the MTB prevalence among HIV positives is unknown in HCMC, we admit that our assumption about a well-mixed population may not reflect the TB transmission among people in G2 group. It may be the case that both HIV and TB more co-circulate a specific group (such as low income people [39–42]) in HCMC. At this point, the force of TB infection imposed to people in G2 group should be modelled as $s.\lambda(t)$. The parameter s in this situation represents for the force of TB infection enhancement. Even in the situation that the enhancement is absent ($s = 1$), the 95%CIs of $k1$ is huge. The lower bound is close to zero. In other words, if we assume that the (re-)infection process has no impact on hyper-susceptible people, we still can explain our data by the (re-)activation process. This points out that introducing a new parameter (s) to transmission process of people in G2 does not improve the identifiability of the analysis. This argument suggests that (re-)infection process and (re-)activation process confounds each other among people in G2. Therefore, whether the trend of the (re-)infection process among people in G2 is going down like in G1 is difficult to verify from this analysis.

The enhancement of force of TB infection among people in HIV high-risk group ($s > 1$) intuitively reduces the estimate of ω_{h1} and ω_{h2}. In case that s is fixed at 1.5, the estimate of reactivation rate of people in Rh (ω_{h2}) is still significant lower than reactivation rate in Lh (ω_{h1}) (Section 6 and Additional file 1: Table S3 in supplement). In other words, it is likely that people in Rh are still more protected than Lh despite the fact that our model may not give reliable evaluation of (re-)infection and (re-)activation processes among people in G2. We have to emphasize that if people in Rh are more protected than people in Lh does require further investigation and verification with a different model and data set that at least includes information about CD4 cell count and HIV progression. Several papers [30, 43, 44] indicate that the risk of TB increase after CD4 cell counts starts to decline. Therefore, modeling for a short period of HIV infection in this paper overestimates the TB risk of people in Lh. If the risk of TB were very high in early stages of HIV infection, our assumption that AIDS is representative for TB hyper-susceptible people is unrealistic. In this situation, the people in Lh would be more protected than people in Rh. However, if this were the case, we would observe many TB cases with high CD4 cell count that was contradicted by [30, 44] that showed that about 90% of co-infected patients have CD4 cell count lower than 400 cells/μl and the risk of TB increases exponentially with the decline of CD4.

If that people in Rh is more protected than Lh is the case, we hypothesize that the underlying reason is the use of ART in HCMC's population. Much work [11, 15, 45–47] showed that widespread use of ART has strong beneficial impacts on TB mortality and morbidity in the population. The positive impact of ART on TB dynamics is due to ART preventing the decline of CD4 cell count among HIV positives. In Vietnam, ART use started in 2004. From 2004 to 2015 in Vietnam, according to the HIV guidelines, only HIV infected people in clinical stage 3 and 4 were recommended for ART (See Section 2, 3, 4, and 5 of supplement). Once an HIV positive individual starts to use ART, they continue to use ART for the rest of their life. Therefore, for individuals in Uh and Lh, it is unlikely that they have used ART before. Many people start their HIV treatment at the time they are diagnosed with active TB. For the individuals in Rh, it is likely that they had already started their HIV treatment before. Hence, they have greater protection against relapses of TB. Therefore, the delay in HIV treatment may impose a considerable TB burden on HCMC which could be avoided by starting ART earlier, and the number of TB cases in HCMC benefited little from the HIV program from 1996 to 2015.

One limitation of our work is the expected survival time of people in G2. Although this parameter is shown to have considerable variation within the population, the *est* is assumed to be homologous throughout the analysis. The heterogeneity of *est* comes from variation in the kind of high risk groups, the type of opportunistic infection, and especially ART status. However, these kinds of information were not recorded in our data. Another limitation of our work is how we simulate our dynamical system. Because the expected survival time of people in G2 group is relatively short, year by year simulation in this work may result a crude approximation of

TB dynamics. One improvement is that instead of using year-to-year simulation, month-to-month simulation could be applied. However, it is important to emphasize that month-to-month simulation requires that the hyper-susceptibility data set is available by month which is a the limitation of the available data. Misclassification of TB patients is also a disadvantages of the model. It is believed that misclassification always happens and varies in time as the community awareness and TB diagnosis technique are improved. Nevertheless, the model is not designed to capture this fact. Thus, it may bias the reporting rate and reactivation rates.

One criticism that can be made about our TB transmission model is the assumption that the average infectious period of all TB patients is only six months. The infectious period of a TB patient is defined as the period that this patient can spread TB to others. Note that the behaviour of our TB model may not change if we decrease the infectious period and increase the transmission parameter at the same time. Therefore, our analysis appears to be robust with respect to this parameter. In the literature, there is a significant variation of TB infectious period used. The paper [20] suggest that this period is six months that equals to the duration of TB treatment. Another example can be seen in [48]. This paper suggests that period of infectivity (of adult) ranges from 30 days to 120 days. The paper [21] suggest this period is two years. For untreated TB patients, the paper [49] assume this duration is five years. However, this quantity in [10] is fixed at two years. The paper [50] does systematic review and conclude that this period is about 3 years (with very high mortality rate). From clinical viewpoint, this period for TB should be considered as the period that TB patients have symptoms such as coughing. It is likely that patients without symptoms is believed to have very low infectivity. This period is fixed at six months in our analysis through two data set. First, the clinical data (unpublished) of TB treatment in Vietnam indicates that more than 95% TB patients are smear-negative and symptom-free after three to four months of treatment. Second, the delay time for finding TB treatment since symptom appearance in HCMC about 43 days (see Additional file 1: Figure S6). Further investigation on infectious period may shed new light to the relationship between this factor and the persistence of TB in the population.

Another criticism is about the population-representa tiveness of our data sets. Overall, pediatric TB is under-reported in Vietnam [34]. Majority of reported cases used in this study (data set D1) is also from adult. Consequently, whether the prevalence of HIV among TB patients (data set D3) is population representative is unclear. Furthermore, the data set D1 just records TB patients in public sector only (We used this number as *TB notifications*). TB patients that receive similar TB treatment in private sector are not recorded. The number of TB patients in private sector is believed to be considerable. Moreover, the IGRA data set D2 – a small data set with only 78 samples - was collected from people in working age. One important point is that we have to emphasize that after comparing the estimate of true incidence and our reporting data set D1, the proportion of active TB cases that goes to public sector in HCMC for TB treatment ranges from 58 to 66% which is very consistent with the estimate presented by WHO [7, 51] for Vietnam (about 65%). In other words, this model likely reflects the true TB dynamics in HCMC. At this point, it is unclear that if the model only represents the adult population or the whole population.

Although this paper shows that the TB transmission of HCMC was going down from 1996 to 2015, we need to mention some confounding factors. In order to describe the change of the transmission process, we assume that the contact parameter is time-varying. However, the change in infectious time of TB patient (we do not have data on this factor) may reduce the TB prevalence and give the same result. In general, the TB dynamics is very slow [17, 31] compared to other acute infectious disease such as influenza or hand foot mouth disease. One TB epidemics may last for a couple centuries [17]. Thus, any changes in non-linear terms (such as contact parameter) can be approximated by changes in linear term (such as reactivation rate or infectious period) for a couple of decades. For this reason, it is unclear the underlying mechanism of the declining TB transmission. Over the past 20 years, there was a significant change in all aspects of social economy that may have positive impact on TB transmission in HCMC. For example, the Vietnam government decided to open the country and changed from communist economy to market economy. The Gross Domestic Product (per capita) of Vietnam changed from 323 USD in 1996 to 2171 USD in 2015 [52]. People spend more money on health care. Furthermore, the awareness of people about TB also changed as the NTP ran many public engagement campaigns and adopted new policies to educate people. The urbanization may also have positive impact as it reduced the over-crowding in big cities such as HCMC. Furthermore, in order to keep our analysis simple, we assume that the TB dynamics in 1992 was endemic and the contact parameter varied linearly from 1996 to 2015. However, these assumptions may be violated in reality. If this is a case, this violation may have negative impact on our estimate of TB transmission reduction quantitatively.

The main focus of this paper is evaluating the impact of HIV/AIDS to TB dynamics in HCMC. In order to achieve this target with our data set, we constructed a mathematical model with very simple HIV/AIDS structure. Note that our result shows that HIV/AIDS has limited effect on TB transmission in population which is consistent with [11]. Although this result indicates that the simple HIV/AIDS structure of our model appears not to have negative impact on the main target of the paper, it is important to emphasize that this simple structure does not give us a satisfied answer on the TB epidemiology of hyper-susceptible individuals. The risk of active TB increases exponentially with CD4 cell count reduction [29, 30]. Therefore, assuming this risk is homologous among hyper-susceptible individuals and using only people with AIDS to depict the hyper-susceptible individuals may not give us a full picture of TB infection and reactivation among HIV positives. As a result, some findings of this paper can serve as new hypotheses for further investigating TB epidemiology of hyper-susceptible individuals in a suitable model with better HIV/AIDS structure and data.

The multi-drug resistant (MDR) topic in TB is receiving more and more interest from the scienctific community. The true mechanism of MDR in Vietnam is still a large unanswered question because the prevalence of MDR among people with and without AIDS are very different (4% and > 20% respectively). Future developments of this modeling work will concentrate on answering understanding mechanisms to explain the strong correlation between AIDS and MDR in Vietnam.

Conclusion

This paper is the first paper that quantitatively investigates the TB dynamics of HCMC using a mathematical model to intergrating many data sources. It contributes to our knowledge of TB dynamics in HCMC from 1996 to 2005 – the period in which HIV/AIDS widely spread in Vietnamese population. As the HIV/AIDS widely spread in the population, the number of hyper-susceptible individuals inevitably increased. Therefore, despite the declining trend of TB (re-)infection process among people in G1, the number of TB notifications in HCMC increased sharply from 1996 to 2008.

For co-infected patients, this paper indicates that their infectivity is very low. In other words, how we model TB dynamics in G2 has almost no impact to G1. Furthermore, this paper shows that (re-)infection and (re-)activation processes of G2 have very low identifiability. It implises that if (re-)infection process of G2 was declining from 1996 to 2015 (like G1) is impossible to verify with our model and data.The analysis in this paper suggests that to hyper-susceptible individuals, individuals in Rh are likely more protected (in term of TB) than individuals in Lh. We hypothesize that the underlying reason for this is the guidelines about timing of the start of ART. This situation requires further investigation and verification with different data sets and models. If this situation is the case, we suggest HIV treatment policy in Vietnam should be reconsidered as Vietnam is a high TB burden country.

Abbreviations

AIC: Akaike Information Criterion; ART: Antiretroviral Therapy; CI: Confidence Interval; DOTS: The Direct Observed Treatment, Short Course; DTU: District Tuberculosis Unit; ExPTB: Extra-pulmonary Tuberculosis; GSO: General Statistics Office of Vietnam; HCMC: Ho Chi Minh City; IGRA: Interferon-Gamma Release Assay; MDR: Multi-drug Resistant; MTB: Mycobacterium Tuberculosis; NTP: National Tuberculosis Control Program; PTB: Pulmonary Tuberculosis; TB: Tuberculosis

Acknowledgements

Thanks to Nguyen Thi Mai Thu for important conversation about HIV/AIDS program in Vietnam.

Funding

This work was supported by TDModNet Seed Funding Program [to D.N.V], the Wellcome Trust [110179/Z/15/Z to G.T, 206724/Z/17/Z to N.T.T.T]. The funders had no role in study design, data collection and analysis, decision to publish, or preparation of the manuscript.

Availability of data and materials

Reporting TB data set (D1) analyzed during this study are included in this published article and its Additional files 1, 2, 3, 4, 5.
IGRA data set (D2) analyzed during this study are included in this published article and its supplementary information files.
Co-infected data set (D3) analyzed during this study are included in this published article and its supplementary information files.
AIDS data set analyzed during this study is included in this published article, its supplementary information files, and two following links:

1. http://www.aidsdatahub.org/sites/default/files/publication/An_annual_update_on_HIV_epidemic_in_Viet_Nam_2014.pdf (page 10 - the number of AIDS reported cases for Vietnam from 1993 to 2013).
2. http://vaac.gov.vn/Cms_Data/Contents/Vaac/Folders/Solieubaocao/Solieu/~contents/BCG2DGP6NQ77KBCX/Bao-cao-2015_so-lieu_Final.pdf (the number of AIDS reported cases for Vietnam in 2015).

Demographic data analyzed during this study are available at General Statistics Office of Vietnam's website: https://gso.gov.vn/default_en.aspx?tabid=774

Authors' contributions

DNV, MFB, GT, and NTTT contributed to setting up the study. DNV, NTH, and DTMH collected data. DNV performed data analysis. DNV, MFB, GT, and HC interpreted the findings and wrote the manuscript. All authors have read and approved this manuscript.

Consent for publication

Not applicable.

Competing interests

The authors declare that they have no competing interests.

Author details
[1]Wellcome Trust Major Overseas Programme, Hospital for Tropical Diseases, Oxford University Clinical Research Unit, 764 Vo Van Kiet Street, District 5, Ho Chi Minh City, Vietnam. [2]Pham Ngoc Thach Hospital, Ho Chi Minh City, Vietnam. [3]Centre for Tropical Medicine and Global Health, Nuffield Department of Medicine, University of Oxford, Oxford, UK. [4]Center for Infectious Disease Dynamics, Department of Biology, Pennsylvania State University, Pennsylvania, USA.

References

1. Rampatige R, Gilks CF. Autopsies and better data on causes of death in Africa. Lancet Infect Dis [internet]. 2015;15:492–4 Elsevier Ltd . Available from: http://linkinghub.elsevier.com/retrieve/pii/S1473309915700964.
2. Ngo AD, Rao C, Hoa NP, Adair T, Chuc NTK. Mortality patterns in Vietnam, 2006: findings from a national verbal autopsy survey. BMC Res Notes [Internet]. 2010;3:78 Available from: http://www.pubmedcentral.nih.gov/articlerender.fcgi?artid=2851717&tool=pmcentrez&rendertype=abstract.
3. World Health Organization. Treatment of tuberculosis guidelines. 4th. 2009.
4. World Health Organization. Treatment of tuberculosis: Guidelines for national programmes. 2003.
5. Huong NT, Duong BD, Co N V., Quy HT, Tung LB, Bosman M, et al. Establishment and development of the National Tuberculosis Control Programme in Vietnam. Int J Tuberc Lung Dis. [internet]. 2005;9:151–156. Available from: http://www.ncbi.nlm.nih.gov/pubmed/15732733.
6. World Health Organization. Global Tuberculosis Report - 2011. 2011;
7. World Health Organization. Global Tuberculosis Report - 2015; 2015. p. 1.
8. Nguyen TA, Oosterhoff P, Hardon A, Tran HN, Coutinho RA, Wright P. A hidden HIV epidemic among women in Vietnam. BMC Public Health [Internet]. 2008;8:37. Available from: http://www.pubmedcentral.nih.gov/articlerender.fcgi?artid=2248180&tool=pmcentrez&rendertype=abstract.
9. Vietnam Ministry of Health. Annual Report of HIV Epidemic - 2015. 2015;
10. Bacaër N, Ouifki R, Pretorius C, Wood R, Williams B. Modeling the joint epidemics of TB and HIV in a south African township. J Math Biol [Internet]. 2008;57:557–93 Available from: http://link.springer.com/10.1007/s00285-008-0177-z.
11. Williams BG, Gouws E, Somse P, Mmelesi M, Lwamba C, Chikoko T, et al. Epidemiological trends for HIV in southern Africa: implications for reaching the elimination targets. Curr HIV/AIDS Rep. 2015;12:196–206.
12. Pretorius C, Menzies NA, Chindelevitch L, Cohen T, Cori A, Eaton JW, et al. The potential effects of changing HIV treatment policy on tuberculosis outcomes in South Africa: results from three tuberculosis-HIV transmission models. AIDS [Internet]. 2014;28 Suppl 1:S25–S34. Available from: http://www.ncbi.nlm.nih.gov/pubmed/24468944
13. Kunkel A, Crawford FW, Shepherd J, Cohen T. Benefits of continuous isoniazid preventive therapy may outweigh resistance risks in a declining tuberculosis/HIV coepidemic. AIDS [Internet]. 2016;30:2715–23 Available from: https://www.ncbi.nlm.nih.gov/pmc/articles/PMC5089846/pdf/nihms814768.pdf.
14. Heymann SJ. Modelling the efficacy of prophylactic and curative therapies for preventing the spread of tuberculosis in africa. Trans R Soc Trop Med Hyg. 1993;87:406–11.
15. Williams BG, Gupta S, Wollmers M, Granich R. Progress and prospects for the control of HIV and tuberculosis in South Africa: a dynamical modelling study. Lancet Public Heal [Internet]. The Author(s). Published by Elsevier Ltd. This is an Open Access article under the CC BY-NC-ND license; 2017;2:e223–e230. Available from: https://doi.org/10.1016/S2468-2667(17)30066-X.
16. Cain K, Kanara N, Laserson K, Vannarith C, Sameourn K, Samnang K, et al. The epidemiology if HIV associated tuberculosis in rural Cambodia. Int J Tuberc Lung Dis. 2007;11:1008–13.
17. Blower SM, Mclean AR, Porco TC, Small PM, Hopewell PC, Sanchez MA, et al. The intrinsic transmission dynamics of tuberculosis epidemics. Nat Med [Internet]. 1995;1:815–821. Available from: http://www.nature.com/doifinder/10.1038/nm0895-815.
18. Gomes MGM, Franco AO, Gomes MC, Medley GF. The reinfection threshold promotes variability in tuberculosis epidemiology and vaccine efficacy. Proc R Soc B Biol Sci [Internet]. 2004;271:617–23 Available from: http://www.pubmedcentral.nih.gov/articlerender.fcgi?artid=1691632&tool=pmcentrez&rendertype=abstract.
19. Ahmadin, Fatmawati. Mathematical modeling of drug resistance in tuberculosis transmission and optimal control treatment. Appl Math Sci. [Internet]. 2014;8:4547–4559. Available from: http://www.m-hikari.com/ams/ams-2014/ams-89-92-2014/fatmawatiAMS89-92-2014.pdf.
20. Rodrigues P, Gomes MGM, Rebelo C. Drug resistance in tuberculosis—a reinfection model. Theor Popul Biol [Internet]. 2007; 71:196–212 Available from: https://www.sciencedirect.com/science/article/pii/S0040580906001316?via%3Dihub.
21. Vynnycky E, Fine PEM. The natural history of tuberculosis: the implications of age-dependent risks of disease and the role of reinfection. Epidemiol Infect [Internet]. 1997;119:S0950268897007917. Available from: https://www.ncbi.nlm.nih.gov/pmc/articles/PMC2808840/pdf/9363017.pdf.
22. Abu-Raddad LJ, Sabatelli L, Achterberg JT, Sugimoto JD, Longini IM, Dye C, et al. Epidemiological benefits of more-effective tuberculosis vaccines, drugs, and diagnostics. Proc Natl Acad Sci USA. [Internet]. 2009;106: 13980–13985. Available from: http://www.pnas.org/content/pnas/106/33/13980.full.pdf.
23. Bhunu CP, Garira W, Mukandavire Z. Modeling HIV/AIDS and tuberculosis coinfection. Bull Math Biol [Internet]. 2009;71:1745–80 Available from: http://link.springer.com/10.1007/s11538-009-9423-9.
24. Bolarin G. Omatola IU. A Mathematical analysis of HIV/TB co-infection model. Proc. 2006 winter Simul. Conf. 2006. p. 459–465.
25. Naresh R, Tripathi A, Omar S. Modelling the spread of AIDS epidemic with vertical transmission. Appl Math Comput [Internet]. 2006;178:262–72 Available from: http://linkinghub.elsevier.com/retrieve/pii/S0096300305009720.
26. Roeger L-IW, Feng Z, Castillo-Chavez C. Modeling TB and HIV co-infections. Math Biosci Eng [Internet]. 2009;6:815–837. Available from: http://www.ncbi.nlm.nih.gov/pubmed/19835430
27. Wang X, Yang J, Zhang F. Dynamic of a TB-HIV coinfection epidemic model with latent age. J Appl Math [Internet]. 2013;2013:1–13 Available from: http://www.hindawi.com/journals/jam/2013/429567/.
28. Yaesoubi R, Cohen T. Identifying dynamic tuberculosis case-finding policies for HIV/TB coepidemics. Proc Natl Acad Sci [Internet]. 2013;110:9457–62 Available from: http://www.pnas.org/lookup/doi/10.1073/pnas.1218770110.
29. Jones BE, Young SMM, Antoniskis D, Davidson PT, Kramer F, Barnes PF. Relationship of the manifestations of tuberculosis to CD4 cell counts in patients with human immunodeficiency virus infection. Am Rev Respir Dis [Internet]. 1993;148:1292–7 Available from: http://www.atsjournals.org/doi/abs/10.1164/ajrccm/148.5.1292.
30. Gupta RK, Lawn SD, Bekker L-G, Caldwell J, Kaplan R, Wood R. Impact of human immunodeficiency virus and CD4 count on tuberculosis diagnosis: analysis of city-wide data from Cape Town, South Africa. Int J Tuberc Lung Dis [Internet]. 2013;17:1014–22 Available from: http://openurl.ingenta.com/content/xref?genre=article&issn=1027-3719&volume=17&issue=8&spage=1014.
31. Ozcaglar C, Shabbeer A, Vandenberg SL, Yener B, Bennett KP. Epidemiological models of Mycobacterium tuberculosis complex infections. Math Biosci. 2012;236:77–96.
32. General Statistics Office of Vietnam. Population and Employment Statistics [Internet]. Stat Handb. Vietnam. 2016 [cited 2017 Mar 13]. Available from: https://gso.gov.vn/default_en.aspx?tabid=774
33. Vietnam Authority of HIV/ AIDS Control. An Annual Update on The HIV Epidemic in Vietnam. 2014;
34. Blount RJ, Tran B, Jarlsberg LG, Phan H, Thanh Hoang V, Nguyen NV, et al. Childhood tuberculosis in northern Viet Nam: a review of 103 cases. PLoS One. 2014;9.
35. Immunotec O. T-Spot TB Package Insert - For In Vitro Diagnostic Use Only; 2003. p. 2.
36. Nelder JA, Mead R. A simplex method for function minimization. Comput J [Internet]. 1965;7:308–13 Available from: https://pdfs.semanticscholar.org/da24/280dfcd767524fb1a1702f50f388ca0d4082.pdf.
37. Gelman A, Carlin J, Stern H, Dunson D, Vehtari A, Rubin D. Bayesian data analysis, third edition (Chapman & Hall/CRC texts in statistical science). Third edit. London: Chapman and Hall/CRC; 2014.
38. Garfein RS, Laniado-laborin R, Rodwell TC, Lozada R, Deiss R, Burgos JL, et al. Latent Tuberculosis among Persons at Risk for Infection with HIV. Emerg Infect Dis. 2010;16:757–63.
39. Oxlade O, Murray M. Tuberculosis and poverty: why are the poor at greater risk in India? PLoS One [Internet]. 2012; 7: e47533. Available from: http://www.ncbi.nlm.nih.gov/pubmed/23185241
40. Gillies P, Tolley K, Wolstenholme J. Is AIDS a disease of poverty? AIDS Care [Internet]. 1996;8:351–64 Available from: https://www.ncbi.nlm.nih.gov/pubmed/8827126.

41. Muniyandi M, Ramachandran R. Socioeconomic inequalities of tuberculosis in India. Expert Opin Pharmacother [Internet]. 2008;9:1623–8 Available from: http://www.tandfonline.com/doi/full/10.1517/14656566.9.10.1623.
42. Grange J, Zumla A. Tuberculosis and the poverty-disease cycle. J R Soc Med [Internet]. 1999;92:105–107. Available from: https://www.ncbi.nlm.nih.gov/pmc/articles/PMC1297096/pdf/jrsocmed00011-0007.pdf.
43. Sonnenberg P, Glynn JR, Fielding K, Murray J, Godfrey-Faussett P, Shearer S. How soon after infection with HIV does the risk of tuberculosis start to increase? A retrospective cohort study in south African gold miners. J Infect Dis [Internet]. 2005;191:150–158. Available from: http://www.ncbi.nlm.nih.gov/pubmed/15609223
44. Ellis PK, Martin WJ, Dodd PJ. CD4 count and tuberculosis risk in HIV-positive adults not on ART: a systematic review and meta-analysis. PeerJ [Internet]. 2017;5:e4165. Available from: https://peerj.com/articles/4165
45. Nanoo A, Izu A, Ismail NA, Ihekweazu C, Abubakar I, Mametja D, et al. Nationwide and regional incidence of microbiologically confirmed pulmonary tuberculosis in South Africa, 2004–12: a time series analysis. Lancet Infect Dis. [Internet]. Elsevier Ltd. 2015;15:1066–76 Available from: http://linkinghub.elsevier.com/retrieve/pii/S1473309915001474.
46. Van Rie A, Westreich D, Sanne IM. Tuberculosis in patients receiving antiretroviral treatment: incidence, risk factors, and prevention strategies. J Acquir Immune Defic Syndr. 2011;56:349–55.
47. Kaplan R, Caldwell J, Middelkoop K, Bekker L-G, Wood R. Impact of ART on TB case fatality stratified by CD4 count for HIV-positive TB patients in Cape Town, South Africa (2009–2011). JAIDS J Acquir Immune Defic Syndr [Internet]. 2014;66:487–494. Available from: https://www.ncbi.nlm.nih.gov/pubmed/24820105.
48. Wood R, Johnstone-Robertson S, Uys P, Hargrove J, Middelkoop K, Lawn SD, et al. Tuberculosis transmission to young children in a south African community: modeling household and community infection risks. Clin Infect Dis [Internet]. 2010;51:401–8 Available from: http://cid.oxfordjournals.org/lookup/doi/10.1086/655129.
49. Cohen T, Murray M. Modeling epidemics of multidrug-resistant M. tuberculosis of heterogeneous fitness. Nat Med [Internet]. 2004;10:1117–1121. Available from: http://www.nature.com/doifinder/10.1038/nm1110
50. Tiemersma EW, van der Werf MJ, Borgdorff MW, Williams BG, Nagelkerke NJD. Natural history of tuberculosis: duration and fatality of untreated pulmonary tuberculosis in HIV negative patients: a systematic review. PLoS One [Internet]. 2011;6:e17601. Available from: http://www.ncbi.nlm.nih.gov/pubmed/21483732
51. World Health Organization. Global Tuberculosis Report - 2012. 2012;
52. Worldbank. GDP per capita (current US$) | Data [Internet]. [cited 2018 Apr 19]. Available from: https://data.worldbank.org/indicator/NY.GDP.PCAP.CD?locations=VN
53. Andrews JR, Noubary F, Walensky RP, Cerda R, Losina E, Horsburgh CR. Risk of progression to active tuberculosis following reinfection with Mycobacterium tuberculosis. Clin Infect Dis [Internet]. 2012;54:784–91 Available from: https://academic.oup.com/cid/article-lookup/doi/10.1093/cid/cir951.
54. Shea KM, Kammerer JS, Winston CA, Navin TR, Horsburgh CR. Estimated Rate of Reactivation of Latent Tuberculosis Infection in the United States, Overall and by Population Subgroup. Am J Epidemiol [Internet]. 2014;179:216–25 Available from: http://aje.oxfordjournals.org/cgi/doi/10.1093/aje/kwt246.

5

Current treatment of multidrug resistant tuberculosis in Ethiopia: an aggregated and individual patients' data analysis for outcome and effectiveness of the current regimens

Setegn Eshetie[1*], Animut Alebel[2], Fasil Wagnew[2], Demeke Geremew[3], Alebachew Fasil[4] and Ulrich Sack[5]

Abstract

Background: The programmatic management of Multidrug-resistant tuberculosis (MDR-TB) is entirely based on a WHO recommended long-term, 18–24 month lasting treatment regimen. However, growing evidence shows that low treatment success rate and high rates of adverse events are associated with this regimen. Up to date, the MDR-TB treatment outcome is not sufficiently understood in Ethiopia. Therefore, this analysis aimed to determine the pooled estimates of successful (cure, completed, or both), and poor outcomes (death, failure, and lost to follow ups).

Method: A systematic search was performed to identify eligible studies reporting MDR-TB treatment outcomes in Ethiopia. Relevant studies for our analysis were retrieved from PubMed database search, Google Scholar and institutional repository sites of Ethiopian universities up to March 15, 2018. The primary outcome was treatment success, referring to a composite of cure and treatment completion. A random effect model was used to calculate pooled estimates.

Results: Six studies reporting treatment outcome on the 1993 MDR-TB patients were included in this analysis. Of the cases, the 1288 and 442 patients had a successful and poor outcome, respectively. In the pooled analysis, treatment success was observed in 59.2% (95%CI, 48.1–70.4) of patients, while 23.3% (95%CI, 19.7–27.0%) of patients had a poor outcome. in sub-group analysis,46.1% (95%CI, 34.2–58.0) were cured, 12.8% (5.7–20.0) treatment completed, 14.3% (11.5–17.2) died, 7.5% (3.7–11.3) lost to follow up, and 1.6% (1.1–2.2%) experienced treatment failure. The 25.0% (14.6–35.5) patients whose treatment outcome was not assessed (on treatment or transfer-out).

Conclusion: The result of this study highlight treatment success among MDR-TB is below acceptable range. To update the current treatment regimen, the levels of evidence need to be replicated through meticulous surveillance systems.

Keywords: Ethiopia, MDR-TB, Treatment success

* Correspondence: wolet03.2004@gmail.com
[1]Department of Medical Microbiology, School of Biomedical and Laboratory Sciences, College of Medicine and Health Sciences, University of Gondar, Gondar, Ethiopia
Full list of author information is available at the end of the article

Background

Multidrug-resistant tuberculosis (MDR-TB) is defined by resistance to at least the two most powerful first line anti-tuberculosis drugs, isoniazid, and rifampicin [1]. MDR-TB remains a major public health crisis, with an estimated 490, 0000 new cases are emerging globally each year [2]. The increasing incidence of drug resistant TB is mainly reported from resource-limited countries where TB care programs are compromised. Globally, 3.9% (95% CI 2.7–5.1%) of new cases and 21% (95% CI 15–28%) of previously treated TB cases were in MDR-TB cases. It is also estimated that each year 580,000 and 250,000 deaths reported among new and previously treated MDR-TB cases [3], respectively. According to the recent global report, 2900 (1800–4000) MDR-TB cases were estimated among notified pulmonary TB in Ethiopia [2]. A latest meta-analysis study also reported that 2% of new cases and 17% among previously treated cases were MDR-TB patients [4].

Programmatic management of drug-resistant TB treatment is based on conventional or longer MDR/ rifampicin resistant (RR)-TB treatment regimens, which lasts for 20–24 months and achieved a success rate nearly in 50% of patients, worldwide [5]. The low successful treatment outcome might be due to prolonged treatment period, low drug efficacy and toxic regiments. Recent advances show that high treatment success was achieved by using a short course treatment regimen. To date, few studies have been conducted to reveal the effectiveness of short-course MDR/or RR-TB treatment regimen. The recent meta-analysis studies showed that the treatment success rate using a shorter MDR/RR-TB treatment regimen was ranged from 83.0–83.7% [6–8], which is significantly higher than a meta-analysis reported a success rate for conventional, longer MDR/RR-TB treatment regimen (54%) [9]. Moreover, the effectiveness of shorter course MDR/RR-TB treatment was also explored in other institutional and observational studies. A study from nine African countries revealed that the treatment success and cure rate of short MDR/RR-TB regimen was 81.6% and 72.4%, respectively [10]. Similarly, promising reports for short course MDR/RR-TB treatment were also noted in Bangladesh, Niger, and Cameron [11–14].

Generally, the existing facts asserted that the safety and effectiveness of the shorter MDR/RR-TB regimen are superior compared to the previously appreciated reports for the longer MDR/RR-TB regimen. Even more, a 9–12 month regimen for MDR/RR-TB was also recommended by World Health Organization (WHO) [15]. But, prior to putting this regimen in place or before this regimen can be prescribed for the MDR/RR-TB patients in a given country, the level evidence in both regimens needs to be replicated and supported through rigorous research and with a large number of patients, in order to conclude that this most effective treatment for MDR/RR-TB. Besides, still findings are based on observational design, and therefore future researches need to be focus on high-level designs such as randomized controlled trials (RCTs) to generate highly relevant evidence in this regard. Most importantly, this short course treatment should not completely replace the conventional treatment approach since the fact that patients with fluoroquinolones or other 2nd line drug resistance, extra-pulmonary tuberculosis, pregnancy and with severe clinical problems are known not to be considered for shorter MDR/RR-TB regimen. In this case, the national TB control program (NTPs) in need to maintain the conventional treatment approaches.

The MDR-TB treatment in Ethiopia is mainly based on a standard or long course treatment, which is known as less effective to achieve high levels of successful outcome. The Ethiopian Federal Ministry of Health adopted a standardized regimen consists of an 8-month intensive phase with a combination of pyrazinamide, capreomycin, levofloxacin and prothionamide or ethionamide and cycloserine, a 12-month continuation phase with a combination of pyrazinamide, levofloxacin,prothionamide or ethionamide and cycloserine [16].

By far, few observational studies have been conducted to reveal treatment outcomes among MDR-TB patients, and even the findings are inconsistent and representing only local information. Hence, the effectiveness of the standard MDR-TB treatment was not fully assessed in Ethiopia. Therefore, we report here a meta-analysis of observational studies of regimens of 18–24 months in duration whose composition was based on a standardized longer term regimen. The purpose of the study was first, to determine the pooled successful and unfavorable treatment outcome measures. Secondly, the sub-group analysis was also done to estimate the proportion of cured and treatment completed cases among successfully treated cases, and to evaluate poor treatment outcomes including treatment failures, deaths, and lost to follow ups.

Methods

Studies/setting

Studies that reported the treatment outcome among MDR-TB patients in Ethiopia were included for this analysis. However, studies focused on non-MDR or drug-susceptible TB patients were not eligible for this study.

Study protocol registration

The study has been registered in PROSPERO database with protocol number, CRD42018090711.

Intervention

The original studies reported an outcome from patients treated with a longer, 18–24 months MDR-TB treatment regimen.

Comparison

MDR-TB treatment in Ethiopia is largely based on a standardized longer regimen. Therefore, no comparison was undertaken for this analysis.

Outcomes

MDR-TB treatment outcomes were evaluated as treatment success and unfavorable outcome. Successful outcomes described as patients meeting the definition of Cure or treatment completed. Poor treatment outcomes refer to patients meeting the definition of death, lost to follow up, and treatment failed.

Search strategy and quality evaluation

The PubMed database was employed to retrieve the available research reports in Ethiopia. A highly sensitive search strategy was developed using the combination of the following Keywords; treatment outcome AND multidrug-resistant tuberculosis OR drug-resistant tuberculosis OR MDR-TB AND Ethiopia, both as exploded as MESH headings and free-text terms. Manual searching was also done from the institutional repository websites of Ethiopian universities (such as Addis Ababa University, and University of Gondar) to include unpublished reports. Besides, grey literature searching was also performed using Google Scholar database to collect non-PubMed indexed articles. Electronic database searches were conducted in February and March 2018. Two authors (SE, AE) reviewed all abstracts and a full-text article, with the final decision, was made through consensus. In cases of disagreement, the consensus was achieved through arbitration of other authors.

Studies were potentially acceptable if they report the treatment outcome on at least 100 MDR-TB patients within a defined study design approach, retrospective, and prospective cohorts. The original studies were also rated as good quality when the average treatment duration was 12 months and above. However, treatment outcome other than MDR-TB was not examined in our meta-analysis. The overall quality score of the included studies was measured using the Newcastle-Ottawa quality assessment scale for observational studies (Additional file 2: Table S2).

Data extraction and statistical analysis

Two investigators (SE, AA) extracted data using a standard abstraction form. In the case of disagreement, other investigators (FW, US) took part to resolve the differences through discussion. Data abstraction was carried out with regard treatment outcomes. The primary outcome of this study was treatment success included cure, treatment completed, or both. The secondary outcome of the study was poor outcomes (such as, lost to follow up, death and failure). Moreover, for each included study the following information was also collected; HIV status, and previous history of anti-TB treatment.

The pooled proportions of the treatment outcomes with 95%CI were statistically measured using Stata version 11.0 software (College Station, TX: StataCorp LP). A Freeman-Tukey-type arcsine square-root transformation and DerSimonian and Laird random-effects model were used to stabilize variances and calculate pooled estimates [17].The sensitivity analysis on primary outcome was done using a Bayesian random-effects model with Monte Carlo Markov chain simulations of variability [18]. The I^2 statistic was used to assess the proportion of overall variation attributable to between-study heterogeneity [19].

Results

Selection process and description of the included studies

The selection process is depicted in Fig. 1, a total of 132 abstracts were identified from an initial electronic database search. Following title and abstract evaluation, 100 citations were excluded and the remaining 32 were subjected to full-text evaluation. After full-text review, 2 studies were found to be eligible for the analysis and a further 4 studies were obtained through manual searching, institutional repository sites of Addis Ababa University and email contact from the primary investigator. Finally, 6 studies were found to be acceptable for our analysis [20–25].

The baseline characteristics of the studies were indicated Table 1, of the included studies, three were retrospective cohorts, and the remaining were descriptive retrospective chart reviews and prospective cohort studies. All studies reported the patients' previous history of anti-TB drug treatment and HIV co-infection. The included studies reported treatment outcome among 1993 MDR-TB patients representing Northwestern, Northeastern, Central, Eastern and Southern Ethiopia, MDR-TB care centers. Of the patients, successful treatment outcome was observed in 1288 patients, while 442 were poorly treated cases (Table 2). However, the treatment outcome of 263 patients was not evaluated; this was due to either the transfer out or patients on the course of treatment. Relatively high treatment success rate was reported in Meressa et al. (78.6%) [25] followed by Tolera et al. (65.9%) [24] and Alene et al. (63.6%) [22]. On the other hand, a high proportion of patients with poor outcome was observed in Tolera et al. (34.1%) [24], followed by Alene et al. (25.6%) [22] and Baye et al. (22.7%) [20].

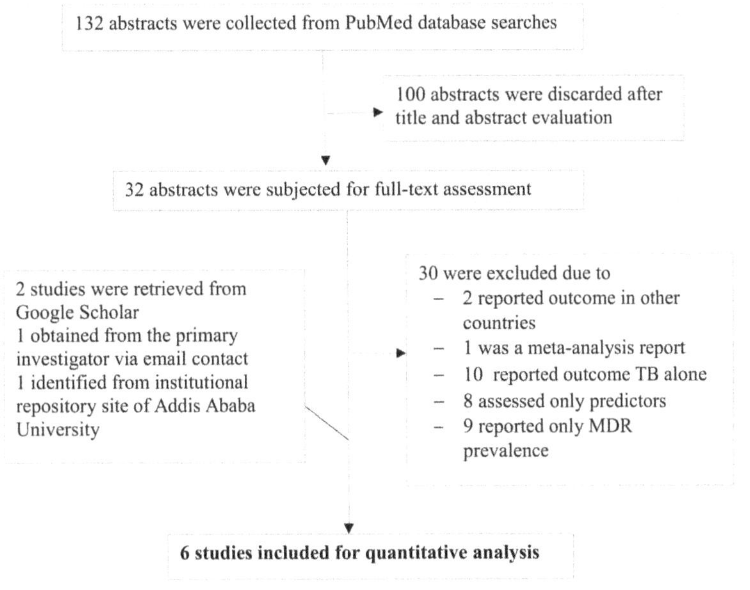

Fig. 1 Study selection process

MDR-TB treatment outcomes

In the present analysis, the pooled treatment success was estimated as 59.2% (95%CI, 48.1–70.4). The high heterogeneity between studies was observed (I^2, 96.3%) (Fig. 2), but evaluation of the publication bias is not recommended for a meta-analysis of lower than 10 studies. Likewise, the overall poor treatment outcome was also determined, as seen in Fig. 3, 23.3% (95%CI, 19.7–27.0%) of the patients were unsuccessfully treated. High heterogeneity was also indicated (I^2, 70.7%).

In sub-group analysis, 46.1% (95%CI, 34.2–58.0) and 12.8% (95%CI, 5.7–20.0) of MDR-TB patients were cured and treatment completed, respectively (Fig. 4). Moreover, the pooled proportion of poor treatment outcomes was also presented in Fig. 5, 14.3% (95%CI, 11.5–17.2) died, 7.5%(95%Cl, 3.7–11.3) lost to follow up, and 1.6% (95%Cl, 1.1–2.2%) were patients with treatment failure. In Fig. 5, 25.0% (95%Cl, 14.6–35.5) of the MDR-TB patients whose treatment outcome was not examined, as noted in the original studies, these were patients on treatment or transfer-out.

Discussion

Though the WHO task force set a strategic plan to target of 75% successful treatment outcome of MDR-TB by the end of 2015 in global bases [26], many countries including Ethiopia have not yet achieved this ambitious aim. Maximizing the favorable treatment outcome in MDR-TB is a global health priority and one of the key performance indicators of WHO's End TB strategy [27]. Ethiopia has made the treatment of MDR-TB a national health priority [28].

The national MDR-TB treatment program based on the recommendations from the 2011 update of Guidelines for the programmatic management of drug-resistant tuberculosis [29].The treatment of MDR-TB requires a long lasting drug exposure, and is also significantly associated with high rates of adverse drug events. Recent meta-analysis report documented a lower treatment success rate among patients treated with a longer MDR-TB regimen compared to those treated with a short course MDR-TB treatment [9].

To our knowledge, this is the first combined analysis to evaluate the effectiveness of the currently used MDR-TB treatment program in Ethiopia. In the present analysis, the pooled estimate of successful treatment was 59.2% (95%CI, 48.1–70.4), while 23.3% (95%CI, 19.7–27.0%) had poor treatment outcome. The treatment success observed in this analysis is comparable with the results of recently published meta-analyses of the outcomes of MDR-TB treatment with conventional drug regimens. Notably, a 54% treatment success rate for conventional MDR-TB treatment regimen was found in a meta-analysis conducted by Ahuja et al. [9]. Similar MDR treatment outcome was estimated in a meta-analysis conducted by Orenstein et al. [30], and pooled analysis from 21 countries [31], showed 62% successful outcome. Thus, it is suggested that the need to modify the duration and the composition of the current MDR-TB treatment regimens. Because of the lengthy therapy, toxicity and fewer efficacies of second-line anti-TB drugs resulting high rates of an unfavorable outcome subsequently lead to the rapid emergence of the extensively drug-resistant TB.

Table 1 The baseline characteristics of the included studies

Study area	First author, year of publication	Study period	Study design	No of MDR-TB cases	Types of cases	Method	Treatment category	HIV status
Northeastern Ethiopia	Baye et al, 2018 [20]	2012–2016	RC	141	Pulmonary tuberculosis (96.5%) Extra-pulmonary tuberculosis (3.5%)	Line probe assay Culture Xpert MTB/RIF	New (8.5%) Relapse (13.5%) After lost to follow up (2.1%) Failure of a new regimen (30.5%) After the failure of retreatment (42.6%) Transfer in from other sites (1.4%) Other (1.4%)	HIV co-infected, 38 (27%), the majority of the patients have received ART (84.2%)
Southern Ethiopia	Girum et al, 2017 [21]	2009 to 2014	RC	154	Pulmonary tuberculosis (94%) Extra-pulmonary tuberculosis (6%)	Culture Xpert MTB/RIF	History of previous treatment (90%) New cases (10%)	HIV co-infection, 11 (7.2%), of them 9 have had a history of previous treatment
Northwest Ethiopia	Alene et al, 2017 [22]	2010 to 2015	RC	242	Pulmonary tuberculosis (94%) Extra-pulmonary tuberculosis (6%)	Culture Xpert MTB/RIF	History of previous treatment (93%) New cases (7%)	HIV co-infection, 51 (21.1%)
Central Ethiopia	Mequanint et al., 2014 [23]	2011 to 2013	DRC	680	Pulmonary tuberculosis (84%) Extra-pulmonary (15.6%) Both, 0.4%	Culture	History of previous treatment, 35%	HIV co-infection, 193 (28.4%)
Eastern Ethiopia	Tolera et al. 2018 [24]	2005 to 2016	DRC	164	Pulmonary tuberculosis (98.2%) Extra-pulmonary tuberculosis (1.8%)	–	Retreated cases, 97%	HIV co-infection, 41 (25%), the majority of the patients have received ART (97.6%)
Central and Northwest Ethiopia	Meressa et al., 2015 [25]	2009 to 2014	PC	612	Pulmonary tuberculosis (93%) Extra-pulmonary tuberculosis (7%)	Culture Line probe assay	History of previous treatment (98.5%) HIV infection (21.7%)	HIV co-infection, 133 (21.7%), the median CD4 count was 239 cells/ml^3, the majority of the patients have received ART (90.2%)

Key: *RC* retrospective cohort study, *DRC* descriptive retrospective cross-sectional study, *PC* prospective cohort study

Table 2 MDR-TB treatment outcome extracted from the original studies

First author and year of publication	Study area	Successful outcome			Unfavorable outcome				Not evaluated		
		Cured, n (%)	Treatment completed, n (%)	Total, N (%)	Died, n (%)	Lost to follow up, n (%)	Treatment failed, n (%)	Total, N (%)	Transfer out, n (%)	On treatment, n (%)	Total, N (%)
Baye et al., 2018 [20]	Northeastern Ethiopia	55 (39.0)	3 (2.1)	58 (41.1)	22 (68.8)	8 (15.6)	2 (1.4)	32 (22.7)	–	–	51 (36.2)
Girum et al, 2017 [21]	Southern Ethiopia	39 (25.3)	26 (16.9)	65 (42.2)	13 (8.4)	20 (13.0)	0	33 (21.4)	5 (3.2)	50 (32.5%)	56 (36.4)
Alene et al, 2017 [22]	Northwest Ethiopia	131 (54.1)	23 (9.5)	154 (63.6)	31 (12.8)	27 (11.2)	4 (1.7)	62 (25.6)	6 (2.5)	20 (8.3)	26 (10.7)
Mequanint et al., 2014 [23]	Central Ethiopia	274 (40.3)	148 (21.8)	422 (62.1)	105 (15.4)	9 (1.3)	14 (2.1)	128 (18.8)	8 (1.2)	122 (17.9)	130 (19.1)
Tolera et al., 2018 [24]	Eastern Ethiopia	86 (52.4)	22 (13.4)	108 (65.9)	37 (22.6)	17 (10.4)	2 (1.2)	56 (34.1)	0	0	0
Meressa et al., 2015 [25]	Central and Northwest Ethiopia	396 (64.7)	85 (13.9)	481 (78.6)	85 (13.9)	36 (5.9)	10 (1.6)	131 (21.4)	0	0	0

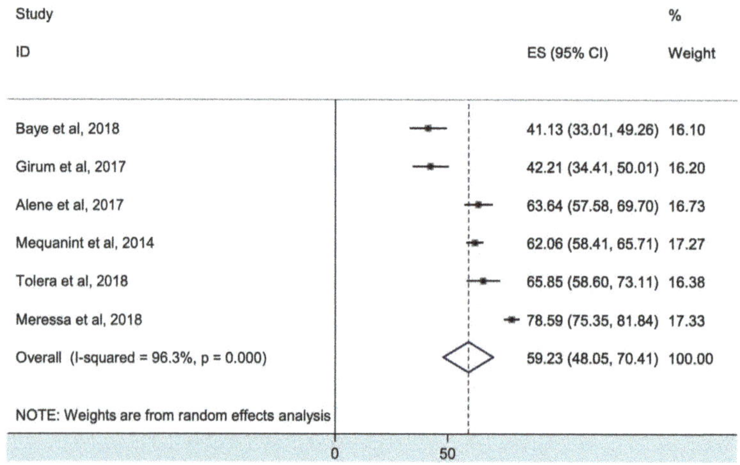

Fig. 2 Pooled estimates of successful treatment outcome

Most recently, an effective standardized treatment regimen lasting less than 12 months has been adopted in countries like Bangladesh, Benin, Burkina-Faso, Burundi, Cameroon, Central African Republic, Côte d'Ivoire, DR Congo, Guinea, Niger, Rwanda, Senegal, Swaziland, and Uzbekistan [10–14]. The regimen composed of the initial phase of 4 months therapy with kanamycin, moxifloxacin, prothionamide, clofazimine, isoniazid, pyrazinamide and ethambutol, and followed by 5 months of treatment with moxifloxacin, clofazimine, pyrazinamide, and ethambutol. Based on the data from recent studies, high treatment success has been achieved in above-mentioned countries. Most importantly, meta-analysis studies revealed that the treatment success rate using shorter MDR/RR-TB treatment regimens was ranged from 83.0–83.7% [6, 7], which higher than previously appreciated treatment outcome. Furthermore, an observational survey of nine African countries also noted promising results of using 12-month regimen [10].

Of note, the latest advancement asserted that the effectiveness of the shorter treatment regimen, in May 2016 WHO moves one step forward to update drug-resistant TB treatment guideline, and underscored the recommendation on the use of the 9–12 month treatment regimen [15]. This encouraged the National Tuberculosis Program (NTP) of Ethiopia need to test and implement a similar 12-month regimen. Though there are several positives with this regimen, its use could be restricted by the fact that patients with fluoroquinolones or other 2nd line drug resistance, extra-pulmonary tuberculosis, pregnancy and with severe clinical problems are known not to be considered for shorter MDR/RR-TB regimen. In this case, the NTPs need to preserve the conventional treatment approaches.

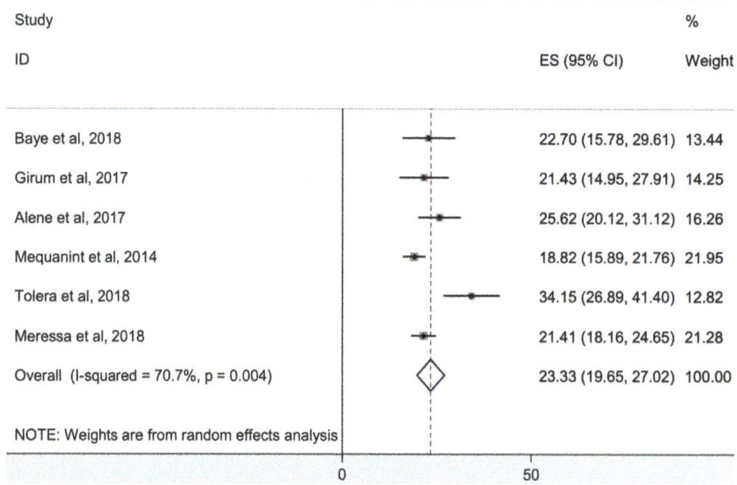

Fig. 3 A pooled estimate of poor treatment outcome

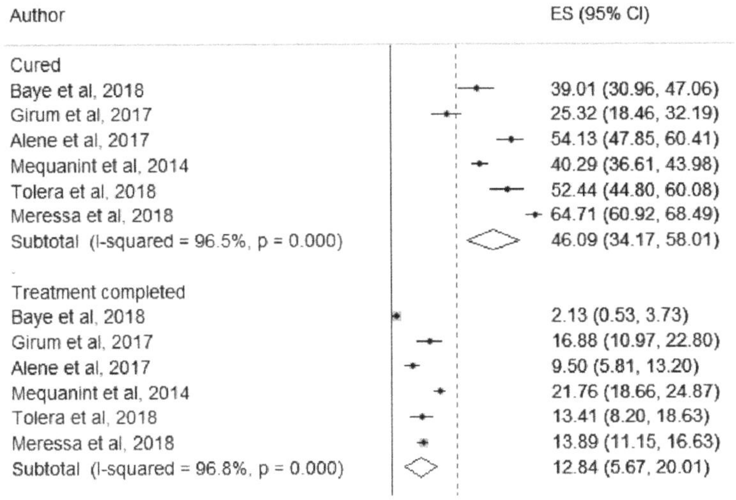

Fig. 4 The pooled proportion of cured and treatment completed cases

In sub-group analysis, it also estimated that 46.1% (34.2–58.0) cured, 12.8% (5.7–20.0) treatment completed, 14.3% (11.5–17.2) died, 7.5% (3.7–11.3) lost to follow uped, 1.6% (1.1–2.2%) experienced treatment failure and 25.0% (14.6–35.5) of the patients whose treatment outcome was not evaluated. Particularly, the cure rate indicated in our analysis is substantially inferior to the results reported with a shorter MDR-TB regimen [15]. Aside from the drug-resistant nature of the infection, the low cure rate might be due to lack of sufficient MDR-TB care centers, poor patient adherence, the low performance of NTPs at central and regional levels, poor efficacy and prolonged duration of the treatment. According to WHO 2017 report [2], achieving high cure rate one of the key pillars of End TB strategy. The result of this study informs the NTPs to update the current treatment approaches as per recently recommended treatment guideline. However, prior to this prospective

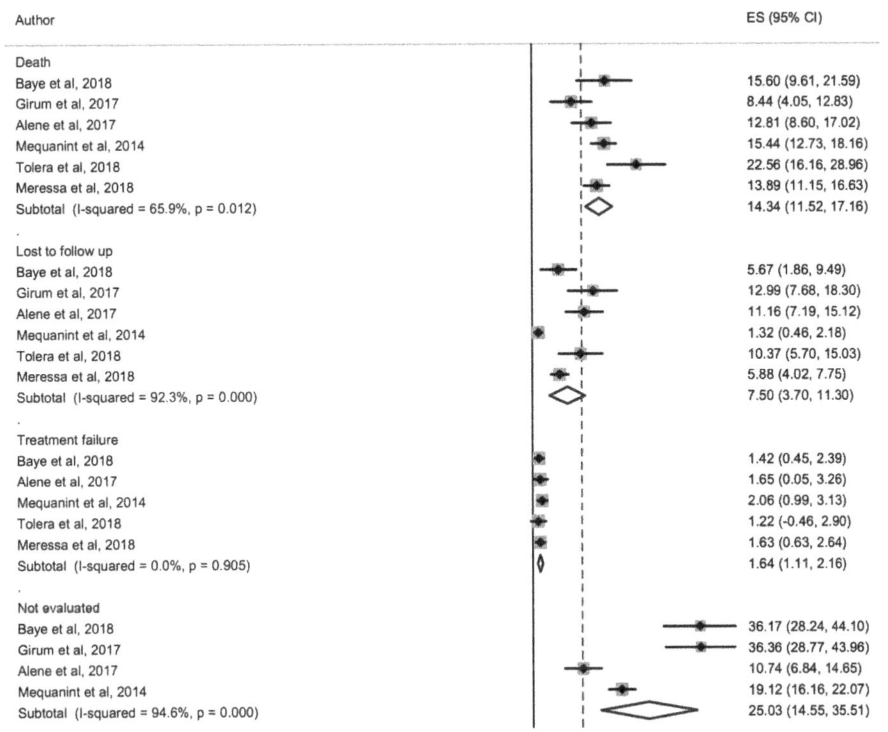

Fig. 5 The pooled proportion of died, lost to follow up, patients experienced treatment failure, and patients whose outcome was not evaluated

cohort analysis of a large number of patients required to support the evidence detailed above. Additionally, the Ethiopian Federal Ministry of Health should design smooth platforms to facilitate surveillance data on culture-based drug susceptibility testing; it may be used to identify a population of eligible patients for Short course MDR/RR-TB treatment.

Limitations of the study

One of the limitations of this analysis was observational and few studies have been included to measure MDR-TB treatment outcome. Potential predictors of poor treatment outcome Such as HIV infection and history TB treatment was not evaluated because the association was not measured in the original studies. Besides, sub-group analysis of the MDR-TB outcome was not done based on the mode of patient treatment (hospital and/or ambulatory) because lack of clear information in the reports.

Conclusion

The results suggest that low treatment success rate was estimated among MDR-TB patients whose composition of the treatment was based on a conventionally used treatment regimen. Therefore, our analysis remarks the need to test and implement recently adopted a shorter MDR-TB treatment regimen. Prior to implementation the levels of evidence need to be supported through rigorous institutional and national-wide studies.

Abbreviations

CI: Confidence interval; HIV: Human immuno-deficiency virus; MDR-TB: Multidrug resistant Tuberculosis; NTPs: National Tuberculosis Control Programs; TB: Tuberculosis; WHO: World Health Organization

Authors' contributions

SE: Conception of study idea, study design, literature review, data collection, data extraction, data analysis and interpretation, and drafting manuscript. AA, FW, DG & AF: Data collection and extraction, reviewing manuscript. US: Supervision, analysis and interpretation, and reviewing manuscript. All authors have read and approved the manuscript.

Consent for publication

Not applicable.

Competing interests

The authors declare that they have no competing interests.

Author details

[1]Department of Medical Microbiology, School of Biomedical and Laboratory Sciences, College of Medicine and Health Sciences, University of Gondar, Gondar, Ethiopia. [2]Department of Clinical Nursing, College of Health Sciences, Debre Markos University, Debre Marqos, Ethiopia. [3]Department of Immunology and Molecular Biology, College of Medicine and Health Sciences, University of Gondar, Gondar, Ethiopia. [4]Department of Clinical Chemistry, College of Medicine and Health Sciences, University of Gondar, Gondar, Ethiopia. [5]Institute of Clinical Immunology, Medical Faculty, University of Leipzig, Leipzig, Germany.

References

1. Adhvaryu M, Vakharia B. Drug-resistant tuberculosis: emerging treatment options. Clin Pharmacol. 2011;3:51–67.
2. World Health Organization. Global tuberculosis report 2017. Geneva: WHO; 2017.
3. World Health Organization. Global tuberculosis report. Geneva: WHO; 2016.
4. Eshetie S, Gizachew M, Dagnew M, Kumera G, Woldie H, Ambaw F, Tessema B, Moges F. Multidrug resistant tuberculosis in Ethiopian settings and its association with previous history of anti-tuberculosis treatment: a systematic review and meta-analysis. BMC Infect Dis. 2017;17(1):219.
5. Uplekar M, Weil D, Lonnroth K, Jaramillo E, Lienhardt C, Dias HM, Falzon D, Floyd K, Gargioni G, Getahun H. WHO's new end TB strategy. Lancet. 2015;385(9979):1799–801.
6. Khan FA, Salim MH, du Cros P, Casas EC, Khamraev A, Sikhondze W, Benedetti A, Bastos M, Lan Z, Jaramillo E. Effectiveness and safety of standardised shorter regimens for multidrug-resistant tuberculosis: individual patient data and aggregate data meta-analyses. Eur Respir J. 2017;50(1):1700061.
7. Bastos ML, Lan Z, Menzies D. An updated systematic review and meta-analysis for treatment of multidrug-resistant tuberculosis. Eur Respir J. 2017;49(3):1600803.
8. Fox GJ, Benedetti A, Cox H, Koh WJ, Viiklepp P, Ahuja S, Pasvol G, Menzies D. Group 5 drugs for multidrug-resistant tuberculosis: individual patient data. Eur Respir J. 2017;49(1):00993–2016.
9. Ahuja SD, Ashkin D, Avendano M, Banerjee R, Bauer M, Bayona JN, Becerra MC, Benedetti A, Burgos M, Centis R, et al. Multidrug resistant pulmonary tuberculosis treatment regimens and patient outcomes: an individual patient data meta-analysis of 9,153 patients. PLoS Med. 2012;9(8): e1001300.
10. Trebucq A, Schwoebel V, Kashongwe Z, Bakayoko A, Kuaban C, Noeske J, Hassane S, Souleymane B, Piubello A, Ciza F, et al. Treatment outcome with a short multidrug-resistant tuberculosis regimen in nine African countries. Int J Tuberc Lung Dis. 2018;22(1):17–25.
11. Aung KJ, Van Deun A, Declercq E, Sarker MR, Das PK, Hossain MA, Rieder HL. Successful '9-month Bangladesh regimen' for multidrug-resistant tuberculosis among over 500 consecutive patients. Int J Tuberc Lung Dis. 2014;18(10):1180–7.
12. Van Deun A, Maug AK, Salim MA, Das PK, Sarker MR, Daru P, Rieder HL. Short, highly effective, and inexpensive standardized treatment of multidrug-resistant tuberculosis. Am J Respir Crit Care Med. 2010;182(5):684–92.
13. Kuaban C, Noeske J, Rieder HL, Ait-Khaled N, Abena Foe JL, Trebucq A. High effectiveness of a 12-month regimen for MDR-TB patients in Cameroon. Int J Tuberc Lung Dis. 2015;19(5):517–24.
14. Piubello A, Harouna SH, Souleymane MB, Boukary I, Morou S, Daouda M, Hanki Y, Van Deun A. High cure rate with standardised short-course multidrug-resistant tuberculosis treatment in Niger: no relapses. Int J Tuberc Lung Dis. 2014;18(10):1188–94.
15. Falzon D, Schunemann HJ, Harausz E, Gonzalez-Angulo L, Lienhardt C, Jaramillo E, Weyer K. World health organization treatment guidelines for drug-resistant tuberculosis, 2016 update. Eur Respir J. 2017;49(3):1–12.
16. Federa Ministry of Health. Guidelines on programmatic management of drug resistant tuberculosis in Ethiopia. Addis, Ababa: MOH; 2013.
17. Borenstein M, Hedges LV, Higgins JP, Rothstein HR. A basic introduction to fixed-effect and random-effects models for meta-analysis. Res Synth Methods. 2010;1(2):97–111.
18. Smith TC, Spiegelhalter DJ, Thomas A. Bayesian approaches to random-effects meta-analysis: a comparative study. Stat Med. 1995;14(24):2685–99.

19. Rucker G, Schwarzer G, Carpenter JR, Schumacher M. Undue reliance on I(2) in assessing heterogeneity may mislead. BMC Med Res Methodol. 2008;8:79.
20. Baye AM, Sarhie WD, Endalew BT. Treatment outcomes of multi-drug-resistant tuberculosis and its determinants in Boru Meda hospital, Northeast Ethiopia. J Infect Dis Ther. 2018;6(350):1–5.
21. Girum T, Tariku Y, Dessu S. Survival status and treatment outcome of multidrug resistant tuberculosis (MDR-TB) among patients treated in treatment initiation centers (TIC) in South Ethiopia: a retrospective cohort study. Ann Med Health Sci Res. 2017;7:331–3.
22. Alene KA, Viney K, McBryde ES, Tsegaye AT, Clements AC. Treatment outcomes in patients with multidrug-resistant tuberculosis in north-West Ethiopia. Trop Med Int Health. 2017;22(3):351–62.
23. Mequanint G, Mengistu Z. Prevalence of MDR-TB and treatment outcome among tuberculosis patients attending at St. Peter TB Specialized Hospital. Addis Ababa: Addis Ababa University; 2014. Available at http://etd.aau.edu.et/bitstream/handle/123456789/7091/Gashaw%20Mequanint.pdf?sequence=1&isAllowed=y.
24. Tolera M, Dessie Y, Oljira L, Geleto A. Treatment outcome of multi drug resistant tuberculosis patients and its associated factors in Eastern Ethiopia. Ethiopia: Haramaya University; 2018.
25. Meressa D, Hurtado RM, Andrews JR, Diro E, Abato K, Daniel T, Prasad P, Prasad R, Fekade B, Tedla Y, et al. Achieving high treatment success for multidrug-resistant TB in Africa: initiation and scale-up of MDR TB care in Ethiopia--an observational cohort study. Thorax. 2015;70(12):1181–8.
26. World Health Organization. Towards universal access to diagnosis and treatment of multidrug-resistant and extensively drug-resistant tuberculosis by 2015: WHO progress report 2011. Geneva: WHO; 2011.
27. World Health Organization. The End TB Strategy. Geneva: WHO; 2017.
28. Federa Ministry of Health. Annual Tuberculosis Bulletin: Health Promotion and Diseases Prevention Directorate. Addis Ababa: MOH; 2013.
29. World Health Organization. Guidelines for the programmatic management of drug-resistant tuberculosis. Geneva: WHO; 2011.
30. Orenstein EW, Basu S, Shah NS, Andrews JR, Friedland GH, Moll AP, Gandhi NR, Galvani AP. Treatment outcomes among patients with multidrug-resistant tuberculosis: systematic review and meta-analysis. Lancet Infect Dis. 2009;9(3):153–61.
31. Johnston JC, Shahidi NC, Sadatsafavi M, Fitzgerald JM. Treatment outcomes of multidrug-resistant tuberculosis: a systematic review and meta-analysis. PLoS One. 2009;4(9):e6914.

Outcomes and prognostic factors of non-HIV patients with pneumocystis jirovecii pneumonia and pulmonary CMV co-infection

Qing Yu[1], Peng Jia[1], Li Su[1], Hong Zhao[2] and Chengli Que[1*]

Abstract

Background: *Pneumocystis jirovecii* pneumonia (PJP) and pulmonary cytomegalovirus (CMV) infection are common opportunistic infections among immunocompromised patients. However, few studies have evaluated their co-infection, especially among non-HIV patients. Therefore, we aimed to evaluate the outcomes and prognostic factors among non-HIV patients with PJP according to their CMV infection status.

Methods: This retrospective study evaluated non-HIV patients who were diagnosed with PJP between January 2009 and January2016.The patients were classified and compared according to their pulmonary CMV infection status (positive infection: bronchoalveolar lavage fluid [BALF] CMV DNA loads of >500copies/mL).

Results: Among 70 non-HIV patients with PJP, we identified 38 patients (54.3%) with pulmonary CMV infection. There was no significant difference in the mortality rates for the two groups ($p = 0.15$). Pulmonary CMV infection was significantly more common among patients who were receiving glucocorticoids and immunosuppressants, compared to corticosteroids only ($p = 0.02$). Pulmonary CMV infection was also significantly associated with severe dyspnea, a lower PaO_2/FiO_2, and the presence of centrilobular nodules ($p = 0.008$). Higher CMV DNA loads in the BALF were positively associated with mortality ($p = 0.012$).

Conclusions: Combined therapy using corticosteroids and other immunosuppressants may be a risk factor for pulmonary CMV co-infection among patients with PJP. In addition, CMV pneumonia should be considered when centrilobular nodules and/or severe hypoxemia are observed in non-HIV patients with PJP. Furthermore, antiviral treatment should be promptly initiated for patients with a high CMV DNA load in BALF, based on their poor prognosis.

Keywords: *Pneumocystis jirovecii*pneumonia, Cytomegalovirus, CMVDNA load, Prognosis

Background

Pneumocystis jirovecii pneumonia (PJP) is a common opportunistic infection among immunocompromised patients, and especially among patients with human immunodeficiency virus (HIV) infection. In addition, autoimmune diseases, malignancy, organ transplantation, and treatment using immunosuppressants and antineoplastic drugs increase the risk of *P. jirovecii* infection [1–5]. Cytomegalovirus (CMV) infection is another common cause of pneumonia in immunocompromised hosts, and CMV co-infection can be observed in patients who are infected with other pathogens (especially *P. jirovecii*) [6]. Previous studies have reported that 28–69% of HIV-infected patients also exhibit co-infection with *P. jirovecii*andCMV [7–10]. However, CMV can also be found in the respiratory secretions of patients without clear signs of pneumonia [11], and the pathogenesis and prognosis of pulmonary CMV infection with PJP in non-HIV patients is poorly understood.

In an animal model, CMV altered the host's immune environment by modulating molecules that are involved

* Correspondence: quechengli@bjmu.edu.cn
[1]Department of Respiratory and Critical Care Medicine, Peking University First Hospital, Beijing 100034, China
Full list of author information is available at the end of the article

in immune recognition and inflammation [12]. Moreover, CMV infection can alter the host's immune response by suppressing the function of helper T-cells and antigen-presenting cells, which are essential for achieving PJP resolution [12]. Nevertheless, researchers have not found any significant differences in the morbidity and mortality rates among HIV-infected patients with PJP according to their pulmonary CMV infection status [7, 9, 13]. Although the clinical characteristics and prognosis of PJP are different in HIV-infected and non-HIV patients [14, 15], there are few reports regarding PJP and CMV co-infection among non-HIV patients, despite a reported incidence of 29.2% (31/106) in a study by Tark et al. [13].

The present study aimed to evaluate the outcomes and prognostic factors among non-HIV patients with PJP according to their pulmonary CMV infection status.

Methods

Patients

For this study, we retrospectively identified non-HIV patients who were diagnosed with PJP between January 2009 and January 2016. These patients had undergone bronchoalveolar lavage using a flexible bronchoscope and the standard techniques [16]. The bronchoalveolar lavage fluid (BALF) specimens were processed and stained using Gomori methenamine silver (GMS), and the BALF specimens were also evaluated for the presence of pneumocystis cysts. The results of these evaluations and the patient's clinical manifestations were used to confirm a diagnosis of PJP. In this study, we also compared the demographic characteristics, clinical characteristics, and rates of morbidity and mortality among non-HIV patients with PJP according to their pulmonary CMV infection status.

Microbiological methods

The BALF specimens were also sent to microbiological laboratory using Gram staining, acid-fast staining, and culture for bacterial and fungal infection. Real-time quantitative polymerase chain reaction (PCR) was used to evaluate the BALF loads of CMV DNA for all patients, and a cut-off value of ≥500copies/mL(about 125 IU/ml) was considered positively identify pulmonary CMV infection, based on the manufacturer's instructions (Human Cytomegalovirus Fluorescence Quantitative Polymerase Chain Reaction Diagnostic Kit; Da An Gene Company, Guangzhou, China).

Statistical analysis

All analyses were performed using SPSS software (version 19.0; SPSS Inc., Chicago, IL). Categorical variables were compared using the chi-square test or Fisher's exact test. Continuous variables were analyzed by median IQR and compare them using the Mann–Whitney U-test. The rank sum test was used to analyse the association between mortality and the BALF loads of CMV DNA. Differences with a p-value of <0.05 were considered statistically significant.

Results

During the study period, we identified 70 non-HIV patients who were diagnosed with PJP (43 men, 27 women; median age: 50 years, range: 21–81 years). And all patients with PJP had undergone BALF testing for CMV-DNA. Thirty-eight patients (54.3%) exhibited pulmonary CMV infection (CMV DNA loads of ≥500copies/mL in their BALF). Twenty-eight patients exhibited bacterial co-infection and nineteen patients exhibited fungal co-infection. In our study, the PJP patients co-infection with CMV was significantly associated with combined use of glucocorticoids and T-cell immunosuppressants (p = 0.02). There was no significant difference in the mortality rates when we compared the patients with and without pulmonary CMV infection(17/38 [44.7%] vs.9/32 [28.2%], respectively; p = 0.15)(Table 1).

In terms of C-reactive protein levels, CD4 + T-lymphocyte count, and lactate dehydrogenase levels, no significant differences were found between patients co-infected with or without CMV. However, patients with both PJP and CMV co-infection exhibited a significantly higher frequency of having a $PaO_2/FiO_2$of < 100(p = 0.04) (Table 2). We also analysed the patients' clinical and radiographic manifestations (Table 3). Fever (84.3%) and dyspnea (65.7%) were the two most common symptoms, and patients with PJP and CMV co-infection exhibited a significantly higher rate of dyspnea (p = 0.04). Ground-glass opacities were observed during the chest computed tomography (CT) for all patients, with upper lobe predominance in15 cases and consolidation in 33 cases. However, there were no association between the lesion's location or consolidation and pulmonary CMV infection (both, p > 0.05). Centrilobular nodules were identified on the CT scan in17 patients, and 14 of these patients had pulmonary CMV infection; this association was statistically significant (p = 0.008).

We also measured the serum loads of CMV DNA and found that 21 patients had detectable CMV DNA in their serum and BALF specimens. Seventeen patients exhibited positive BALF specimens, but negative serum specimens. None of the 32 patients with negative BALF specimens exhibited detectable CMV DNA in their serum. We observed a positive association between BALF loads of CMV DNA and mortality among the 38 patients with PJP and pulmonary CMV co-infection (Table 4).

Discussion

Among HIV-infected patients, PJP and pulmonary CMV co-infection is relatively common (28–69% of all cases)

Table 1 The demographic characteristics, underlying diseases, and mortality rates among non-HIV patients with PJP according to pulmonary CMV infection status

	CMV-DNA positive in BALF (n = 38)	CMV-DNA negative in BALF(n = 32)	p
Demographics			
Age, yr., median	51(21–77)	48(22–81)	0.48
Gender ratio(male:female)	23:15	20:12	0.87
Underlying diseases,n(%)			
Solid organ transplantation	3(7.9)	3(9.4)	1.00
Hematologic malignancy	4(10.5)	9(28.2)	0.06
Hematopoietic stem cell transplantation	3(75)	4(44.4)	
Non-hematologic malignancy	2(5.3)	2(6.3)	1.00
Dermatologic diseases	4(10.5)	5(15.6)	0.78
Kidney disease	12(31.5)	5(15.6)	0.12
Interstitial lung disease	0(0)	1(3.1)	1.00
Connective tissue disease	9(23.7)	5(15.6)	0.40
Idiopathic thrombocytopenia	2(5.3)	1(3.1)	1.00
Others	2(5.3)	1(3.1)	1.00
Immunosuppressive agents,n(%)			
Steroids	37(97.4)	31(96.9)	1.00
Dosage of steroid, recent 1 month(mg)	40(10–100)	45(10–300)	0.54
Steroid + T-cell immunosuppressants	28(73.7)	15(65.2)	0.02
Steroid +Anti-CD20+ monoclonal antibody[a]	1(2.6)	6(18.8)	0.06
Chemotherapy/Radiotherapy	2(5.3)	3(9.4)	0.84
Treatment for PJP			
TMP-SMZ(%)	33(86.8)	31(96.9)	0.29
Treatment duration, days, median	15(4–31)	21(2–23)	0.051
Shift to second-line therapy[b](%)	23(60.5)	12(37.5)	0.055
Due to treatment failure	18(47.4)	11(34.4)	0.27
Due to adverse reaction[c]	5(13.2)	1(3.1)	0.29
Morbidity,n(%)			
Admitted to ICU	16(42.1)	9(28.2)	0.22
Mechanical ventilation	14(36.8)	8(25.0)	0.29
Mortality	17(44.7)	9(28.2)	0.15

[a]Rituximab
[b]second-line therapy: primaquine plus clindamycin and caspofungin
[c]Adverse reactions included thrombocytopenia, bone marrow suppression, and drug allergy (2 cases)
PJP Pneumocystis jirovecii pneumonia, *CMV* cytomegalovirus, *BALF* bronchoalveolar lavage fluid, *TMP-SMZ* sulfamethoxazole and trimethoprim, *ICU* intensive care unit

[7–10], and the CMV infection is often related to the patient's non-specific immunosuppression. Although PJP is a relatively indolent process in HIV-infected patients, it is usually a potentially life-threatening infection among immunocompromised non-HIV patients. Thus, although there is no significant difference in mortality among HIV-infected patients with PJP according to their CMV infection status [7, 9, 13], we cannot extrapolate it to non-HIV counterparts.

In the present study, we observed that 54.3% of our non-HIV patients with PJP exhibited CMV co-infection, with subgroup analyses revealing co-infection rates of 31.5% among patients with kidney disease and 20% among patients with hematological malignancies who had not received hematopoietic stem cells (Table 1). Tark et al. attributed the different rates of CMV co-infection to the use of T-cell immunosuppressants, as they found that the use of these agents was significantly associated with CMV pneumonia [13]. Our findings support their conclusions, as CMV co-infection in the present study was significantly associated with the combined use of glucocorticoids and T-cell immunosuppressants (p = 0.02). We found the significant association between the use of T-cell immunosuppressants and the

Table 2 The laboratory test results according to pulmonary CMV infection status

	CMV-DNA positive in BALF	CMV-DNA negative in BALF	*p*
WBC count (10^9/L)	7.67 ± 3.56	10.16 ± 5.51	0.08
ALT elevation, n (%)	15(39.5%)	6(18.8%)	0.06
CRP, mg/L	31.1(0.21–266)	69.1(5.18–314)	0.24
LDH, IU/L	400(151–1167)	398(181–1918)	0.79
CD4 + T lymphocyte count,/ul	223.0 ± 171.6	319.4 ± 277.9	0.13
Neutrophils in BALF, %	33(0–96)	17(3–97)	0.41
Lymphocyte in BALF,%	17(0–76)	32(0–80)	0.12
Pulmonary co-infection, n (%)			
Bacteria	18 (47.4%)	10 (31.3%)	0.17
Fungus	12 (31.6%)	7 (21.9%)	0.36
PaO2/FiO2,n(%)			
PaO2/FiO2 > 300	8(21.1%)	11 (34.4%)	0.21
200 < PaO2/FiO2 ≤ 300	10 (26.3%)	9 (28.1%)	0.86
100 < PaO2/FiO2 ≤ 200	7 (18.4%)	8 (25.0%)	0.50
PaO2/FiO2 ≤ 100	13(34.2%)	4 (12.5%)	0.04

CMV cytomegalovirus, *BALF* bronchoalveolar lavage fluid, *WBC* white blood cell, *ALT* alanine aminotransferase, *CRP* C-reactive protein, *LDH* lactate dehydrogenase

morbidity among patients with PJP and CMV co-infection (p = 0.02). Therefore, it appears that the use of T-cell immunosuppressants may be a risk factor for CMV co-infection in PJP patients (odds ratio [OR]: 3.32,95% confidence interval [CI]: 1.19–9.29). Furthermore, a PaO_2/FiO_2 of ≤100 was significantly more common among patients with PJP and pulmonary CMV co-infection(p = 0.035), which suggests that this form of co-infection causes more severe lung injuries, compared to PJP alone, in non-HIV patients. Therefore, when non-HIV patients with PJP present with severe hypoxemia, the possibility of pulmonary CMV co-infection should be excluded.

The initial symptoms of PJP are non-specific and including fever, dyspnea, cough, and ground-glass opacities on chest CT. If it is left untreated, PJP it will quickly progress to respiratory failure, especially among non-HIV patients [17]. In the present study, dyspnea was significantly more common among patients with PJP and CMV co-infection, compared to PJP alone (p = 0.04, odds ratio [OR]: 2.84,95% confidence interval [CI]: 1.03–7.89). Besides, patients with PJP and pulmonary CMV co-infection are more likely to exhibit lower PaO_2/FiO_2.

Among non-HIV patients with immunosuppression, the radiographical evidence of CMV pneumonia typically includes poorly-defined ground-glass opacities, small nodules, the tree-in-bud pattern, and the halo sign during high-resolution computed tomography (HRCT). These findings are predominantly distributed in the middle and lower lung fields, while thickening of the bronchovascular bundles and pleural effusion arerare [18, 19]. However, ground-glass opacities with an apical-predominant distribution, the mosaic pattern, the crazy-paving pattern, and cystic changes are common HRCT findings in cases of PJP [20–22]. In the present study, we found that PJP and CMV co-infection was significantly associated with the presence of centrilobular nodules (p = 0.008,OR: 5.64, 95%CI: 1.45–21.95), which

Table 3 The patients' clinical and radiographic manifestations according to pulmonary CMV infection status

	CMV-DNA positive in BALF	CMV-DNA negative in BALF	*p*
Symptoms, n (%)			
fever	31 (81.6%)	28 (87.5%)	0.50
dyspnea	29 (76.3%)	17 (53.1%)	0.04
CT findings			
ground-glass opacities	38/38 (100.0%)	32/32 (100.0%)	1.00
consolidations	18/38 (47.4%)	15/32 (46.9%)	0.97
centrilobular nodules	14/38 (36.8%)	3/32 (9.4%)	0.008
upper lobe predominance	7/38 (18.4%)	8/32 (25.0%)	0.50

CMV cytomegalovirus, *BALF* bronchoalveolar lavage fluid, *CT* computed tomography

Table 4 The association between mortality and CMV DNA in bronchoalveolar lavage fluid

CMV-DNA load in BALF(copies/ml)	Prognosis		*p*
	survivor (n)	non-survivor(n)	
$\leq 1 \times 10^4$	10	3	0.012
$1 \times 10^4 \sim 1 \times 10^5$	6	2	
$\geq 1 \times 10^5$	5	12	

CMV cytomegalovirus, *BALF* bronchoalveolar lavage fluid

indicates that CMV pneumonia should be considered in the differential diagnosis of non-HIV patients with PJP who exhibit centrilobular nodules.

CMV infection may manifest as a primary infection, latent infection, reactivated infection, or reinfection. The most common form in the general population is a latent infection, and patients with a latent infection may transmit the infection to other individuals through their bodily fluids. In addition, latent infections typically have no clinical effects unless the host becomes immunocompromised. As with other herpes viruses, latent CMV can be reactivated during periods of stress, and especially in immunocompromised adults with a critical illness [23]. Nichols et al. has found that the human CMV reactivation is common in these cases due to the immunocompromised state of patients [24]. And Peres et al. has reported that monitoring the CMV reactivation and preemptive or prophylactic treatment are critical for these patients [25]. The emergence of rapid PCR detection methods has facilitated the accurate, rapid, and quantitative detection of CMV DNA in the patient's bodily fluids [26]. Furthermore, PCR can be used to detect CMV reactivation, although some researchers have reported that CMV reactivation could simply be an indicator of immunecompromise status and illness severity, and may not require diagnostic procedures and treatment [27]. Nevertheless, Yu et al. found that in the immunocompromised patients with rheumatic diseases can be diagnosed with CMV pneumonia based on serum CMV DNA loads of $>1.75 \times 10^4$copies/mL [28]. Moreover, Madi N et al. found in renal transplant patients with symptomatic CMV infection the CMV-DNA in serum were all more than 6.5×10^4copies/mL. While at present, only a few studies have evaluated a cut-off value for CMV-DNA in BALF [29, 30]. Drew et al. has reported that CMV DNA levels of $>5 \times 10^5$copies/mL in the patient's BALF confirmed the presence of CMV pneumonia [31], and Boeckh et al. found that CMV viral load > 500 IU/ml in BALF was likely to represent CMV pneumonia in hematopoietic stem cell transplantation patients [32]. Therefore, based on the absence of standardized CMV DNA assays, additional studies are needed to identify an accurate and reliable cut-off values for CMV DNA in BALF to identify CMV infection and pneumonia.

In our study, the 38 patients with pulmonary CMV co-infection received intravenous ganciclovir combined with anti-pneumocystis therapy, while the patients with only PJP received anti-pneumocystis treatment alone. There was no significant difference in mortality between these two groups ($p = 0.15$). There are two possible explanations for this phenomenon. Firstly, ganciclovirис is considered effective for CMV infection. Secondly, the pulmonary CMV infection that we detected may represent CMV reactivation, rather than CMV pneumonia. Besides, in our patients with CMV-DNA positive in BALF, only 30% were found CMV-DNA positive in their serum, which indicates that the BALF testing provided greater sensitivity. Furthermore, the BALF-positive serum-negative patients exhibited CMV DNA loads of $<1 \times 10^4$copies/mL, which indicates that we cannot exclude the possibilities of local inflammation and/or CMV reactivation. In this context, some researchers have classified CMV infection according to the BALF viral load, with low-level infections referring to a load of $<1 \times 10^4$copies/mL, moderate infections having a load between 1×10^4 to 1×10^5copies/mL, and serious infections with a load of $>1 \times 10^5$copies/mL [33]. Moreover, Bauer et al. has confirmed that higher levels of CMV DNA were detectable in infected tissues [34]. In the present study, we used the above-mentioned grading system to classify the patients' CMV infections and found that higher CMV DNA loads were significantly associated with mortality ($p = 0.012$). Therefore, timely antiviral treatment is likely needed to reduce the risk of mortality in cases that with high loads of CMV-DNA in their BALF.

There are several limitations to our study. First, patients with confirmed CMV infection require antiviral therapy, and patients without CMV infection do not require antiviral therapy, which makes it impossible to create a control group that is CMV-negative and receives antiviral therapy. This lack of a control group may limit our ability to conclusively comment on the association between CMV infection and prognosis. Second, BALF that is positive for CMVDNA could be attributed to latent infection, reactivation, or CMV pneumonia, and many of the patients exhibited severe hypoxemia, which precluded the use of lung biopsy to diagnose CMV pneumonia. Third, the small single-center sample of patients is prone to selection bias.

Conclusions

Our study indicates that pulmonary CMV co-infection was significantly associated with the combined use of glucocorticoids and T-cell immunosuppressants among non-HIV patients with PJP. In addition, CMV pneumonia must be considered when centrilobular nodules and severe hypoxemia are present in non-HIV patients with

PJP. Furthermore, high BALF loads of CMV DNA were positively associated with mortality, which indicates that antiviral treatment should be rapidly administered when these non-HIV patients exhibit PJP and CMV co-infection. Nevertheless, larger scale, well-designed prospective studies are needed to clarify the unanswered questions.

Abbreviations
BALF: Bronchoalveolar lavage fluid; CI: Confidence interval; CMV: Cytomegalovirus; CT: Computed tomography; HIV: Human immunodeficiency virus; HRCT: High-resolution computed tomography; OR: Odds ratio; PCR: Polymerase chain reaction; PJP: *Pneumocystis jirovecii* pneumonia

Acknowledgments
We thank our patients for their cooperation in this study.

Funding
None.

Authors' contributions
QY finished this manuscript, and had full access to all of the data in the study and takes responsibility for the integrity of the data and the accuracy of the data analysis. CLQ contributed substantially to the study's design, data analysis and interpretation, and modified of the manuscript. PJ and LS processed and stained the BALF specimens by using methenamine silver, and evaluated the presence of pneumocystis cysts. HZ evaluated the BALF loads of CMV DNA in the BALF and serum. All authors read and approved the final manuscript.

Competing interests
The authors declare that they have no competing interests.

Consent for publication
Not applicable.

Author details
[1]Department of Respiratory and Critical Care Medicine, Peking University First Hospital, Beijing 100034, China. [2]Department of Infectious Disease, Peking University First Hospital, Beijing 100034, China.

References

1. Thomas CF Jr, Limper AH. Pneumocystis pneumonia. N Engl J med. 2004;350(24):2487–98.
2. Roblot F, Godet C, Le Moal G, Garo B, Faouzi Souala M, Dary M, et al. Analysis of underlying diseases and prognosis factors associated with Pneumocystis carinii pneumonia in immunocompromised HIV-negative patients. Eur J Clin Microbiol Infect Dis. 2002;21(7):523–31.
3. Pagano L, Fianchi L, Mele L, Girmenia C, Offidani M, Ricci P, et al. Pneumocystis carinii pneumonia in patients with malignant haematological diseases: 10 years' experience of infection in GIMEMA centres. Br J Hematol. 2002;117(2):379–86.
4. Sepkowitz KA. Opportunistic infections in patients with and patients without acquired immunodeficiency syndrome. Clin Infect Dis. 2002;34(8):98–107.
5. Zahar JR, Robin M, Azoulay E, Fieux F, Nitenberg G, Schlemmer B. Pneumocystis carinii pneumonia in critically ill patients with malignancy: a descriptive study. Clin Infect Dis. 2002;35(8):929–34.
6. Salomon N, Perlman DC. Cytomegalovirus pneumonia. Semin Respir Infect. 1999;14(4):353–8.
7. Jacobson MA, Mills J, Rush J, Peiperl L, Seru V, Mohanty PK, et al. Morbidity and mortality of patients with AIDS and first-episode Pneumocystis carinii pneumonia unaffected by concomitant pulmonary cytomegalovirus infection. Am rev Respir Dis. 1991;144(1):6–9.
8. Miles PR, Baughman RP, Linnemann CC Jr. Cytomegalovirus in the bronchoalveolar lavage fluid of patients with AIDS. Chest. 1990;97(5):1072–6.
9. Bozzette SA, Arcia J, Bartok AE, McGlynn LM, McCutchan JA, Richman DD, et al. Impact of Pneumocystis carinii and cytomegalovirus on the course and outcome of atypical pneumonia in advanced human immunodeficiency virus disease. J Infect Dis. 1992;165(1):93–8.
10. Benfield TL, Helweg-Larsen J, Bang D, Junge J, Lundgren JD. Prognostic markers of short-term mortality in AIDS-associated Pneumocystis carinii pneumonia. Chest. 2001;119(3):844–51.
11. Angelici E, Contini C, Sebastiani G, Folgori F, Delia S, Serra P, et al. Cytomegalovirus in bronchoalveolar lavage specimens from patients with AIDS: comparison with antigenaemia and viraemia. J med Microbiol. 1996; 45(2):149–52.
12. Freeman RB Jr. The 'indirect' effects of cytomegalovirus infection. Am J Transplant. 2009;9(11):2453–8.
13. Kim T, Moon SM, Sung H, Kim MN, Kim SH, Chio SH, et al. Outcomes of non-HIV-infected patients with Pneumocystis pneumonia and concomitant pulmonary cytomegalovirus infection. Scand J Infect Dis. 2012;44(9):670–7.
14. Ewig S, Bauer T, Schneider C, Pickenhain A, Pizzulli L, Loos U, et al. Clinical characteristics and outcome of Pneumocystis carinii pneumonia in HIV-infected and otherwise immunosuppressed patients. Eur Respir J. 1995;8(9):1548–53.
15. Mansharamani NG, Garland R, Delaney D, Koziel H. Management and outcome patterns for adult Pneumocystis carinii pneumonia, 1985 to 1995: comparison of HIV-associated cases to other immunocompromised states. Chest. 2000;118(3):704–11.
16. Klech H, Pohl W. Technical recommendations and guidelines for bronchoalveolar lavage (BAL). Report of the European Society of Pneumology Task Group. Eur Respir J. 1989;2(6):561–585.
17. Ho M. Cytomegalovirus. In: Mandell GL, editor. Mandell, Douglas, and Benett's principles and practice of infectious disease (vol 2). 4th ed. New York: Churchill Livingstone; 1995. p. 1351–64.
18. Franquet T, Lee KS, Müller NL. Thin-section CT findings in 32 immunocompromised patients with cytomegalovirus pneumonia who do not have AIDS. AJR am J Roentgenol. 2003;181(4):1059–63.
19. Gasparetto EL, Ono SE, Escuissato D, Marchiori E, Roldan L, Marques HL, et al. Cytomegalovirus pneumonia after bone marrow transplantation: high resolution CT findings. Br J Radiol. 2004;77(921):724–7.
20. Webb WR, Müller NL, Naidich DP, editors. High-resolution CT of the lung. 3th ed. Philadelphia: Lippincott-Raven; 2001. p. 71–96.
21. Boiselle PM, Crans CA Jr, Kaplan MA. The changing face of Pneumocystis carinii pneumonia in AIDS patients. AJR am J Roentgenol. 1999;172(5):1301–9.
22. Kuhlman JE, Kavuru M, Fishman EK, Siegelman SS. Pneumocystis carinii pneumonia: spectrum of parenchymal CT findings. Radiology. 1990;175(3):711–4.
23. La Rosa C, Diamond DJ. The immune response to human CMV. Future Virol. 2012;7(3):279–93.
24. Nichols WG, Corey L, Gooley T, Davis C, Boeckh M. High risk of death due to bacterial and fungal infection among cytomegalovirus (CMV)-seronegative recipients of stem cell transplants from seropositive donors: evidence for indirect effects of primary CMV infection. J Infect Dis. 2002;185(3):272–82.
25. Peres RM, Costa CR, Andrade PD, Bonon SH, Albuquerque DM, de Oliveria C, et al. Surveillance of active human cytomegalovirus infection in hematopoietic stem cell transplantation (HLA sibling identical donor): search for optimal cutoff value by real-time PCR. BMC Infect Dis. 2010;10:147.
26. Cinel G, Pekcan S, Ozçelik U, Alp A, Yalçın E, Doğru Ersöz D, et al. Cytomegalovirus infection in immunocompetent wheezy infants: the diagnostic value of CMV PCR in bronchoalveolar lavage fluid. J Clin Pharm Ther. 2014;39(4):399–403.
27. Papazian L, Hraiech S, Lehingue S, Roch A, Chiche L, Wiramus S, et al. Cytomegalovirus reactivation in ICU patients. Intensive Care med. 2015;42(1):28–37.

28. Xue Y, Jiang L, Wan WG, Chen YM, Zhang J, Zhang ZC. Cytomegalovirus pneumonia in patients with rheumatic diseases after immunosuppressive therapy: a single center study in China. Chin med J. 2016;129(3):267–73.
29. Madi N, Al-Nakib W, Mustafa AS, Saeed T, Pacsa A, Nampoory MR. Detection and monitoring of cytomegalovirus infection in renal transplant patients by quantitative real-time PCR. Med Princ Pract. 2007;16(4):268–73.
30. Ljungman P, Boeckh M, Hirsch HH, Josephson F, Lundgren J, Nichols G, et al. Definitions of cytomegalovirus infection and disease in transplant patients for use in clinical trials. Clin Infect Dis. 2017;64(1):87–91.
31. Drew WL. Laboratory diagnosis of cytomegalovirus infection and disease in immunocompromised patients. Curr Opin Infect Dis. 2007;20(4):408–11.
32. Boeckh M, Stevens-Ayers T, Travi G, Huang ML, Cheng GS, Xie H, et al. Cytomegalovirus (CMV) DNA quantitation in bronchoalveolar lavage fluid from hematopoietic stem cell transplant recipients with CMV pneumonia. J Infect Dis 2017. doi: 10.1093/infdis/jix048. [Epub ahead of print].
33. Zhai WJ, Wei JL, Zhao MF, Wang M, Zhou Z, Liu P, et al. Comparison between CMV quantitative PCR and CMV-pp65 antigen test for detection of CMV infection in allogeneic hematopoietic stem cell transplantation. Zhong Guo Shi Yan Xue ye Xue Za Zhi. 2009;17(6):1522–6.
34. Bauer CC, Jaksch P, Aberle SW, Haber H, Lang G, Klepetko W, et al. Relationship between cytomegalovirus DNA load in epithelial lining fluid and plasma of lung transplant recipients and analysis of coinfection with Epstein-Barr virus and human herpesvirus 6 in the lung compartment. J Clin Microbiol. 2007;45(2):324–8.

Persistent adenovirus B3 infections associated with bronchiolitis obliterans treated with cidofovir in a child with mosaic tetrasomy 9p

Rhiannon Ions[1], Manjith Narayanan[1,2], Michael Browning[3], Erol A. Gaillard[1,2], Gary Stiefel[1] and Julian W. Tang[2,4*]

Abstract

Background: Adenoviruses (AdV) are non-enveloped, double-stranded DNA viruses with multiple serotypes, which cause a variety of end-organ disease in both immunocompetent and immunocompromised individuals. Some adenoviruses can become latent in the mucosa-associated lymphoid tissue (e.g. adenoids and tonsils), with the potential to reactivate sporadically, leading to upper or lower respiratory tract infection and disease. Bronchiolitis Obliterans (BO) is a rare chronic lung disorder which usually follows a severe insult to the respiratory tract. In children, it is a complication of severe infections (as post-infectious BO), typically manifesting after a severe respiratory infection, in previously healthy pre-school children. Symptoms and signs of air trapping (hyperinflated chest, expiratory wheeze) with persistent oxygen requirement are characteristic. The presence of the unusual mosaic tetrasomy 9p genotype in this case, despite standard cidofovir therapy for persistent or chronic adenovirus infection, may have impacted on the child's long-term clinical outcomes.

Case presentation: We present a case of persistent AdV B3 infection in a 14-month old boy with mosaic tetrasomy 9p, which persisted for 10 weeks, resulting in radiologically-confirmed BO, requiring cidofovir to control the persistent AdV B3 infection and standard therapy with pulsed steroids. We argue that in the presence of the mosaic tetrasomy 9p, earlier antiviral therapy may have decreased the severity of BO, as this mutation is known to be associated with some degree of immune dysregulation.

Conclusions: Adenovirus infections are common in children and may persist as latent infections, with subsequent reactivations during loss of immune control, related to systemic illness arising from other causes. In chronic, reactivated AdV infection with pneumonia, BO is a recognised complication. However, in this case, with the presence of the mosaic tetrasomy 9p mutation, earlier antiviral therapy may have reduced such longer term complications, due to the immune dysregulatory nature of this mutation.

Keywords: Case report, Adenovirus, Bronchiolitis obliterans, Mosaic tetrasomy 9p, Immune dysregulation, Cidofovir

* Correspondence: julian.tang@uhl-tr.nhs.uk
[2]Infection, Immunity and Inflammation, University of Leicester, Leicester, UK
[4]Clinical Microbiology and Virology, University Hospitals of Leicester NHS Trust, Level 5 Sandringham Building, Leicester Royal Infirmary, Infirmary Square, Leicester LE1 5WW, UK
Full list of author information is available at the end of the article

Background

Adenoviruses (AdV) are non-enveloped, double-stranded DNA viruses with multiple serotypes, which cause a variety of end-organ disease in both immunocompetent and immunocompromised individuals [1, 2]. There is growing evidence that some adenoviruses can become latent in the mucosa-associated lymphoid tissue (e.g. adenoids and tonsils), with the potential to reactivating sporadically, leading to upper or lower respiratory tract infection and disease [2, 3].

Bronchiolitis Obliterans (BO) is a rare chronic lung disorder which usually follows a severe insult to the respiratory tract [4–8]. In children, it is a common sequel of severe infections, often termed as post-infectious BO. The natural history of this condition is persistence of chronic respiratory symptoms for longer than 4–8 weeks following an acute severe respiratory infection, in children who were previously healthy. Though this can happen at any age, the incidence is highest in infancy/pre-school children. Symptoms and signs of air trapping (hyperinflated chest, expiratory wheeze) and persistent oxygen requirement are typical features.

Mosaic tetrasomy 9p is a rare somatic mutation that has been known about for the past 20 years [9, 10]. It manifests clinically with various congenital abnormalities, including severe intellectual impairment and delayed growth and dysmorphic features (e.g. hypertelorism, ear abnormalities, microretrognathia, bulbous nose, microcephaly, growth retardation, joint dislocation and scoliosis). Genetically, it is due to the presence of an additional chromosome that incorporates two copies of the 9p arm in either an isodicentric or pseudodicentric manner. In patients living with this genotype, the two forms are usually present in a mosaic state, hence the term mosaic tetrasomy 9p [11]. More recently, it has been associated with some degree of immune dysregulation [12], which may demonstrate a potential to impact on host responses to infections, though no specific immunodeficiency syndrome has yet been linked to this mutation [13].

We present a case of persistent AdV B3 infection in an infant with mosaic tetrasomy 9p, which persisted for 10 weeks, resulting in BO, requiring treatment with steroids and cidofovir, to control the persisting AdV B3 infection. We suggest that, in the presence of the mosaic tetrasomy 9p mutation, that earlier antiviral therapy may have decreased the onset and severity of the BO.

Case presentation

A 14-month old boy presented with respiratory distress, wheeze and hypoxia. This was preceded by 24 h of coryza, fever and reduced feeding. He was admitted directly to intensive care, where he was diagnosed with pneumonia. Treatment was started with empirical antibiotics. He was intubated and ventilated for 4 days, after which he was extubated and stepped down to high dependency unit (HDU) on continuous positive airways pressure (CPAP) ventilation. He continued to have persistently increased work of breathing, persistent expiratory wheeze and symptoms and signs of air trapping.

Though he did not progress to respiratory failure, weight gain and oxygenation was achieved only by initiation of Heated Humidified High Flow Nasal cannula therapy (HHHFNC).

Polymerase chain reaction (PCR) testing of nasopharyngeal aspirates (NPAs) revealed the persistence of rhinovirus and adenovirus for 10 weeks in both NPAs and bronchoalveolar lavages (BALs), with parainfluenza type 3 found in just one NPA sample. Adenovirus was also found in blood by PCR testing. Rhinovirus is not normally tested for in blood samples and there was no validated assay available for this. One BAL and one urine sample were screened for cytomegalovirus (CMV) by PCR also, and found to be negative. One stool sample was tested and found to be negative for rotavirus and adenovirus (despite the persistence of adenovirus in the respiratory samples at this time).

There was no significant family history of any genetic diseases and the patient was born at term. Mum is a smoker but states that she did not smoke during her pregnancy. During pregnancy, intrauterine growth restriction was identified. At the time of admission his weight was < 0.4th centile, but this was increasing. His parents report poor feeding since birth and an increased work of breathing from 5 months old. He is known to the allergy services for severe eczema and faltering weight, and has been diagnosed with cow's milk protein allergy. His eczema medications have included topical tacrolimus, moderately potent topical steroids and emollient therapy.

His other medical history includes two previous episodes of bronchiolitis, three and 1 month prior to this admission (including one overnight stay during a trip to Australia). Prior to admission, he had only received two courses of antibiotics in his life – once for an infected BCG vaccine site and once for an ear infection.

During his inpatient stay, he had 2 further intercurrent bacterial respiratory infections, treated by broad spectrum antibiotics. Immunological investigations revealed an IgG and IgM hypogammaglobunemia but a normal IgA. He was up-to-date with his childhood immunisations prior to admission, but has had a poor response to tetanus and twice to haemophilus B, demonstrated by low IgG levels to both. He was also found to have near absent B-cells and a reduced number of T-cells, and prophylaxis for *Pneumocystis jiroveci* was commenced. HIV testing was negative on two occasions. We withheld any further live virus vaccinations, in view of his immunodeficiency (Table 1, Fig. 1).

Table 1 Immunological results at presentation

Serology	Patient results	Age-related normal range
IgG	1.8 g/L	3.0–9.0
IgA	0.33 g/L	0.20–0.70
IgM	0.42 g/L	0.60–2.1
Anti-tetanus toxoid	0.03 IU/ml	> 0.15 (protective level)
Anti-Haemophilus type B	< 0.11 mg/L	> 1.0 (protective level)
Lymphocyte subsets		
Absolute lymphocyte count	1.04×10^9/L	3.4–9.0
CD3+ (T cells)	0.95×10^9/L	1.90–5.9
CD3 + CD4+ (helper T)	0.74×10^9/L	1.40–4.3
CD3 + CD8+ (cytotoxic T)	0.20×10^9/L	0.50–1.70
CD16 + CD56+ (NK cells)	0.03×10^9/L	0.16–0.95
CD19+ (B cells)	0.01×10^9/L	0.61–2.60

At this stage, a CT chest was performed (Fig. 2). The findings (mosaic pattern attenuation of both lung fields with a combination of air trapping and oligaemia, more pronounced in expiratory images) were consistent with BO which was believed to be secondary to the persistent adenovirus rather than the rhinovirus infection. Reasons for this were mainly that rhinoviruses are predominantly upper respiratory tract infections, whereas AdVs can cause more systemic infections and AdV DNA was detected in the blood. No biopsy or histopathological investigation was performed in order to confirm BO.

A flexible bronchoscopy showed structurally normal airways. Screening for tuberculosis was negative.

After a multidisciplinary team discussion, it was decided to commence pulse methyl-prednisolone therapy (3 daily doses of 10 mg/kg given every month) and long-term azithromycin (10 mg/kg 3 doses every week) for management of BO. Prior to commencing the steroids, cidofovir was administered to control the adenovirus replication and reduce the dissemination of the adenovirus.

Cidofovir (5 mg/kg, intravenously, with probenecid) was given on fortnightly basis for 4 months, during which he his renal function was monitored weekly. All the patient's renal function test results remained within our institutional laboratory's normal ranges (sodium 133–146 mmol/L; potassium 3.5–5.0 mmol/L; urea 1.5–5.0 mmol/L; creatinine 15–31 μmol/L) throughout the treatment period with cidofovir, indicating good tolerance to the drug. Since commencing steroid therapy, it was possible to gradually wean him off his HHHFNC, and he has since been thriving well. He was discharged on supplemental oxygen, which was weaned off over the next 12 months.

An array comparative genomic hybridisation (CGH) revealed mosaic tetrasomy of short arm of chromosome 9. There are no reports yet of immunodeficiency in association with mosaic tetrasomy 9p, nor any specific vulnerability to any particular viral infections [13], but has previously been associated with auto-immune conditions associated with IFN-1 dysregulation (predisposing to inflammatory myositis and lupus-like syndrome) [12].

A conclusive diagnosis of a specific immunodeficiency/immunomodulation is yet to be made in this case, as this profile does not fit any primary immune deficiency. Molecular genetic testing for mutations in 82 genes associated with primary immunodeficiency and gastrointestinal disorders (TIGER panel, Great Ormond Street Hospital, London) did not identify any clearly pathogenic variants. The patient is currently being given weekly supplemental immunoglobulins.

Most recently, the child has now cleared the long-term rhinovirus and adenovirus infections, and has been weaned off steroids and long term oxygen therapy. His weight gain has been adequate on air, and he is still too young for spirometry testing. Ongoing problems

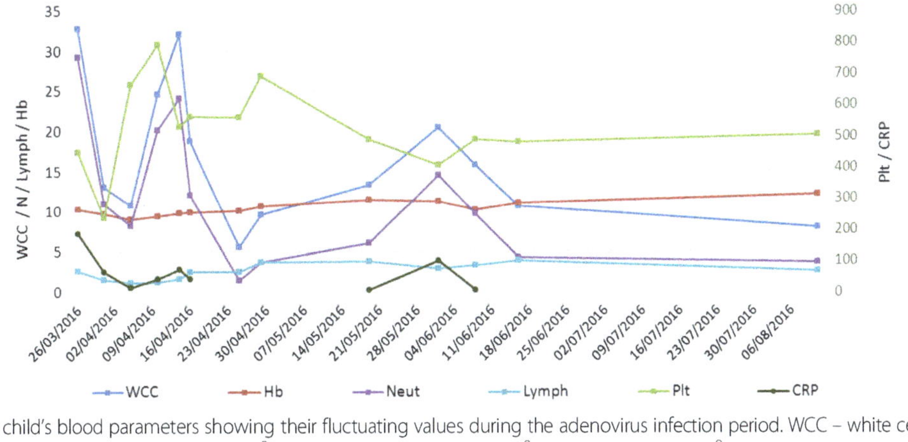

Fig. 1 Plots of the child's blood parameters showing their fluctuating values during the adenovirus infection period. WCC – white cell count ($\times 10^9$/L); Hb – haemoglobin (g/dL); Neut – neutrophils ($\times 10^9$/L); Lymph – lymphocytes ($\times 10^9$/L); Plt – platelets ($\times 10^9$/L); CRP – C-reactive protein (mg/L)

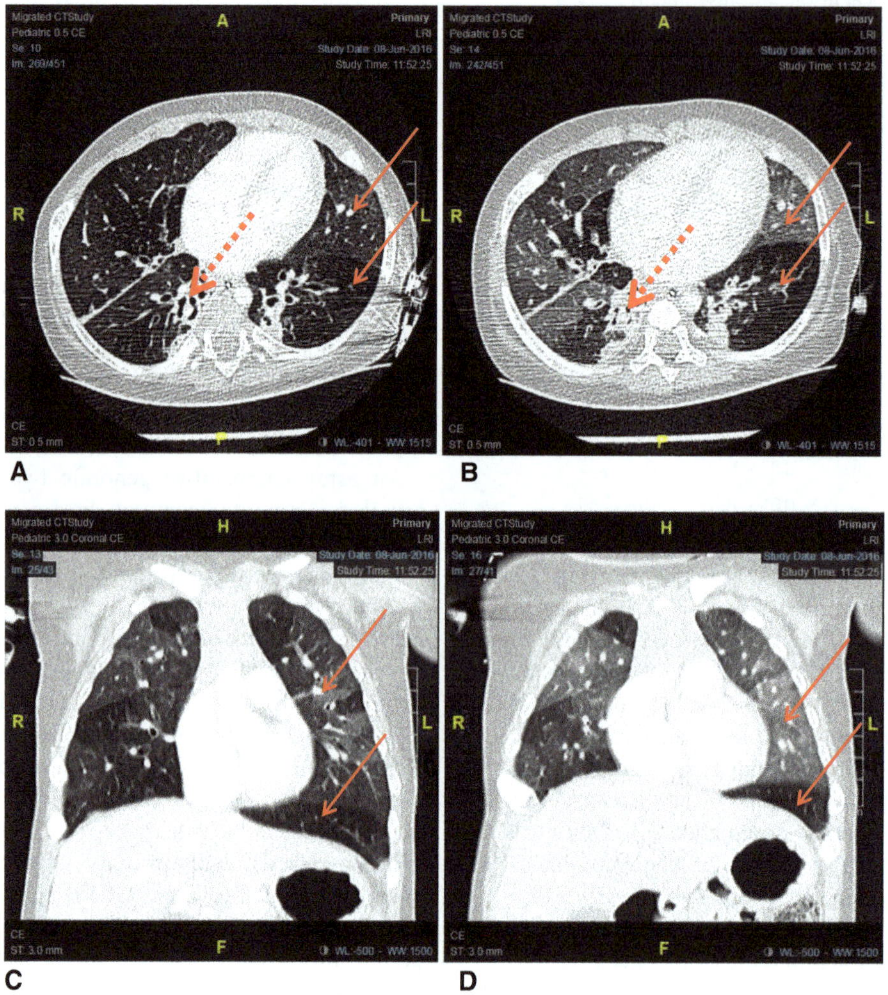

Fig. 2 a Inspiratory cross-sectional; **b** Expiratory cross-sectional; **c** Inspiratory coronal; **d** Expiratory coronal. Areas of hypo- and hyper-attenuation (thin arrows), which are more evident on expiratory scans, showing mosaic perfusion. Traction bronchiectasis is also shown (thick dotted arrows). The images show features recognised to be associated with bronchiolitis obliterans, including: mosaic perfusion, air trapping, vascular attenuation, bronchiectasis and peribronchial thickening, as seen in the mosaic pattern of attenuation of both lung fields

include recent *Pseudomonas aeruginosa* infection, with a wet cough, which is likely due to the bronchiectasis component of the BO disease.

Discussion and conclusion

This case demonstrates the long-term shedding (for 10 weeks) of rhinovirus and Adv B3, as detectable by the PCR testing of respiratory secretions, in a young boy who developed post-adenoviral bronchiolitis obliterans on the background of a potential, as yet undefined, immunodeficiency and chromosomal anomaly (mosaic tetrasomy 9p).

It is likely that chronic AdV B3 infection contributed to persistent inflammation which may have contributed to the development of BO. This may have been further exacerbated by a dysregulated IFN-1 response, which has been described previously in association with tetrasomy 9p [12]. The relatively benign course and response to steroid therapy suggests a mild disease, and it is possible that cidofovir therapy acted as a disease modifying agent by reducing the viral load and associated immune stimulus during the active inflammation phase.

Adenovirus B3 is well-recognised to cause respiratory infections, particularly in children [1, 2, 4]. Persistent adenovirus infections with latency in children have been described [2, 3]. Post-infective BO is an uncommon complication of adenoviral infection [4–8].

In particular, Chung et al. [4] describe nine severe cases of adenovirus infection, all of whom had severe symptoms – similar to the case described here. Of these nine cases, one died and five of the survivors went on to develop BO. None of these patients appeared to have been treated with cidofovir or other antiviral drugs. In a case control study of 109 consecutive cases from Argentina with BO (compared against a control population of bronchiolitis without BO), Colom et al. [8] suggested a link between severity of bronchiolitis and progression to BO. The odds ratio of children on mechanical ventilation with bronchiolitis who then went on to develop BO was 11 on multivariate regression analysis.

The general consensus among pediatric pulmonologists is that lung biopsy is now not usually required for the diagnosis of post-infectious BO [14], with chest HRCT being the preferred investigation, currently [15].

Cidofovir is an antiviral used against DNA viruses – particularly human herpesviruses and adenoviruses. It acts by binding irreversibly to the viral DNA polymerase, as a false substrate, inhibiting viral replication, and is therefore virostatic not virucidal by this mechanism of action. It is given intravenously, and needs to be given with probenecid to reduce its nephrotoxicity. Adverse effects include mainly nephrotoxicity, but also nausea and vomiting, headache, neutropenia, hair loss, eye problems (uveitis, iritis) – and more rarely deranged liver function and anemia. Although there have been no formal clinical trials of cidofovir or its related lipid-soluble form (Brincidofovir), numerous case reports/series and reviews have supported its use in transplant/immunosuppressed paediatric patients with adenovirus infections [16–21].

It is possible that cidofovir therapy can mitigate the progression to bronchiolitis obliterans by reducing the viral load. As far as we are aware cidofovir therapy has not been reported, specifically, to decrease risk of BO in children with severe adenoviral lung infection. However, since cidofovir is well-known to reduce the viral load of AdV in AdV-infected immunocompromised children [19], it is not unreasonable to propose that earlier treatment with cidofovir, in a patient with some immune dysregulation resulting from the presence of the mosaic tetrasomy 9p mutations, should reduce onset and severity of adenoviral infection and the risk of developing BO.

Adenovirus infections are common in children and may persist as latent infections, with subsequent reactivations during loss of immune control, related to systemic illness arising from other causes. In chronic, reactivated AdV infection with pneumonia, teams should be aware that BO is one of the possible complications. In the presence of somatic host mutations that may give rise to some immune dysregulation, like mosaic tetrasomy 9p, earlier treatment chronic AdV infections with antiviral drugs may reduce this risk. Further studies would be useful, but may be difficult with such rare genetic mutations.

Abbreviations

AdV: Adenovirus; BAL: Bronchoalveolar lavage; BO: Bronchiolitis obliterans; CGH: Comparative genomic hybridisation; CPAP: Continuous positive airways pressure; CT: Computed tomography; HDU: High dependency unit; HHHFNC: Heated Humidified High Flow Nasal cannula therapy; NPA: Nasopharyngeal aspirate; PCR: Polymerase chain reaction

Acknowledgements
None

Funding
No funding was required for the writing of this case report.

Authors' contributions

RI, MN, EAG, GS – participated in the clinical care of the patient on the ward or in clinic. MB, JWT – supervised the immunological (MB) and virological (JWT) laboratory testing, interpretation and reporting, and advised on related clinical management. RI – wrote the first draft of the paper, which was further edited for content, style and accuracy by MN, MB, EAG, GS and JWT. All authors critically reviewed the manuscript for publication. All authors have read and approved the final version of this manuscript.

Consent for publication

Written consent to publish this case report and any accompanying images has been obtained from the patient's parents.

Competing interests

JWT is one of the Virology Section Editors for the journal. The other authors declare that they have no competing interests.

Author details
[1]Children's Hospital, University Hospitals of Leicester, NHS Trust, Leicester, UK. [2]Infection, Immunity and Inflammation, University of Leicester, Leicester, UK. [3]Immunology, University Hospitals of Leicester, NHS Trust, Leicester, UK. [4]Clinical Microbiology and Virology, University Hospitals of Leicester NHS Trust, Level 5 Sandringham Building, Leicester Royal Infirmary, Infirmary Square, Leicester LE1 5WW, UK.

References

1. James L, Vernon MO, Jones RC, Stewart A, Lu X, Zollar LM, et al. Outbreak of human adenovirus type 3 infection in a pediatric long-term care facility--Illinois, 2005. Clin Infect Dis. 2007;45:416–20.
2. Kalu SU, Loeffelholz M, Beck E, Patel JA, Revai K, Fan J, et al. Persistence of adenovirus nucleic acids in nasopharyngeal secretions: a diagnostic conundrum. Pediatr Infect Dis J. 2010;29:746–50.
3. Garnett CT, Talekar G, Mahr JA, Huang W, Zhang Y, Ornelles DA, et al. Latent species C adenoviruses in human tonsil tissues. J Virol. 2009;83:2417–28.
4. Chuang Yu CCH, Wong KS, Huang JG, Huang YC, Chang LY, et al. Severe adenovirus infection in children. J Microbiol Immunol Infect. 2003;36:37–40.
5. Jeon JS, Yi HA, Ki SY, Jeong SW, Uh ST, Jin SY, et al. A case of bronchiolitis obliterans organizing pneumonia associated with adenovirus. Korean J Intern Med. 1997;12:70–4.
6. de Blic J, Deschildre A, Chinet T. [Post-infectious bronchiolitis obliterans]. Rev Mal Respir 2013;30:152–160. [Article in French].
7. Li YN, Liu L, Qiao HM, Cheng H, Cheng HJ. Post-infectious bronchiolitis obliterans in children: a review of 42 cases. BMC Pediatr. 2014;14:238.
8. Colom AJ, Teper AM, Vollmer WM, Diette GB. Risk factors for the development of bronchiolitis obliterans in children with bronchiolitis. Thorax. 2006;61:503–6.

9. Stumm M, Tönnies H, Mandon U, Götze A, Krebs P, Wieacker PF. Mosaic tetrasomy 9p in a girl with multiple congenital anomalies: cytogenetic and molecular-cytogenetic studies. Eur J Pediatr. 1999;158:571–5.
10. Eggermann T, Rossier E, Theurer-Mainka U, Backsch C, Klein-Vogler U, Enders H, et al. New case of mosaic tetrasomy 9p with additional neurometabolic findings. Am J Med Genet. 1998;75:530–3.
11. El Khattabi L, Jaillard S, Andrieux J, Pasquier L, Perrin L, Capri Y, et al. Clinical and molecular delineation of Tetrasomy 9p syndrome: report of 12 new cases and literature review. Am J Med Genet A. 2015;167:1252–61.
12. Frémond ML, Gitiaux C, Bonnet D, Guiddir T, Crow YJ, de Pontual L, et al. Mosaic Tetrasomy 9p: a Mendelian condition associated with pediatric-onset overlap myositis. Pediatrics. 2015;136:e544–7.
13. Genetic and Rare Diseases Information Centre (GARD). Tetrasomy 9p. https://rarediseases.info.nih.gov/diseases/42/tetrasomy-9p. Accessed 14 Jun 2018.
14. Chang AB, Masel JP, Masters B. Post-infectious bronchiolitis obliterans: clinical, radiological and pulmonary function sequelae. Pediatr Radiol. 1998; 28(1):23–9.
15. Champs NS, Lasmar LM, Camargos PA, Marguet C, Fischer GB, Mocelin HT. Post-infectious bronchiolitis obliterans in children. J Pediatr (Rio J). 2011; 87(3):187–98.
16. Carter BA, Karpen SJ, Quiros-Tejeira RE, Chang IF, Clark BS, Demmler GJ, et al. Intravenous Cidofovir therapy for disseminated adenovirus in a pediatric liver transplant recipient. Transplantation. 2002;74:1050–2.
17. Neofytos D, Ojha A, Mookerjee B, Wagner J, Filicko J, Ferber A, et al. Treatment of adenovirus disease in stem cell transplant recipients with cidofovir. Biol Blood Marrow Transplant. 2007;13:74–81.
18. Lindemans CA, Leen AM, Boelens JJ. How I treat adenovirus in hematopoietic stem cell transplant recipients. Blood. 2010;116:5476–85.
19. Matthes-Martin S, Feuchtinger T, Shaw PJ, Engelhard D, Hirsch HH, Cordonnier C, et al. European guidelines for diagnosis and treatment of adenovirus infection in leukemia and stem cell transplantation: summary of ECIL-4 (2011). Transpl Infect Dis. 2012;14:555–63.
20. Lopez SMC, Michaels MG, Green M. Adenovirus infection in pediatric transplant recipients: are effective antiviral agents coming our way? Curr Opin Organ Transplant. 2018;23:395–9.
21. Yusuf U, Hale GA, Carr J, Gu Z, Benaim E, Woodard P, et al. Cidofovir for the treatment of adenoviral infection in pediatric hematopoietic stem cell transplant patients. Transplantation. 2006;81:1398–404.

8

Assessing the impact of antiretroviral therapy on tuberculosis notification rates among people with HIV: a descriptive analysis of 23 countries in sub-Saharan Africa, 2010–2015

Diya Surie[1*], Martien W. Borgdorff[2], Kevin P. Cain[3], Eleanor S. Click[1], Kevin M. DeCock[4] and Courtney M. Yuen[5,6]

Abstract

Background: HIV is a major driver of the tuberculosis epidemic in sub-Saharan Africa. The population-level impact of antiretroviral therapy (ART) scale-up on tuberculosis rates in this region has not been well studied. We conducted a descriptive analysis to examine evidence of population-level effect of ART on tuberculosis by comparing trends in estimated tuberculosis notification rates, by HIV status, for countries in sub-Saharan Africa.

Methods: We estimated annual tuberculosis notification rates, stratified by HIV status during 2010–2015 using data from WHO, the Joint United Nations Programme on HIV/AIDS, and the United Nations Population Division. Countries were included in this analysis if they had ≥4 years of HIV prevalence estimates and ≥ 75% of tuberculosis patients with known HIV status. We compared tuberculosis notification rates among people living with HIV (PLHIV) and people without HIV via Wilcoxon rank sum test.

Results: Among 23 included countries, the median annual average change in tuberculosis notification rates among PLHIV during 2010–2015 was -5.7% (IQR -6.9 to -1.7%), compared to a median change of -2.3% (IQR -4.2 to -0.1%) among people without HIV (p-value = 0.0099). Among 11 countries with higher ART coverage, the median annual average change in TB notification rates among PLHIV was -6.8% (IQR -7.6 to -5.7%) compared to a median change of -2.1% (IQR -6.0 to 0.7%) for PLHIV in 12 countries with lower ART coverage (p = 0.0106).

Conclusion: Tuberculosis notification rates declined more among PLHIV than people without HIV, and have declined more in countries with higher ART coverage. These results are consistent with a population-level effect of ART on decreasing TB incidence among PLHIV. To further reduce TB incidence among PLHIV, additional scale-up of ART as well as greater use of isoniazid preventive therapy and active case-finding will be necessary.

Keywords: Tuberculosis, HIV infections, Incidence, Epidemics, Africa, Risk factors

* Correspondence: dsurie@cdc.gov
[1]Division of Global HIV and TB, Centers for Disease Control and Prevention, Atlanta, GA, USA
Full list of author information is available at the end of the article

Background

Human immunodeficiency virus (HIV) infection is the most powerful known risk factor for tuberculosis (TB). HIV increases both the risk of reactivation of latent TB infection and the risk of rapid progression to active TB disease [1–4]. At the population level, the increased risk of TB among people living with HIV (PLHIV) has resulted in the resurgence of TB epidemics worldwide [5, 6]. Nowhere has this convergence of epidemics been more pronounced than in sub-Saharan Africa where HIV remains a major driver of the TB epidemic [7–9]. While only 10% of 10.4 million new TB cases reported worldwide in 2016 were among PLHIV, almost three quarters of these cases occurred in sub-Saharan Africa [9]. Successful TB control in this region requires addressing the disproportionate burden of TB among PLHIV.

In the last decade, the use of antiretroviral therapy (ART) in sub-Saharan Africa has greatly increased [10]. By helping to restore the immune system, ART has been shown to have a substantial effect on preventing TB in PLHIV [11–14]. In a meta-analysis of 11 studies, participants receiving ART had a 65% reduction in the development of TB compared to participants receiving no ART, regardless of their baseline CD4 count [11]. Given its proven individual-level effect, one would expect that the expansion of ART coverage would lead to the population-effect of declining TB incidence among PLHIV. Indeed, in Kenya, South Africa, and Malawi, TB notification rates among people with HIV are estimated to have declined substantially more than TB notification rates among people without HIV, concurrent with the expansion of ART coverage [15–18]. However, the extent to which this is true across the sub-Saharan African region is unclear.

To examine whether there is evidence of a population-level effect of ART on TB across sub-Saharan Africa, we estimated TB case notification rates stratified by HIV status for countries in the WHO African region. We then sought to compare trends in case notification rates among PLHIV and people without HIV, assessing both in the context of changing ART coverage.

Methods

Data sources

We estimated TB case notification rates stratified by HIV status using several existing, publicly available data sources. We obtained the number of total notified TB cases in each country, the number with HIV test results, and the number with positive HIV test results, by year, from WHO [19]. We obtained HIV prevalence estimates among adults aged 15–49 years, by year, from the Joint United Nations Programme on HIV/AIDS (UNAIDS) [20], and population estimates among adults aged 15–49 years, by year, from the United Nations Population Division (UNPD) [21].

To describe trends in ART coverage, we obtained ART coverage estimates, by year, from UNAIDS [22]. Coverage is defined as the percentage of all adults and children living with HIV who are currently receiving ART [23]. At the time of publication, ART coverage estimates from UNAIDS were available from 2010 onwards, and population estimates from UNDP were available through 2015; the period of our analysis was therefore from 2010 through 2015.

Inclusion and exclusion criteria

All 47 countries in the WHO African region were considered for this analysis. We considered data quality for each country and each year to determine inclusion. A year of data was considered to be of adequate quality if an HIV prevalence estimate was available and if ≥75% of notified TB cases had been tested for HIV. Any country with <4 years of data meeting these criteria was excluded from analysis. After estimating HIV-stratified TB notification rates, we excluded countries that showed greater than 50% year-to-year variation in the estimated notification rates, suggesting either data quality issues or too few patients with TB to make rate calculations meaningful.

Estimating TB notification rates stratified by HIV status

To estimate TB notifications among PLHIV, we estimated a numerator based on TB notifications and a denominator based on population-level HIV-prevalence estimates (Fig. 1a). For the numerator, we estimated the annual number of notified TB cases in PLHIV in a country in a given year by multiplying the number of total notified TB cases in the country by the proportion of TB cases with an HIV-positive test result. We therefore assumed that TB cases who did not receive an HIV test had an equal likelihood of being HIV-positive as those who did; we believe this assumption to be reasonable for the countries included in our analysis given that routine HIV testing for TB patients has been recommended since 2004 [24] and that we only included countries where ≥75% of TB patients had been tested. We used aggregate TB case notifications instead of age-stratified TB case notifications due to inconsistencies in the age-stratified data. For the denominator, we calculated the number of PLHIV in each country by multiplying UNAIDS HIV prevalence estimates among adults aged 15–49 years by the UNPD population estimate for this age group. We restricted this population denominator to adults aged 15–49 years, as the HIV prevalence estimates are more robust for this age group than for children or older adults. To address the mismatch between the age groups in the numerator and denominator, we

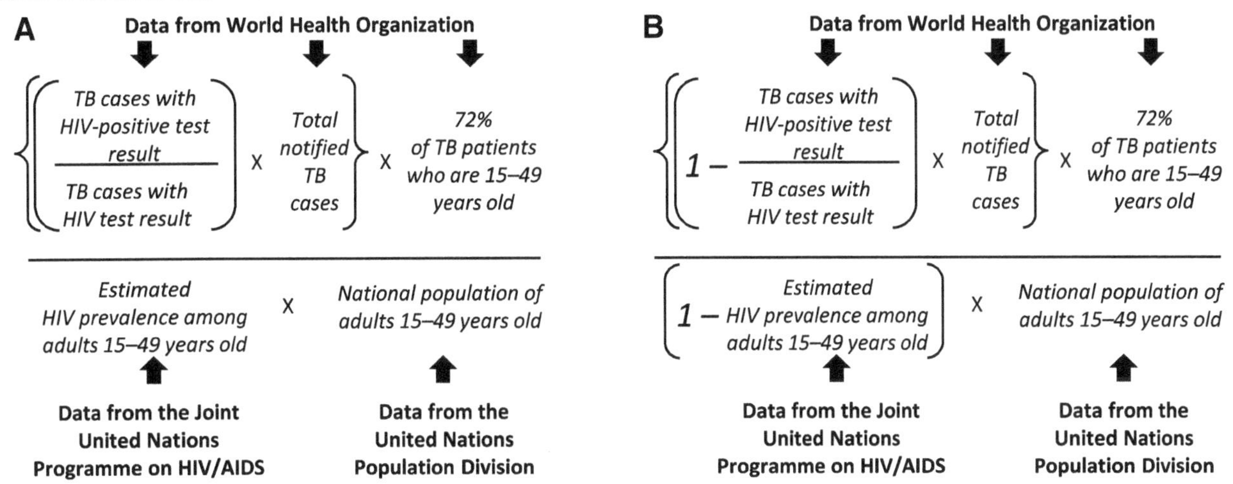

Fig. 1 a and **b** Calculation of estimated annual TB notification rates for (**a**) people living with HIV and (**b**) people without HIV

multiplied the numerator by the median average proportion of notified TB cases that were aged 15–49 years old among 19 countries in which the sum of all reported TB cases with a known age was ≥90% of all reported TB during 2010–2015 (median: 72%, interquartile range [IQR]: 69–75%).

A similar process was used to estimate TB notification rates among people without HIV (Fig. 1b). We subtracted the calculated TB/HIV cases from total notified TB cases to obtain the numerator, multiplying by 72% to correct for the mismatch in age groups between numerator and denominator. We subtracted the population of adults 15–49 years old with HIV from the total population in this age group to form the denominator.

Trends in TB notification rates

To describe trends in TB notification rates during 2010–2015, we calculated for each country the average annual percent change in TB notification rate among PLHIV and the average annual percent change in TB notification rate among people without HIV. These calculations were based on the corresponding 2010 and 2015 notification rates and assumed a constant annual percent change during this period. That is:

$$N = M \times (1 + A)^4$$

Where:
N = case notification rate in 2015
M = case notification rate in 2010
A = average annual percent change in case notification rate

For countries that lacked data for either 2010 or 2015, we performed an analogous calculation using notification rates for the terminal years of the date range.

Because of the potential error introduced by the assumptions we made in estimating TB case notification rates stratified by HIV status, we focused our analysis on assessment of trends over time, reasoning that even if the estimates for a country were inaccurate in a systematic way, the relationship between estimates in different years would remain robust. We used the Wilcoxon rank sum test with exact *p*-values to compare whether average annual changes in TB notification rates among PLHIV were significantly different from average annual changes in TB notification rates among people without HIV across all countries. To determine whether declines in TB notification rates among PLHIV were greater in countries with higher ART coverage, we compared the countries with greater-than-average ART coverage to those with lower-than-average ART coverage using the Wilcoxon rank sum test. The same comparison was made for declines in TB notification rates among people without HIV. Data were analyzed using SAS version 9.3 (SAS Institute, Cary, NC).

Results

Countries included in analysis

Of 47 countries in the WHO African region, 23 (49%) met inclusion criteria (Figs. 2 and 3) with 156 individual years of data included across the 23 included countries. In 2010, the median HIV prevalence in these countries was 5.6% (IQR 1.9–14.2%) and median WHO estimated TB incidence was 219 cases per 100,000 population (IQR 133–633 cases per 100,000 population; Table 1). In 2010, the median ART coverage was 26% (IQR 16–33%). From 2010 to 2015, the median absolute increase in ART coverage, defined as the difference between ART coverage in 2015 and ART coverage in 2010, was 25% (IQR 16–31%). Across all 156 years of included data, the median HIV testing coverage among TB cases was 96% (IQR 90–99%).

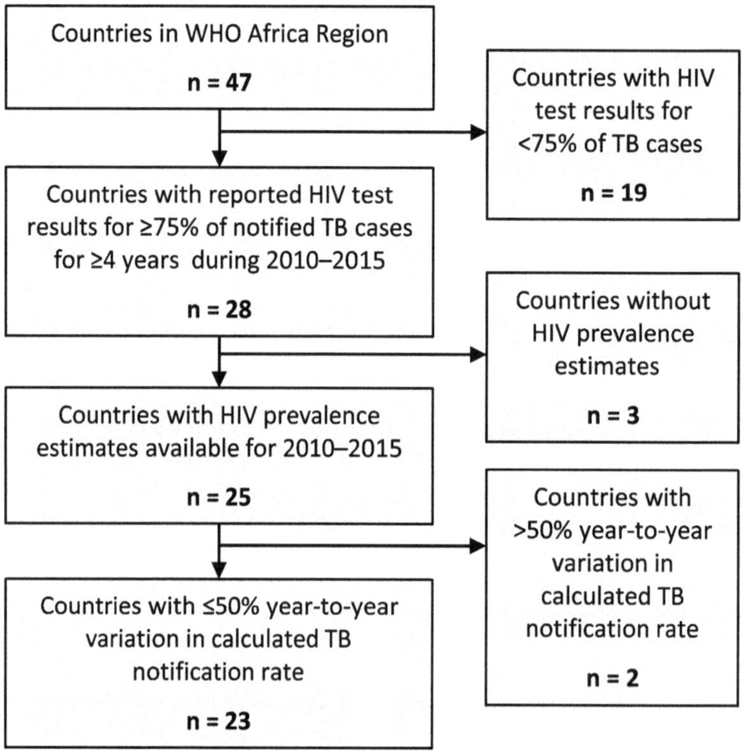

Fig. 2 Flowchart depicting selection of countries for this analysis

Trends in TB notifications

Among 19 countries with sufficient data to make HIV-stratified TB case notification estimates for 2010, the median estimated TB case notification rate among PLHIV (rounded to the nearest 10) was 1420 cases per 100,000 population (IQR 910–2410 cases per 100,000 population, Fig. 4a). In 2015, all 23 countries had sufficient data, and the median estimated TB notification rate among PLHIV was 1250 cases per 100,000 population (IQR 780–1580 cases per 100,000 population). By contrast, the median estimated TB case notification rate among people without HIV in 2010 was 130 cases per 100,000 population (IQR 70–220 cases per 100,000 population, Fig. 4b). In 2015, it was 120

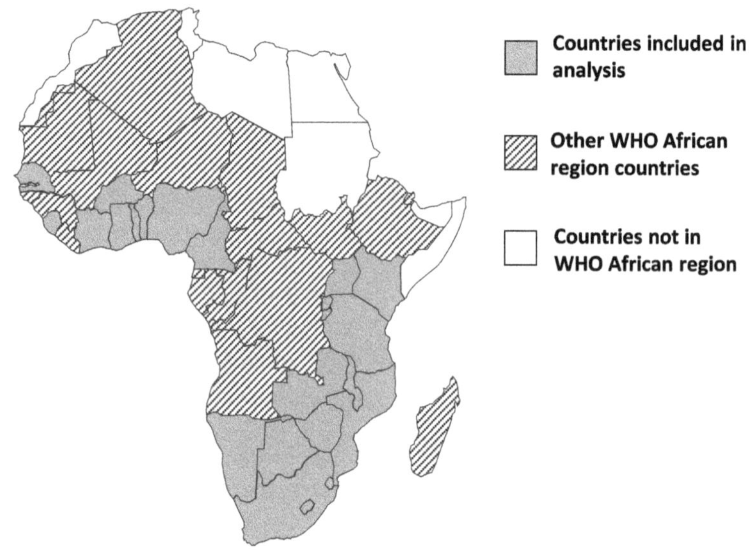

Fig. 3 Countries included in analysis — sub-Saharan Africa, 2010-2015, ($n = 23$)

Table 1 TB and ART trends: comparative summary statistics — 23 countries, sub-Saharan Africa, 2010–2015

	2010 estimated adult HIV prevalence, % (95% CI)	2010 estimated TB incidence per 100,000 (95% CI)	2010 ART coverage,%	Absolute increase in ART coverage[b], %	Average ART coverage, %	Average annual percent change in TB notification rate[a]	
						People with HIV (%)	People without HIV (%)
Central Africa							
Cameroon	4.6 (4.0–5.1)	274 (226–327)	16	14	23	−1.7	+ 1.2
Eastern Africa							
Burundi	1.5 (1.1–1.8)	144 (127–163)	25	25	36	−6.2	−0.9
Kenya	6.1 (5.5–6.8)	298 (286–311)	29	28	42	−6.8	−3.9
Rwanda	3.5 (2.9–4.0)	106 (94–118)	47	27	61	−5.7	−4.1
Tanzania	5.6 (4.7–6.4)	177 (166–189)	18	37	36	−1.4	−2.3
Uganda	7.4 (6.9–7.8)	209 (169–253)	20	40	39	−5.5	−0.1
Southern Africa							
Botswana	23.0 (20.3–24.4)	500 (449–560)	50	27	63	−6.8	−4.7
Lesotho	23.3 (21.1–24.5)	633 (553–719)	29	11	33	−8.3	−5.1
Malawi	10.9 (9.9–11.3)	219 (203–236)	26	32	43	−6.9	−4.2
Mozambique	14.0 (12.3–15.6)	544 (377–741)	13	31	25	+ 1.4	+ 9.3
Namibia	14.2 (12.5–15.5)	867 (686–1070)	43	20	55	−7.6	−0.1
South Africa	18.3 (15.9–20.5)	981 (809–1170)	20	29	36	−8.1	−1.3
Swaziland	27.2 (24.8–28.5)	1290 (1060–1530)	33	36	49	−10.9	−7.4
Zambia	12.7 (12.1–13.3)	462 (418–509)	34	30	49	−6.3	−3.7
Zimbabwe	15.8 (13.5–18.2)	633 (489–795)	29	39	49	−7.6	−5.0
Western Africa							
Benin	1.1 (0.8–1.5)	69 (57–82)	33	18	42	−0.5	−1.8
Burkina Faso	1.1 (0.8–1.3)	58 (49–67)	31	24	42	−6.3	+ 1.9
Côte d'Ivoire	3.8 (3.2–4.2)	190 (165–217)	16	18	24	−2.5	−2.8
Ghana	1.9 (1.5–2.4)	86 (75–97)	13	15	23	−2.0	−3.4
Nigeria	3.4 (2.4–4.6)	133 (64–225)	11	15	18	−5.2	−0.1
Senegal	0.6 (0.5–0.7)	137 (113–163)	28	16	34	−2.2	+ 2.7
Sierra Leone	1.7 (1.3–2.1)	660 (540–791)	11	10	15	+ 2.0	−4.2
Togo	2.9 (2.1–4.2)	73 (60–87)	19	20	28	+ 3.3	−2.2

[a]Average annual percent change is calculated by assuming a constant annual percent change between the first and last years of TB case notification rate estimates based on available high-quality data during 2010–2015; positive values indicate an increase in TB incidence while negative numbers indicate a decrease

[b]Absolute increase in ART coverage is defined as the difference between ART coverage in 2015 and ART coverage in 2010

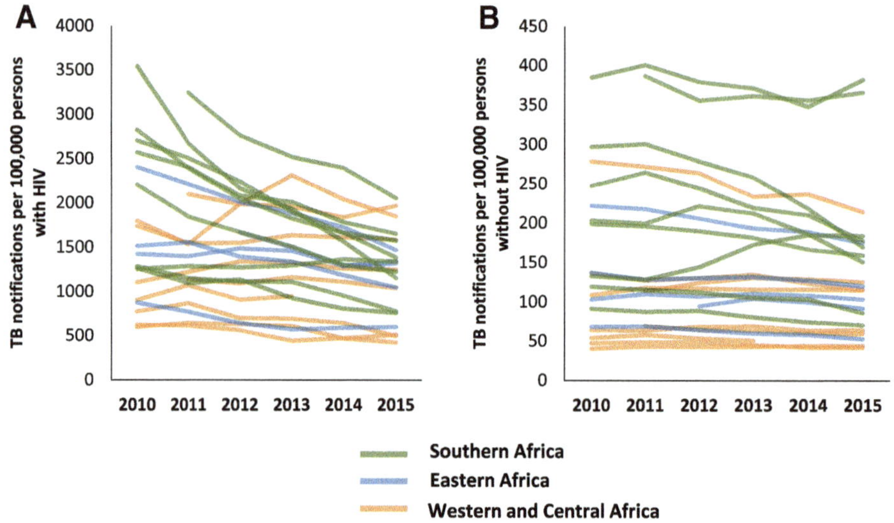

Fig. 4 a and **b** Trends in estimated TB notification rates among (**a**) PLHIV and (**b**) people without HIV by region in Africa — 23 countries, sub-Saharan Africa, 2010–2015

cases per 100,000 population (IQR 60–180 cases per 100,000 population).

Among all countries in the analysis, the median annual average change in estimated TB notification rates among PLHIV was -5.7% (IQR -6.9 to -1.7%; range -10.9 to +3.3%) compared to a median change of -2.3% (IQR -4.2 to -0.1%; range -7.4 to +9.3) for people without HIV (Table 1). This difference was statistically significant ($p = 0.0099$). TB notification rates declined more among PLHIV than among people without HIV in 16 (70%) countries; in 1 (4%) country, TB notification rates increased in both populations, but the increase was smaller for PLHIV than with people without HIV. In 6 (26%) countries, TB notification rates either decreased less or increased more than TB notification rates in people without HIV; 5 (83%) out of these 6 countries were located in western Africa.

Among 11 countries whose average ART coverage during the analytic period was greater than the median of 36%, the median annual average change in TB notification rates among PLHIV was -6.8% (IQR -7.6 to -5.7%) compared to a median change of -2.1% (IQR -6.0 to 0.7%) for PLHIV in 12 countries whose average ART coverage was less than or equal to the median. This difference was statistically significant ($p = 0.0106$). By contrast, the median annual average change in TB notification rates among people without HIV in the 11 countries with higher ART coverage was -3.9% (IQR -4.7 to -0.1%) compared to a median change of -1.8% (IQR -3.3 to 0.9) for people without HIV in the 12 countries with lower ART coverage. This difference was not statistically significant ($p = 0.1693$).

Discussion

Based on estimated HIV-stratified TB case notification rates in 23 sub-Saharan African countries, TB notification rates among PLHIV have declined more than among people without HIV, concurrently with the expansion of ART. Additionally, TB notification rates among PLHIV declined more in countries with higher ART coverage. While this analysis was descriptive and could not explore causality, these results are consistent with a population-level effect of ART on decreasing TB incidence among PLHIV.

To our knowledge, this analysis is the first attempt to broadly examine the relationship between ART coverage and TB notification rates among PLHIV across sub-Saharan Africa. Reports from a few countries in eastern and southern Africa [15–17] had previously shown greater declines in TB notification rates among PLHIV than among people without HIV in the era of ART scale-up. Our results suggest this to be the case in other eastern and southern African countries as well. However, in most of the western African countries in our analysis, TB notification rates among PLHIV decreased less than among people without HIV, or actually increased. One possible contributor to this worrisome trend is the low ART coverage in several western African countries; there may be a threshold of ART coverage that is required before population-level declines in TB are observed. Another possible contributor is the fact that western African countries tend to have concentrated rather than generalized HIV epidemics, which leads to greater uncertainty in their adult HIV prevalence estimates. Furthermore, the marginalization of key populations with HIV in these countries may exacerbate their susceptibility to TB despite the availablity of ART [25]. Thus, without more information about the overlap of TB and HIV epidemiology in these settings, estimates made based only on population-level data are more difficult to interpret. Nonetheless, improving the accessibility and acceptability of HIV testing and ART to key populations in these countries may be critical to decreasing TB among PLHIV.

As countries move toward implementing the "Test and Start" policy [26] to treat all PLHIV with ART regardless of CD4 cell count, monitoring the impact of ART scale-up on TB trends will become increasingly important. The ability to do so depends on being able to stratify TB trends by HIV status. As our study demonstrates, it is possible to make crude estimates based on the types of data that are currently available. However, only half the countries in the region had sufficient data of adequate quality, with insufficient HIV testing coverage among TB patients being the most common reason for excluding countries from our analysis. Prioritizing HIV testing for TB patients is thus not only important to ensure appropriate clinical management, but also for monitoring trends in TB incidence among PLHIV.

Although ART is expected to play a critical role in reducing TB incidence among PLHIV, it is not the only important factor. For example, isoniazid preventive therapy (IPT) has been shown to reduce the development of TB, independent of ART, and is increasingly considered an integral component of routine care for PLHIV [27–29]. As scale-up of IPT also occurs across sub-Saharan Africa, monitoring the population-level impact of both ART and IPT on reducing TB incidence will be needed. Furthermore, focusing interventions only on PLHIV will not be sufficient to halt the incidence of TB among PLHIV. People without HIV tend to be a reservoir for TB transmission to PLHIV [1, 6, 30–32], so investment in general TB elimination strategies such as active case-finding to find and treat all cases are crucial to reducing TB incidence among PLHIV. Finally, to better understand the contribution of different factors on reducing TB incidence among PLHIV, research is needed that goes beyond analyzing population-level indicators. For instance, long-term cohort studies of PLHIV can help quantify the impact of IPT and ART delivered in programmatic settings, while molecular epidemiology studies can provide insight into transmission of TB from people without HIV to PLHIV.

Our study was subject to limitations that affect the conclusions that can be drawn from our results. Inherent in a descriptive analysis is the limitation that causal inferences cannot be made. Therefore, although TB incidence declined more among PLHIV than people without HIV, and although the declines in TB incidence were greater among PLHIV in countries with the highest ART coverage, we cannot claim that ART caused the declines. Other factors such as improved nutrition or housing conditions, as well as improved TB programs or health system improvements that occurred in the process of building stronger programs to deliver ART, may have affected TB incidence. It is also possible that increasing IPT coverage could have contributed to the greater declines in TB notification rates observed among PLHIV compared to people without HIV. However, we were unable to assess the potential impact of IPT, or even describe its scale-up, as notification data for the number of people receiving IPT were completely missing for a third of the countries in this analysis, and missing for two thirds of countries for the early years of the analytic period [19].

Our study was also subject to limitations related to the data that were available for analysis. Because we were limited to publicly available country-level data, adequate data were unavailable for over half of the countries in the WHO African region. As a result, our analysis was relatively complete in its coverage of eastern and southern African countries, but highly incomplete for the countries of western and central Africa. This limitation highlights the need to strengthen data in major public domains if we are to assess the impact of recent policy changes moving forward.

Finally, as with all analyses based on TB case notifications, we were unable to account for potential changes in case detection rates over time, or differences in case detection between PLHIV and people without HIV. While we do not know for sure how case detection rates have changed over time, it is likely that improvements in national reporting systems over time have led to increases in the likelihood of people with TB being notified to WHO; therefore, our analysis could underestimate the declines in case notification rates that have occurred. In addition, TB case detection among PLHIV and people without HIV may differ, but the direction of this difference is unknown. For example, given that HIV is a stigmatized disease and the majority of new HIV cases tend to present with advanced immunosuppression [33], delays in TB diagnosis (or missed TB diagnoses altogether) occur more frequently than for people without HIV. By contrast, PLHIV who are in care are routinely screened for TB, while people without HIV are generally not, so case detection among PLHIV may be higher than among people without HIV in some settings. Thus, the quantitative comparison between the case notification rates we estimate for PLHIV and people without HIV must be interpreted with these limitations in mind.

Conclusion

This analysis suggests encouraging trends that TB notification rates have declined more among PLHIV than among people without HIV from 2010 to 2015. We believe that the expansion of ART has likely contributed to this decline. To further reduce TB incidence among PLHIV, additional scale-up of ART, as well as active case-finding in the general population will be necessary. To monitor the impact of these activities, it will be important to collect data on each intervention as well as routinely assess TB case notification rates stratified by HIV status. And finally, to better understand the factors contributing to changes in TB epidemiology among PLHIV, long-term cohort studies will be important to help interpret trends in programmatic data.

Abbreviations

ART: Antiretroviral therapy; HIV: Human immunodeficiency virus; IPT: Isoniazid preventive therapy; PLHIV: People living with HIV; TB: Tuberculosis; UNAIDS: Joint United Nations Programme on HIV/AIDS; UNDP: United Nations Development Programme; WHO: World Health Organization

Acknowledgements

We thank Ray Shiraishi for his help with merging datasets from the data sources used in this analysis.

Funding

This research has been supported by the President's Emergency Plan for AIDS Relief (PEPFAR) through the Centers for Disease Control and Prevention (CDC). The funders had no role in study design, data collection, analysis, interpretation of data, decision to publish, or preparation of the manuscript.

Disclaimer

The findings and conclusions in this report are those of the authors and do not necessarily represent the official position of the Centers for Disease Control and Prevention.

Authors' contributions

Conceptualization: CMY, KDC, and KPC. Methodology: CMY, MWB, KPC, and ESC. Data analysis: DS and CMY. Original draft preparation: DS and CMY. Review and edits: All. Supervision: CMY. All authors read and approved the final manuscript.

Consent for publication

Not applicable.

Competing interests

The authors declare that they have no competing interests.

Author details

[1]Division of Global HIV and TB, Centers for Disease Control and Prevention, Atlanta, GA, USA. [2]Center for Global Health, Office of the Director, Centers for Disease Control and Prevention, Kisumu, Kenya. [3]Division of Global HIV and TB, Centers for Disease Control and Prevention, Kisumu, Kenya. [4]Division of Global HIV and TB, Centers for Disease Control and Prevention, Nairobi, Kenya. [5]Division of Global Health Equity, Brigham and Women's Hospital, Boston, MA, USA. [6]Department of Global Health and Social Medicine, Harvard Medical School, Boston, MA, USA.

References

1. Selwyn PA, Hartel D, Lewis VA, Schoenbaum EE, Vermund SH, Klein RS, et al. A prospective study of the risk of tuberculosis among intravenous drug users with human immunodeficiency virus infection. N Engl J Med. 1989; 320:545–50. https://doi.org/10.1056/NEJM198903023200901.
2. Horsburgh CRJ. Priorities for the treatment of latent tuberculosis infection in the United States. N Engl J Med. 2004;350:2060–7. https://doi.org/10.1056/NEJMsa031667.
3. Centers for Disease Control and Prevention. Guidelines for prevention and treatment of opportunistic infections in HIV-infected adults and adolescents: recommendations from CDC, the National Institutes of Health, and the HIV medicine Association of the Infectious Diseases Society of America. MMWR. 2009;58(RR-04):1–198.
4. Sonnenberg P, Glynn JR, Fielding K, Murray J, Godfrey-Faussett P, Shearer S. How soon after infection with HIV does the risk of tuberculosis start to increase? A retrospective cohort study in south African gold miners. J Infect Dis. 2004;191:150–8. Epub Dec 13 2004. https://doi.org/10.1086/426827.
5. Centers for Disease Control and Prevention. Tuberculosis morbidity — United States, 1992. MMWR. 1993;42:696–7 703–4.
6. Kwan CK, Ernst JD. HIV and tuberculosis: a deadly human syndemic. Clin Microbiol Rev. 2011;24:351–76. https://doi.org/10.1128/cmr.00042-10.
7. Corbett EL, Watt CJ, Walker N, Maher D, Williams BG, Raviglione MC, et al. The growing burden of tuberculosis: global trends and interactions with the HIV epidemic. Arch Intern Med. 2003;163:1009–21. https://doi.org/10.1001/archinte.163.9.1009.
8. Lawn SD, Zumla AI. Tuberculosis. Lancet. 2011;378:57–72. https://doi.org/10.1016/ S0140-6736(10)62173-3.
9. World Health Organization. Global tuberculosis report 2017. Geneva: World Health Organization; 2017. Available from: http://www.who.int/tb/publications/2017/en/. [cited 2017 Jan 28]
10. Joint United Nations Programme on HIV/AIDS. Together we will end AIDS. Geneva: Joint United Nations Programme on HIV/AIDS; 2012. Available from: http://files.unaids.org/en/media/unaids/contentassets/documents/epidemiology/2012/JC2296_UNAIDS_TogetherReport_2012_en.pdf. [cited 2016 Sep 12]
11. Suthar AB, Lawn SD, del Amo J, Getahun H, Dye C, Sculier D, et al. Antiretroviral therapy for prevention of tuberculosis in adults with HIV: a systematic review and meta-analysis. PLoS Med. 2012;9(7):e1001270. https://doi.org/10.1371/journal.pmed.1001270.
12. Badri M, Wilson D, Wood R. Effect of highly active antiretroviral therapy on incidence of tuberculosis in South Africa: a cohort study. Lancet. 2002;359:2059–64.
13. Lawn SD, Kranzer K, Wood R. Antiretroviral therapy for control of the HIV-associated tuberculosis epidemic in resource-limited settings. Clin Chest Med. 2009;30:685–99, viii. https://doi.org/10.1016/j.ccm.2009.08.010.
14. Lawn SD, Wood R, De Cock KM, Kranzer K, Lewis JJ, Churchyard GJ. Antiretrovirals and isoniazid preventive therapy in the prevention of HIV-associated tuberculosis in settings with limited health-care resources. Lancet Infect Dis. 2010;10:489–98. https://doi.org/10.1016/S1473-3099(10)70078-5.
15. Yuen CM, Weyenga HO, Kim AA, Malika T, Muttai H, Katana A, et al. Comparison of trends in tuberculosis incidence among adults living with HIV and adults without HIV — Kenya, 1998–2012. PLoS One. 2014;9(6). https://doi.org/10.1371/journal.pone.0099880.
16. Hermans S, Boulle A, Caldwell J, Pienaar D, Wood R. Temporal trends in TB notification rates during ART scale-up in Cape Town: an ecological analysis. J Int AIDS Soc. 2015;18:20240. https://doi.org/10.7448/IAS.18.1.20240.
17. Middelkoop K, Bekker LG, Myer L, Johnson LF, Kloos M, Morrow C, et al. Antiretroviral therapy and TB notification rates in a high HIV prevalence south African community. J Acquir Immun Defic Syndr. 2011;56:263–9. https://doi.org/10.1097/QAI.0b013e31820413b3
18. Kanyerere H, Girma B, Mpunga J, Tayler-Smith K, Harries AD, Jahn A. Scale-up of ART in Malawi has reduced case notification rates in HIV-positive and HIV-negative tuberculosis. Public Health Action. 2016;6:247–51. https://doi.org/10.5588/pha.16.0053.

19. World Health Organization. Global tuberculosis report database. Available from: http://www.who.int/tb/country/data/download/en/. Accessed 23 Dec 2017
20. Joint United Nations Programme on HIV/AIDS. HIV estimates with uncertainty bounds 1990–2016. Available from: http://www.unaids.org/en/resources/documents/2017/HIV_estimates_with_uncertainty_bounds_1990-2016. Accessed 23 Dec 2017.
21. United Nations Population Division. World population prospects, the 2015 revision. Available from: https://esa.un.org/unpd/wpp/Download/Standard/Population/. Accessed 23 Dec 2017.
22. Joint United Nations Programme on HIV/AIDS. Coverage of people receiving ART. Available from: http://aidsinfo.unaids.org/#. Accessed 23 Dec 2017.
23. Joint United Nations Programme on HIV/AIDS. Global AIDS Response Progress Reporting 2016. Geneva: Joint United Nations Programme on HIV/AIDS; 2016. Available from: https://aidsreportingtool.unaids.org/static/docs/GARPR_Guidelines_2016_EN.pdf. Accessed 22 Sep 2016.
24. World Health Organization. Interim Policy on Collaborative TB/HIV Activities. Geneva: World Health Organization; 2004. Available from: http://www.who.int/hiv/pub/tb/tbhiv/en/. Accessed 2 Feb 2017.
25. Papworth E, Geesay N, An L, Thiam-Niangoin M, Ky-Zerbo O, Holland C, et al. Epidemiology of HIV among female sex workers, their clients, men who have sex with men and people who inject drugs in west and Central Africa. J Int AIDS Soc. 2013;16(Suppl 3):18751. https://doi.org/10.7448/IAS.16.4.18751.
26. World Health Organization. Consolidated guidelines on the use of antiretroviral drugs for treating and preventing HIV infection. Recommendations for a public health approach – second edition. Geneva: World Health Organization; 2016. Available from: http://www.who.int/hiv/pub/arv/arv-2016/en/. [cited 2016 Sep 12]
27. Ayele HT, Mourik MS, Debray TP, Bonten MJ. Isoniazid prophylactic therapy for the prevention of tuberculosis in HIV infected adults: a systematic review and meta-analysis of randomized trials. PLoS One. 2015;10(11):e0142290.
28. Golub JE, Saraceni V, Cavalcante SC, Pacheco AG, Moulton LH, King BS, et al. The impact of antiretroviral therapy and isoniazid preventive therapy on tuberculosis incidence in HIV-infected patients in Rio de Janeiro, Brazil. AIDS. 2007;21:1441–8.
29. Group TAS, Danel C, Moh R, et al. A trial of early Antiretrovirals and isoniazid preventive therapy in Africa. N Engl J Med. 2015;373:808–22. https://doi.org/10.1056/NEJMoa1507198.
30. Corbett EL, Charalambous S, Moloi VM, Fielding K, Grant AD, Dye C, et al. Human immunodeficiency virus and the prevalence of undiagnosed tuberculosis in African gold miners. Am J Respir Crit Care Med. 2004;170:673–9. https://doi.org/10.1164/rccm.200405-590OC.
31. Corbett EL, Charalambous S, Fielding K, Clayton T, Hayes RJ, De Cock KM, et al. Stable incidence rates of tuberculosis (TB) among human immunodeficiency virus (HIV)–negative south African gold miners during a decade of epidemic HIV-associated TB. J Infect Dis. 2003;188:1156–63. https://doi.org/10.1086/378519.
32. Middelkoop K, Mathema B, Myer L, Shashkina E, Whitelaw A, Kaplan G, et al. Transmission of tuberculosis in a south African community with a high prevalence of HIV infection. J Infect Dis. 2015;211:53–61. https://doi.org/10.1093/infdis/jiu403.
33. The IeDEA and ART cohort collaborations. Immunodeficiency at the start of combination antiretroviral therapy in low-, middle- and high-income countries. J Acquir Immune Defic Syndr. 2014;65(1):e8–e16. https://doi.org/10.1097/QAI.0b013e3182a39979 PubMed PMID: PMC3894575.

9

Improvement in tuberculosis infection control practice via technical support in two regions of Ethiopia

Asfaw Ayalew[1*], Zewdu Gashu[1], Tadesse Anteneh[1], Nebiyu Hiruy[1], Dereje Habte[1], Degu Jerene[1], Genetu Alem[2], Ilili Jemal[3], Muluken Melese[1] and Pedro G. Suarez[4]

Abstract

Background: Globally recommended measures for comprehensive tuberculosis (TB) infection control (IC) are inadequately practiced in most health care facilities in Ethiopia. The aim of this study was to assess the extent of implementation of TB IC measures before and after introducing a comprehensive technical support package in two regions of Ethiopia.

Methods: We used a quasi-experimental design, whereby a baseline assessment of TB IC practices in 719 health care facilities was conducted between August and October 2013. Based on the assessment findings, we supported implementation of a comprehensive package of interventions. Monitoring was done on a quarterly basis, and one-year follow-up data were collected on September 30, 2014. We used the Student's *t*-test and chi-squared tests, respectively, to examine differences before and after the interventions and to test for inter-regional and inter-facility associations.

Results: At baseline, most of the health facilities (69%) were reported to have separate TB clinics. In 55.2% of the facilities, it was also reported that window opening was practiced. Nevertheless, triaging was practiced in only 19.3% of the facilities. Availability of an IC committee and IC plan was observed in 29.11 and 4.65% of facilities, respectively. Health care workers were nearly three times as likely to develop active TB as the general population. After 12 months of implementation, availability of a separate TB room, TB IC committee, triage, and TB IC plan had increased, respectively, by 18, 32, 44, and 51% ($p < 0.001$).

Conclusions: After 1 year of intervention, the TB IC practices of the health facilities have significantly improved. However, availability of separate TB rooms and existence of TB IC committees remain suboptimal. The burden of TB among health care workers is higher than in the general population. TB IC measures must be strengthened to reduce TB transmission among health workers.

Keywords: TB infection control, TB transmission, TB prevention, Health care workers, Ethiopia

Background

Tuberculosis (TB) is one of the major infectious diseases that have tested the knowledge and wisdom of mankind. Innovations related to TB diagnosis, prevention, and treatment have lagged behind other technological advancements. After isolation of the tubercle bacillus, it took 38 years to invent a preventive vaccine and 61 years to discover the first anti-TB drug [1, 2]. The death toll from TB is enormous, and it continues to claim millions of lives throughout the world, even though simple preventive measures exist. Through airborne transmission, its favored mode of dissemination, TB has managed to sustain itself for millennia [3, 4].

Against all odds, remarkable progress has been made in recent times through formulation and implementation of effective strategies like the Directly Observed Treatment, Short course (DOTS) and Stop TB strategies,

* Correspondence: aayalew@msh.org; asfonium2000@yahoo.com
[1]Management Sciences for Health, Help Ethiopia Address the Low Performance of Tuberculosis (HEAL TB) Project, Bole Sub City, Kebele 02, House Number 708, PO Box 1157, Code 1250 Addis Ababa, Ethiopia
Full list of author information is available at the end of the article

which greatly contributed to meeting the TB-related target of the Millennium Development Goals (MDGs) of halting and beginning to reverse the TB epidemic [5]. On one hand, between 2000 and 2015, TB mortality declined by 34% and the number of deaths averted as a result of TB treatment was estimated at 49 million. On the other hand, TB remained one of the top 10 killer diseases in 2015. Moreover, increasing TB mortality was seen in Congo and the Democratic People's Republic of Korea [6].

Ethiopia is one of the 30 high-TB-burden countries that have shown a substantial reduction in TB incidence and mortality since 2000. The estimated decline in the incidence rate as of 2010 was 6.7%. In 2015, the estimated TB incidence was 191,000, while the actual notified TB cases were 137,960. In the same year, 599 cases of drug-resistant TB (DR-TB) were notified. Of the notified TB cases, 8% were people living with the human immunodeficiency virus (HIV) [6].

In low-income countries such as Ethiopia, patients and visitors tend to congregate in health facilities' corridors and waiting areas. This congestion is due to uncontrolled population growth and an increasing number of health care seekers, on one hand, and a shortage of health care workers (HCWs) and limited number of health care facilities (HCFs), on the other hand [7]. This overcrowding, in turn, supports airborne nosocomial transmission of TB to HCWs, patients, and even visitors [8]. Highly vulnerable people, such as children, undernourished people, and immunocompromised people, are among the health service seekers in HCFs, which is an opportunity for TB to continue its spread. The emergence and rapid spread of drug-resistant mycobacterial strains, as well as its interaction with HIV, have heightened the demand for effective infection control (IC) interventions at all levels [9–11].

IC, in the TB context, aims at reducing the transmission of TB within populations and relies on a set of managerial, administrative, environmental, and personal protective interventions. When such measures are not implemented, the risk of TB (both drug susceptible and drug resistant) dramatically increases, in some circumstances to epidemic proportions. Inpatient outbreaks of DR-TB among people living with HIV have been reported in Africa and Europe [12, 13]. Implementing IC measures, however, is known to reverse the airborne threat [9]. The TB IC hierarchy of measures is so crucial that the World Health Organization (WHO) has issued a standalone policy document and implementation guidelines for member countries' action. TB IC has also been recommended in important global documents [8, 14–16].

Ethiopia developed its first national TB IC guidelines based on international recommendations in 2009—in the same year that the relevant WHO documents were published [5, 9]. The Federal Ministry of Health has trained a number of health care workers using a TB IC curriculum. Still others were trained in comprehensive TB/HIV services as well as programmatic management of DR-TB, both of which have incorporated TB IC topics [17, 18].

The Help Ethiopia Address the Low Performance of TB (HEAL TB) project led by Management Sciences for Health (MSH) implemented a comprehensive TB control program, one of the components being TB IC. Capacity building for health managers and health workers, supportive supervision, and technical and material support were among the interventions geared toward improving TB IC in HCFs. It is evident that there is little research, particularly intervention studies, about TB IC in low-income settings. The objective of this study was to compare the implementation of TB IC measures before and after introduction of a comprehensive technical support package in two regions of Ethiopia.

Methods

Setting

Ethiopia is the second most populous nation in Africa, with a population close to 99 million. It is administratively composed of nine regional states and two city administrations. Under each regional state there are a number of zonal administrations (also called zones), and under each zone are several *woredas* (districts) [19].

In 2017, there were 22,807 TB notified cases out of the 21.1 million population in Amhara, and 43,321 notified TB cases out of 35.8 million population in Oromia Region [20].

The study employed a pre- and post-intervention design built upon project implementation. All of the project HCFs were included in the study.

Funded by the United States Agency for International Development (USAID), the HEAL TB project supported the government of Ethiopia in addressing many of the major challenges posed by TB. The project began in July 2011 in two of the most populous regional states in the country: Oromia and Amhara, with a total population of 57 million. Before the intervention, HEAL TB conducted a baseline assessment in all HCFs of the selected 11 zones. Twenty-two hospitals and 697 health centers were included in the assessment, which ran from August through October 2013. Basic information on TB IC measures was collected.

Intervention

The intervention package consisted of capacity building, provision of standard operating procedures (SOPs), regular supportive supervision, and program review meetings. The project initially trained woreda TB focal persons on the basics of TB IC and on supervisory skills so that they could provide technical support to HCWs. The woreda TB focal person supervises, on average, five HCFs under his/her catchment once every three months, using supervision checklists and TB SOC indicators. Both templates address TB IC issues. Based on the findings of the supervision, the woreda TB focal person gives on-site feedback and subsequently follows the implementation status of the action plan developed during the last visit. In addition to the woreda TB focal persons, HCWs were also trained using a TB IC curriculum. Different SOPs appropriate to the service delivery points were developed and posted on the wall, starting with the triage room continuing all the way to the laboratory. TB program review meetings were held biannually; during the meetings, woreda TB focal points presented the performance of the HCFs in their respective woredas over the previous six months. In such meetings, TB IC is a major topic that is thoroughly discussed, and improvement plans are formulated.

Data collection instruments

Two types of checklists were used, one for baseline assessment and another for quarterly monitoring. The baseline checklist is a comprehensive tool of eight pages with 171 items structured into different thematic areas, including TB IC. The TB IC questionnaire asks about the (1) availability of a separate TB room, (2) opening of windows during consultation hours, (3) presence of cough triage, (4) TB IC committee, (5) TB IC plan, and (6) number of HCWs who developed active TB in the previous year. The quarterly monitoring instrument also contains a subsection on TB IC specifically referring to the presence of a functional multidisciplinary team/infection prevention committee, revised IC plan, triage/cougher prioritization, and separate TB room. Both tools were developed based on consultation with stakeholders and adaptation of international TB standards [21, 22]. Taking into account the large number of HCFs under project support, it was decided that the number of TB IC indicators should be kept to the minimum, while ensuring robustness, for the sake of efficient resource utilization.

Data collectors and data collection procedures

For the baseline assessment, the data collectors were HEAL TB employees who were medical doctors, health officers, and specialist laboratory professionals, all with public health experience. Training on the baseline assessment tools was provided for two days, before their departure to the field. Observation, review of documents, and interviews were the approaches used to collect the baseline data. Information about the number of HCWs who developed active TB was obtained from the TB registers kept in TB rooms. For this purpose, HCWs were defined as all people working in HCFs.

For quarterly monitoring, the trained woreda TB focal persons were in charge of data collection from their respective catchment HCFs. During the visits, they used the SOC tool, which required them to interview HCF TB focal persons about the status of TB IC activities, to review documents (minutes of infection prevention/IC committees), and to observe practices (prioritization of people with cough; status of the TB room).They spent on average half a day in each HCF to collect relevant TB program data. The following four TB IC indicators were monitored every three months: existence of (1) TB IC committee, (2) triage, (3) separate TB room, and (4) revised/updated TB IC plan. Data were collected from all 719 health facilities at baseline and every quarter thereafter.

Data management and analysis

A data entry template in the Census and Survey Processing System (CSPro), version 4.1 (US Census Bureau, ORC Macro International, and Serpro SA), was prepared, and data were entered into the template immediately after data collection. We checked the data for consistency and completeness by running frequency tables and cross-tabulations.

The data entered into CSPro 4.1 were exported to Stata 11 (College Station, TX: StataCorp., LP), where data cleaning, editing, and consistency checking were performed. Frequencies and percentages were computed to describe the data and compare TB IC practices before and after the program was implemented. We used the Student's t-test to determine significant differences between baseline and post-intervention data. The chi-squared test (Table 1) was also utilized to test for associations between the two regions as well as between hospitals and health centers (Tables 2 and 3).

Ethical considerations

We received ethical approval from the ethics committees of Amhara and Oromia Regional Health Bureaus to analyze the routine data and disseminate the findings. We used health facility level reports for this analysis with the consent of the reporting institutions. No patient identifiers were included in the routine reports.

Table 1 Comparison of the TB IC performance before and after intervention

Variables	Before intervention % ($N = 719$)	After intervention % ($N = 719$)	P-value (Before after t-test)
Separate TB room	69.1	87.1	$P < 0.001$
Cough triage	19.3	63.0	$P < 0.001$
IP/TB IC committee	29.1	61.1	$P < 0.001$
TB IC Plan	4.7	56.1	$P < 0.001$

Table 2 TB IC performance at baseline and after intervention by region

Characteristics	Baseline			After Intervention		
	Region		*P*-value (Chi-square)	Region		*P*-value (Chi-square)
	Amhara ($n = 306$)	Oromia ($n = 413$)		Amhara ($n = 306$)	Oromia ($n = 413$)	
% Cough triage	17.4	21.8	0.31	84.2	46.7	< 0.01
% IP/TB IC committee	57	14.7	< 0.01	71.2	53.6	< 0.01
% TB IC Plan	2.9	6.3	0.16	67.3	48.0	< 0.01

Results

At baseline, separate TB clinics existed in the majority of health facilities (69.1%). HCWs assigned to outpatient departments were reported to be working with open windows in 55.2% of the HCFs. However, coughing patients were prioritized for TB services in only 19.41% of the health facilities. Infection prevention committees and TB IC plans existed in only 29.11 and 4.65% of the assessed HCFs, respectively. There were no statistically significant differences between Amhara and Oromia regions regarding the practice of cough triage ($p = 0.31$) and existence of a TB IC plan ($p = 0.16$).However, regional differences in existence of TB IC committees ($p < 0.01$) did attain statistical significance (Table 2). Furthermore, hospitals differed from health centers significantly in terms of cough triage, TB IC committees, and TB IC plan availability ($p < 0.01$) (Table 3).

Sixty-one of the 8667 HCWs had developed active TB in the year preceding this assessment, making the annual incidence rate 704/100,000. Using WHO's 2012 TB incidence estimation for Ethiopia, which was 247/100,000, we calculated the incidence rate ratio to be 2.85 (for all forms of drug-susceptible TB, not only new cases). The incidence risk ratio was not age standardized; the rates were compared to the general population based on the WHO estimate, which is not age standardized.

Health care workers with TB were identified according to the national diagnostic algorithms, which consisted of sputum smear microscopy (the algorithm was recently revised, so that HCWs are tested with GeneXpert assay), radiography, and cytology—as indicated.

After 12 months of implementation, the number of HCFs with TB IC committees increased to 61%, and prioritized service for coughers had been put in place in 63% of the HCFs ($p < 0.001$). Furthermore, 56% of HFs had written TB IC plans, and 87% had designated separate TB rooms, which was significantly higher than the situation before intervention ($p < 0.001$) (Table 1).

Post-intervention, statistically significant differences occurred between Amhara and Oromia regions pertaining to availability of all the TB IC measures ($p < 0.01$). Moreover, with the exception of existence of TB IC committees ($p = 0.10$), hospitals differed from health centers significantly in terms of cough triage ($p < 0.01$) and availability of TB IC plans ($p = 0.01$).

Discussion

Before the technical support and comprehensive package of interventions, the majority of the health facilities lacked basic work procedures and policies to facilitate smooth implementation of TB IC. After intervention, availability of TB IC plans and use of triage showed marked improvement, while existence of TB IC committees and separate TB rooms improved modestly.

When comparing HCFs in Amhara with those of Oromia Region, the former did well post-intervention in availability of TB IC plans and triage, whereas the latter performed better in existence of TB IC committees. In addition, hospitals performed better than health centers in all the TB IC indicators, which can be explained by a relatively good start at baseline, presence of trained HCWs in sufficient number, and extra supervisory support from different stakeholders due to hospitals' physical accessibility.

According to the WHO directive, facility-level TB IC implementation begins with assignment of a coordinating body. Health facility risk assessment, formulation of a TB IC plan, and implementation of the plan should

Table 3 TB IC performance at baseline and after intervention by type of health facility

Characteristics	Baseline			After Intervention		
	Type of Health Facility		*P*-value (Chi-square)	Type of Health Facility		*P*-value (Chi-square)
	Health Center ($n = 697$)	Hospital ($n = 22$)		Health Center ($n = 697$)	Hospital ($n = 22$)	
% Cough triage	18.8	47.8	< 0.01	61.5	91.7	< 0.01
% IP/TB IC committee	28.6	56.5	< 0.01	60.4	79.2	0.10
% TB IC Plan	3.6	34.8	< 0.01	55.2	83.3	0.01

follow in that order [9]. In our baseline assessment, however, this logical order was not evident. Only 29% of the facilities had functional IP committees, meaning that the great majority of the facilities lacked a responsible body to combat TB transmission. Without this committee, it is not possible to do facility assessments and to plan TB IC activities, in line with the guidelines. The literature is scanty regarding availability of infection prevention/TB IC committees. Ogbonnaya et al. reported that 16.7% of the assessed TB/HIV implementing health facilities in Nigeria had IC committees [23]. This figure is lower than what we found at baseline in Ethiopia. A 32% improvement was seen post-intervention.

The least-implemented TB IC measure was the facility-level IC plan, which was found in only 4.7% of the HCFs. This also brings to light that 24.3% of the HCFs reported as having IC committees failed to develop plans, bringing into question their functionality. In sub-Saharan Africa, availability of TB IC plans in health facilities ranges from none to 77% [24, 25]. In Mozambique, it was 48% [26] and in Uganda, 31% [27]. Our baseline finding lies in between and was increased to 56% after intervention. Unavailability of a TB IC plan implies poor managerial activity and attention. It is very difficult to implement what has not been planned.

Close to 80% of the assessed facilities did not provide prioritized services for presumptive TB patients. Functional triage availability is reported from Nigeria [23] and South Africa [28] as 16.7, and 26%, respectively. In a 2012 study involving nine countries in sub-Saharan Africa, it ranged from 5 to 93% [25]. At baseline, triage availability in Ethiopia was a bit higher than the reported figure from Nigeria but modestly lower than in South Africa and within the range of figures in sub-Saharan Africa. In such a situation, generation of infectious droplet nuclei and contamination of the environment are facilitated; HCWs, visitors, and other patients become highly exposed.

Screening of all health facility care-seekers for TB symptoms, with subsequent isolation and/or fast tracking for services are triage functions and an essential component of administrative control. It is generally agreed that triage is the first defense mechanism against TB transmission in HCFs. Rapid diagnosis and effective TB treatment are the hallmarks of TB IC. Establishment of triaging had increased to 63% of the HCFs by the end of the intervention year.

At baseline, HCWs in half of the assessed facilities opened window(s) during consultation hours and thereafter. This practice was indicative of individuals' precautions rather than a concerted IC effort, given the low level of availability of TB IC committees and plans. Moreover, awareness among HCWs has been raised by their attending trainings related to TB, HIV, and DR-TB. Reports of increased awareness of HCWs (clinicians) about IC were recently demonstrated in Addis Ababa and in northwest Ethiopia in a survey of knowledge, attitudes, and practices [29, 30].

In nearly 70% of the health facilities, TB rooms were standalone. This should not be counted as a strength, however, since all service delivery points are required to have separate rooms as a matter of health service standards. It also implies that the remaining one-third of HCFs are providing TB service together with other services, compromising space and ventilation. In South Africa, dedicated TB rooms were available in only 31% of HCFs [25]. Through project support in Ethiopia, it was possible to increase the level from the baseline of 69 to 87%.

Poor implementation of IC measures is reflected in HCWs' acquisition of TB disease, as this study showed. Sixty-one HCWs acquired TB in 1 year. They were about 2.85 times more likely to acquire active TB disease than the general population. Reports of TB among HCWs from sub-Saharan African countries [24] and resource-rich countries [31] show disparities. The TB case notification rate in HCWs of Malawi was 3.2% as compared to 1.8% for primary schoolteachers [32]. In South Africa, Claassens et al. stated that the standardized incidence ratio of smear-positive pulmonary TB in primary health care workers was more than double that of the general population [28]. A study in 2013 in the same country showed a 10% DR-TB rate among physicians with pulmonary TB diagnosis, which the researchers attributed to lack of effective IC work practices combined with negative attitudes of administrators [33]. A recent meta-analysis by Baussano et al. indicated that the stratified pooled estimates for annual TB incidence risk ratio for countries with high TB incidence (> 100 cases/100,000) is 3.68, whereas it is 2.42 for low-incidence (< 50 cases/100,000) and intermediate-incidence (50–99 cases/100,000) countries. The overall estimate of annual TB incidence risk ratio was 2.97, which is comparable to our finding of 2.85. They concluded that HCWs' risk of acquiring TB was higher than that of the general population across the globe and that effective TB IC measures could decrease annual TB incidence among HCWs by as much 81, 27, and 49% in countries with high, intermediate, and low TB incidence, respectively [34]. Most, if not all, countries have long recognized TB as an occupational disease [9, 35].

It is worth noting the following limitations of the study. We were not able to present data regarding the cross-ventilation status of outpatient departments and active TB disease among HCWs to make comparison with the baseline findings, since our quarterly data source did not capture these items. Furthermore, lack of randomization in quasi-experimental design makes it difficult to control for confounding variables, and hence statistical association may not necessarily imply causal association. Similarly, we used Student's *t*- and chi-squared tests, which do not allow adjustment for confounders. Moreover, we relied on facility-level registers to collect data about the number of HCWs with TB, which might miss those being treated outside the HCF; hence there is a possibility of underreporting.

Conclusions

Building the capacity of district TB focal persons to provide supportive supervision to health facilities, together with the other comprehensive TB program support, was instrumental in improving the TB IC situation of health facilities. Huge gaps in implementation of the recommended TB IC practices at health facility level can be narrowed, if systematized basic capacity building can be provided. The burden of TB among HCWs is higher than the prevalence in the general population. There is a need to further strengthen infection prevention/TB IC committees in order to plan and implement the hierarchy of TB IC activities and reduce TB transmission among patients and HCWs.

Abbreviations

DR-TB: Drug-resistant tuberculosis; HCF: Health care facility; HCW: Health care worker; HIV: Human immunodeficiency virus; IP: Infection prevention; SOC: Standard of care; TB IC: Tuberculosis infection control; TB: Tuberculosis; USAID: United States Agency for International Development; WHO: World Health Organization

Acknowledgements

We would like to thank all the data collectors, as well as the Amhara and Oromia Regional Health Bureaus, for facilitating the implementation of the project. We thank the administrative and clinical staff of the health facilities for their cooperation. Dr. Barbara K. Timmons edited the final manuscript, for whom we are very grateful.

Funding

The United States Agency for International Development (USAID) supported this work through Management Sciences for Health – the Help Ethiopia Address Low Tuberculosis Performance Project (HEAL TB), under cooperative agreement number AID-663 -A-11-00011. The contents of the article are the responsibility of the authors alone and do not necessarily reflect the views of USAID or the United States government.

Authors' contributions

AA conceived and designed the study; NH, DH, & AA participated in the acquisition, analysis, and interpretation of data; AA, DJ, and DH drafted the article; ZG, MM, TA, and PS have contributed to inception, design and implementation of the interventions. They also critically reviewed the first and subsequent drafts of the manuscript and provided critical inputs to the interpretation of the findings. IJ and GA have actively participated in the roll out and implementation of the TB IC in the study regions. Moreover, they have contributed to the drafting and subsequent revision of the manuscript. All authors read and approved the final manuscript.

Consent for publication

Not applicable.

Competing interests

The authors declare that they have no competing interests.

Author details

[1]Management Sciences for Health, Help Ethiopia Address the Low Performance of Tuberculosis (HEAL TB) Project, Bole Sub City, Kebele 02, House Number 708, PO Box 1157, Code 1250 Addis Ababa, Ethiopia. [2]Amhara Regional Health Bureau, PO Box 495, Bahir Dar, Ethiopia. [3]Oromia Regional Health Bureau, PO Box 24341, Addis Ababa, Ethiopia. [4]Management Sciences for Health, Health Programs Group, 4301 North Fairfax Drive, Suite 400, Arlington, VA 22203, USA.

References

1. Mandal A. History of tuberculosis. In: News medical. AZoNetwork. 2017. https://www.news-medical.net/health/History-of-Tuberculosis.aspx. Accessed 30 Nov 2017.
2. Rothman S. The white death: a history of tuberculosis. Med Hist. 2001;45(1): 140–1.
3. Daniel TM. The history of tuberculosis. Respir Med. 2006;100(11):1862–70.
4. Schaaf HS, Zumla AI, editors. Tuberculosis: a comprehensive clinical reference. London: Elsevier; 2009.
5. World Health Organization (WHO). Implementing the end TB strategy: the essentials. Geneva: WHO; 2015.
6. World Health Organization (WHO). 2016 global tuberculosis report. Geneva: WHO; 2016.
7. Federal Minstry of Health (FMOH). Guidelines for prevention of transmission of tuberculosis in health care facilities,congregate and community settings in Ethiopia. 1st ed. Addis Ababa: FMOH; 2009.
8. Jensen PA, Lambert LA, Iademarco MF, Ridzon R, Centers for Disease Control and Prevention. Guidelines for preventing the transmission of *Mycobacterium tuberculosis* in health-care settings. MMWR Recomm Rep. 2005;54(RR-17):1–141.
9. World Health Organization (WHO). WHO policy on TB infection control in health-care facilities, congregate settings and households. Geneva: WHO; 2009.
10. World Health Organization (WHO). Implementing the WHO policy on TB infection control in health-care facilities, congregate settings and households: a framework to plan, implement and scale-up TB infection control activities at country, facility and community level. Geneva: WHO; 2009.
11. Nardell E, Dharmadhikari A. Turning off the spigot: reducing drug-resistant tuberculosis transmission in resource-limited settings. Int J Tuberc Lung Dis. 2010;14(10):1233–43.
12. Gandhi NR, Weissman D, Moodley P, Ramathal M, Elson I, Kreiswirth BN, et al. Nosocomial transmission of extensively drug-resistant tuberculosis in a rural hospital in South Africa. J Infect Dis. 2013;207(1):9–17. https://doi.org/10.1093/infdis/jis631.
13. Moro ML, Gori A, Errante I, Infuso A, Franzetti F, Sodano L, et al. An outbreak of multidrug-resistant tuberculosis involving HIV-infected patients of two hospitals in Milan, Italy. AIDS. 1998;12(9):1095–102.
14. World Health Organization (WHO). The stop TB strategy: building on and enhancing DOTS to meet the TB-related millennium development goals. Geneva: WHO; 2006.
15. World Health Organization (WHO). WHO policy on collaborative TB/HIV activities: guidelines for national programmes and other stakeholders. Geneva: WHO; 2012.
16. World Health Organization (WHO). The global task force on XDR-TB: update. Geneva: WHO; 2007.
17. Federal Ministry of Health (FMOH). Guidelines for clinical and programmatic management of TB, TB/HIV and leprosy in Ethiopia. 5th ed. Addis Ababa: FMOH; 2012. https://www.medbox.org/ethiopia/guidelines-for-clinical-and-programmatic-management-of-tb-tbhiv-and-leprosy-in-ethiopia/preview. Accessed 30 Nov 2017.

18. Federal Ministry of Health (FMOH). Guidelines on programmatic management of drug resistant tuberculosis in Ethiopia. 2nd ed. Addis Ababa: FMOH; 2013. https://www.medbox.org/et-guidelines-hiv-tb/guidelines-on-programmatic-management-of-drug-resistant-tuberculosis-in-ethiopia/preview. Accessed 30 Nov 2017.
19. Federal Ministry of Health (FMOH). Health Sector Transformation Plan.2015/16–2019/20. Addis Ababa: FMOH; 2015. https://www.globalfinancingfacility.org/sites/gff_new/files/Ethiopia-health-system-transformation-plan.pdf. Accessed 30 Nov 2017.
20. US Agency for International Development (USAID), KNCV Tuberculosis Foundation, and Challenge TB. Challenge TB year 2 annual report, October 1st 2015-September 30th 2016. The Hague: KNCV Tuberculosis Foundation; 2017. http://www.challengetb.org/reportfiles/Challenge_TB_Annual_Report_Year_2.pdf. Accessed 30 Nov 2017.
21. World Health Organization (WHO). International standards for tuberculosis care. 3rd ed. Geneva: WHO; 2014. http://www.who.int/tb/publications/ISTC_3rdEd.pdf. Accessed 30 Nov 2017.
22. World Health Organization (WHO). Checklist for periodic evaluation of TB infection control in health-care facilities. Geneva: WHO; 2015. http://www.who.int/tb/areas-of-work/preventive-care/checklist_for_periodic_evaluation_of_tb_infection_control_in_health_facilities.pdf. Accessed 30 Nov 2017.
23. Ogbonnaya LU, Chukwu JN, Uwakwe KA, Oyibo PG, Ndukwe CD. The status of tuberculosis infection control measures in health care facilities rendering joint TB/HIV services in "German leprosy and tuberculosis relief association" supported states in Nigeria. Niger J Clin Pract. 2011;14(3):270–5. https://doi.org/10.4103/1119-3077.86765.
24. Robert J, Affolabi D, Awokou F, Nolna D, Manouan BA, Acho YB, et al. Assessment of organizational measures to prevent nosocomial tuberculosis in health facilities of 4 sub-Saharan countries in 2010. Infect Control Hosp Epidemiol. 2013;34(2):190–5. https://doi.org/10.1086/669085.
25. Reid MJA, Saito S, Nash D, Scardigli A, Casalini C, Howard AA. Implementation of tuberculosis infection control measures at HIV care and treatment sites in sub-Saharan Africa. Int J Tuberc Lung Dis. 2012;16(12):1605–12. https://doi.org/10.5588/ijtld.12.0033.
26. Brouwer M, Coelho E, das Dores Mosse C, Van Leth F. Implementation of tuberculosis infection prevention and control in Mozambican health care facilities. Int J Tuberc Lung Dis. 2015;19(1):44–9. https://doi.org/10.5588/ijtld.14.0337.
27. Buregyeya E, Nuwaha F, Verver S, Criel B, Colebunders R, Wanyenze R, et al. Implementation of tuberculosis infection control in health facilities in Mukono and Wakiso districts, Uganda. BMC Infect Dis. 2013;13:360. https://doi.org/10.1186/1471-2334-13-360.
28. Claassens MM, van Schalkwyk C, du Toit E, Roest E, Lombard CJ, Enarson DA, et al. Tuberculosis in healthcare workers and infection control measures at primary healthcare facilities in South Africa. PLoS One. 2013;8(10):e76272. https://doi.org/10.1371/journal.pone.0076272.
29. Tenna A, Stenehjem EA, Margoles L, Kacha E, Blumberg HM, Kempker RR. Infection control knowledge, attitudes, and practices among healthcare workers in Addis Ababa, Ethiopia. Infect Control Hosp Epidemiol. 2013;34(12):1289–96. https://doi.org/10.1086/673979.
30. Temesgen C, Demissie M. Knowledge and practice of tuberculosis infection control among health professionals in Northwest Ethiopia; 2011. BMC Health Serv Res. 2014;14:593. https://doi.org/10.1186/s12913-014-0593-2.
31. Lambert LA, Pratt RH, Armstrong LR, Haddad MB. Tuberculosis among healthcare workers, United States, 1995-2007. Infect Control Hosp Epidemiol. 2012;33(11):1126–32. https://doi.org/10.1086/668016.
32. Harries AD, Hargreaves NJ, Gausi F, Kwanjana JH, Salaniponi FM. Preventing tuberculosis among health workers in Malawi. Bull World Health Organ. 2002;80(7):526–31.
33. Naidoo A, Naidoo SS, Gathiram P, Lalloo UG. Tuberculosis in medical doctors: a study of personal experiences and attitudes. S Afr Med J. 2013;103(3):176–80. https://doi.org/10.7196/samj.6266.
34. Baussano I, Nunn P, Williams B, Pivetta E, Bugiani M, Scano F. Tuberculosis among health care workers. Emerg Infect Dis. 2011;17(3):488–94. https://doi.org/10.3201/eid1703.100947.
35. Chai SJ, Mattingly DC, Varma JK. Protecting health care workers from tuberculosis in China: a review of policy and practice in China and the United States. Health Policy Plan. 2013;28(1):100–9. https://doi.org/10.1093/heapol/czs029.

10

Association between semi-quantitative microbial load and respiratory symptoms among Thai military recruits

Clarence C. Tam[1,2*], Vittoria Offeddu[1], Kathryn B. Anderson[3,4], Alden L. Weg[4], Louis R. Macareo[4], Damon W. Ellison[4], Ram Rangsin[5], Stefan Fernandez[4], Robert V. Gibbons[6], In-Kyu Yoon[7] and Sriluck Simasathien[8]

Abstract

Background: Multiplex real-time polymerase chain reaction assays have improved diagnostic sensitivity for a wide range of pathogens. However, co-detection of multiple agents and bacterial colonization make it difficult to distinguish between asymptomatic infection or illness aetiology. We assessed whether semi-quantitative microbial load data can differentiate between symptomatic and asymptomatic states for common respiratory pathogens.

Methods: We obtained throat and nasal swab samples from military trainees at two Thai Army barracks. Specimens were collected at the start and end of 10-week training periods (non-acute samples), and from individuals who developed upper respiratory tract infection during training (acute samples). We analysed the samples using a commercial multiplex respiratory panel comprising 33 bacterial, viral and fungal targets. We used random effects tobit models to compare cycle threshold (Ct) value distributions from non-acute and acute samples.

Results: We analysed 341 non-acute and 145 acute swab samples from 274 participants. *Haemophilus influenzae* type B was the most commonly detected microbe (77.4% of non-acute and 64.8% of acute samples). In acute samples, nine specific microbe pairs were detected more frequently than expected by chance. Regression models indicated significantly lower microbial load in non-acute relative to acute samples for *H. influenzae* non-type B, *Streptococcus pneumoniae* and rhinovirus, although it was not possible to identify a Ct-value threshold indicating causal etiology for any of these organisms.

Conclusions: Semi-quantitative measures of microbial concentration did not reliably differentiate between illness and asymptomatic colonization, suggesting that clinical symptoms may not always be directly related to microbial load for common respiratory infections.

Keywords: Multiplex PCR diagnostics, Respiratory illness, Upper respiratory tract infection, Asymptomatic infection, Influenza-like illness, Influenza, *Haemophilus influenza*

* Correspondence: clarence.tam@nus.edu.sg
[1]Saw Swee Hock School of Public Health, National University of Singapore and National University Health System, Singapore 117549, Singapore
[2]London School of Hygiene & Tropical Medicine, WC1E7HT, London, UK
Full list of author information is available at the end of the article

Background

Multiplex polymerase chain reaction (PCR)-based diagnostic techniques allow rapid, simultaneous identification of a broad range of respiratory pathogens [1]. Compared to classical microbiological diagnostic methods, PCR-based assays offer higher sensitivity, specificity, and reproducibility [2]. However, the high sensitivity of multiplex PCR diagnostics does not directly translate into clinical utility, because such assays do not distinguish between viable and dead organisms, or acute infection and asymptomatic colonisation [2]. In the clinical setting, the etiological agent is seldom identified and unspecific respiratory symptoms are often treated empirically [3].

Although the quantification of microbial load may vary depending on the presence of co-infections, specimen type, sampling technique, or timing of sampling, quantitative or semi-quantitative microbial load data from real-time PCR assays may help define organism densities that are consistent with colonization or infection and distinguish between symptomatic and asymptomatic states [4]. In this study, we assessed whether semi-quantitative microbial load availab from real-time PCR assays can differentiate between symptomatic and asymptomatic states for common respiratory agents in a cohort of basic military trainees at two Royal Thai Army barracks.

Methods

Study settings and participants

Details of the study setting and procedures have been described previously [5]. Briefly, participants were recruited from six consecutive cohorts of basic military trainees at two Royal Thai Army barracks between May 2014 and July 2015. Trainees entered the camps for a 10-week training period at the start of May and November each year. Individuals aged ≥18 years entering one of the two army barracks involved in the study were eligible for enrolment. Suspected tuberculosis cases or individuals with immune deficiencies, such as acquired immune deficiency syndrome, leukemia or lymphoma, were excluded.

Throat and anterior nasal swab samples were collected using stiff synthetic swabs by trained study staff at the start and end of each training period (non-acute samples) and were placed in viral transport media (Universal Transport Medium C330; Copan Diagnostics) and stored at − 20 °C until time of transfer to the Armed Forces Research Institute of Medical Sciences for further testing. In addition, enrolled participants were asked to consult the camp's medical unit if they experienced respiratory symptoms during the training period. Medical staff took a history, conducted a medical exam, and recorded symptoms of upper respiratory illness (URI) or influenza-like illness (ILI). URI was defined as an illness with at least two of the following: (i) runny nose or sneezing; (ii) nasal congestion; (iii) sore throat, hoarseness or difficulty swallowing; (iv) cough; (v) swollen or tender glands in the neck; and (vi) fever (oral temperature > 38 °C). ILI was defined as a respiratory illness with acute onset presenting with fever and cough or sore throat. Throat and nasal swab samples were collected on average 1.8 days after symptom onset from individuals who developed URI or ILI during the 10-week follow-up (acute samples).

Laboratory investigations

Specimens from two of the six cohorts (total number of individuals = 274) were tested using a commercial multiplex real-time PCR assay comprising 33 bacterial, viral and fungal targets according to the manufacturer's instructions (FTD33 kit, Fast Track Diagnostics, Esch-sur-Alzette, Luxembourg). These two cohorts were selected because they underwent concurrent routine environmental sampling of air and surfaces within the barracks, which were then similarly tested using the FTD33 kit (data not shown). Multiplex testing of specimens from the remaining cohorts was not done due to resource constraints. A cycle threshold (Ct) value below the detection limit of the assay (< 33) was considered a positive result.

Statistical analyses

Non-acute samples collected at the end of the training period from participants who experienced an acute episode during follow-up were excluded from the analysis, as the Ct-value might reflect post-infectious shedding. We used the McNemar test to determine whether target-specific frequencies were significantly different in non-acute baseline samples and acute samples. In addition, we computed the chi-square (χ^2) or Fisher's exact test (for expected values < 5) to assess whether co-detection of specific microbe pairs occurred more frequently than expected by chance in non-acute baseline or acute samples. To account for data censoring at Ct-value = 33, random effects tobit regression models were used to compare Ct-value distributions from non-acute and acute samples, or Ct-value distributions from samples containing a single or multiple organisms. In addition, we used the Kruskal-Wallis test to compare the median delay between illness onset and sample collection between samples containing one or multiple organisms.

All analyses were conducted using Stata 12 software (Stata Corporation).

Ethics, consent and permissions

The study was approved by the Institutional Review Boards of the Royal Thai Army in Bangkok, Thailand, the Walter Reed Army Institute of Research and the London School of Hygiene & Tropical Medicine. All participants provided written informed consent. The investigators have adhered to the policies for protection of human subjects as prescribed in Army Regulation 70–25.

Results

Microbe frequencies

We analyzed a total of 312 non-acute swab samples collected from 211 recruits at the start ($n = 210$) or end ($n = 102$) of the training period, and 145 acute specimens from 137 individuals who developed one or more URI episodes during follow-up. Of 33 targets contained in the respiratory panel, 19 were detected in at least one specimen (Table 1). Viruses were detected in 13.8% (43/312) and bacteria in 93.3% (291/312) of non-acute samples. Among acute samples, viruses were detected in 44.1% (64/145) and bacteria in 94.5% (137/145) of specimens.

Haemophilus influenzae type B (Hi-B) was the most commonly detected microbe (77.9% of non-acute and 64.8% of acute samples). Other frequently detected bacteria included non-type B *Haemophilus influenzae* (Hi-nonB), *Streptococcus pneumoniae*, and *Klebsiella pneumoniae* (Table 1). Rhinovirus was the most prevalent virus, detected in 6.4% of non-acute and 26.9% of acute samples. All other viruses were detected in < 10% of collected specimens (Table 1).

Hi-nonB, rhinovirus, and coronavirus 229 were detected significantly less frequently in non-acute samples collected at the start of the training period than acute samples (p-values < 0.05) (Table 1). Influenza B was identified in none of the non-acute, but 9.7% of acute specimens.

Frequency of microbe co-detection

Multiple microbes were detected in 47.1% (99/210) of non-acute samples collected at the start of the training period. Co-detection of multiple organisms was significantly higher in both non-acute samples taken at the end of the training period (77.5%) and acute specimens (71.7%) (p-values < 0.001; Table 2). Among acute samples, 9 specific organism pairs were co-detected more frequently than expected by chance (p-values < 0.05) (Table 3; Fig. 1). Hi-B was identified together with Hi-nonB or rhinovirus in 32.4% (47/145) and 22.1% (32/145) of acute samples, respectively. Co-detection of influenza B virus and Hi-nonB occurred in 8.3% (12/145) of acute samples, while the remaining organism pairs

Table 1 Median cycle threshold (Ct) values and interquartile range (IQR) for microbes identified in throat and nasal swab samples. Non-acute samples were collected from Royal Thai Army barracks trainees at the start (R0) and at the end (RF) of each 10-week training period. Acute samples were collected from trainees who developed acute upper respiratory tract infection during follow-up. Percentages indicate the proportion of collected samples positive for each organism

	Non-acute ($n = 312$)						Acute ($n = 145$)			p-value[a]
	R0 ($n = 210$)			RF ($n = 102$)						
	% (n)	Median Ct	IQR	% (n)	Median Ct	IQR	% (n)	Median Ct	IQR	
Bacteria										
H. influenzae B	83.8 (176)	28.3	26.5–29.6	65.7 (67)	29.7	28.6–31.4	64.8 (94)	29.4	28.0–31.3	0.297
H. influenzae non-B	31.9 (67)	30.2	28.4–31.1	73.5 (75)	24.9	22.1–27.1	56.6 (82)	26.7	22.0–29.0	< 0.001
S. pneumoniae	8.1 (17)	29.6	27.7–30.7	34.3 (35)	28.0	26.1–31.0	15.2 (22)	27.1	26.5–29.2	0.706
K. pneumoniae	14.3 (30)	31.2	28.3–32.7	9.8 (10)	29.0	26.8–32.0	15.9 (23)	31.4	29.7–32.3	0.706
S. aureus	10.5 (22)	31.3	30.4–32.5	9.8 (10)	31.4	31.1–32.2	6.2 (9)	31.1	30.6–31.6	0.739
M. catarrhalis	2.4 (5)	30.6	27.7–31.5	3.9 (4)	32.6	32.2–32.8	6.2 (9)	29.7	29.5–31.5	0.564
L. pneumophila	2.4 (5)	32.1	31.4–32.4	2.0 (2)	31.3	30.3–32.4	2.8 (4)	32.5	31.2–32.8	0.317
Viruses										
Rhinovirus	1.9 (4)	30.6	28.6–31.8	15.7 (16)	30.2	27.2–31.7	26.9 (39)	28.9	26.9–31.4	< 0.001
Adenovirus	0.5 (1)	27.2	27.2–27.2	9.8 (10)	30.5	29.6–31.4	2.8 (4)	29.3	27.0–31.0	0.083
Influenza B	0 (0)	–	–	0 (0)	–	–	9.7 (14)	25.4	23.6–31.2	–
Coronavirus 229	1 (2)	23.1	18.2–28.0	2.0 (2)	29.3	27.2–31.5	4.8 (7)	26.9	25.2–31.3	0.034
Enterovirus	0.5 (1)	30.7	30.7–30.7	4.9 (5)	30.2	30.1–30.3	0 (0)	–	–	–
Coronavirus 63	1 (2)	28.5	24.5–32.4	1.0 (1)	30.0	30.0–30.0	1.4 (2)	22.6	21.9–23.3	0.157
Coronavirus HKU	0.5 (1)	30.0	30.0–30.0	0 (0)	–	–	2.1 (3)	32.2	31.6–32.9	–
Parainfluenza 2	0.5 (1)	17.4	17.4–17.4	1.0 (1)	25.3	25.3–25.3	1.4 (2)	23.3	20.1–26.5	0.564
Parainfluenza 4	0.5 (1)	32.0	32.0–32.0	0 (0)	–	–	1.4 (2)	30.3	30.0–30.6	0.317
Coronavirus 43	0.5 (1)	28.1	28.1–28.1	0 (0)	–	–	0.7 (1)	32.6	32.6–32.6	–
Bocavirus	0.5 (1)	17.4	17.4–17.4	0 (0)	–	–	0 (0)	–	–	–
Influenza A	0 (0)	–	–	0 (0)	–	–	0.7 (1)	29.9	29.9–29.9	–

[a] p-value for difference in proportion of positive samples in non-acute samples collected at the start (R0) of the training period or acute samples from individuals who developed URI during follow-up, as computed by McNemar test

Table 2 Frequency of single and multiple infections. Non-acute specimens were collected at the start (R0) or end (RF) of the training period. Acute samples were collected from individuals who developed an acute upper respiratory tract infection during follow-up. Percentages indicate proportion of specimens in which no microbe, a single, or multiple microbes were detected

	Non-acute		Acute	Total
	R0 (n = 210)	RF (n= 102)	(n = 145)	(n= 457)
Negative for all microbes	5.2% (11)	6.9% (7)	4.1% (6)	5.3% (24)
1 microbe detected	47.6% (100)	15.7% (16)	24.1% (35)	33.0% (151)
> 1 microbe detected	47.1% (99)	77.5% (79)	71.7% (104)	61.7% (282)

were found in < 5% of acute specimens (Table 3). No microbe pair occurred more frequently than expected by chance among non-acute baseline samples.

Microbial load

Overall, there was a substantial overlap in Ct-value distributions from non-acute samples collected at the start or end of the training period and acute samples collected from symptomatic individuals during follow-up (Fig. 2). This was the case even when considering only samples where a single organism was identified (Fig. 3).

For Hi-nonB and *S. pneumoniae*, our tobit regression models indicated significantly lower microbial load in non-acute baseline compared to acute samples (p-values < 0.05) (Table 4). For Hi-nonB, a coefficient of 5.56 represents a 5.56 higher average Ct-value in non-acute baseline samples compared to acute specimens, which corresponds to an approximately 47-fold lower microbial load in non-acute compared to acute samples. For *S. pneumoniae*, the average microbial load was 8.2-fold lower in non-acute baseline samples compared to acute specimens. Our analysis also indicated a significantly lower average rhinovirus load in non-acute samples collected either at the start or at the end of the training period compared to acute samples (p-values < 0.05) (Table 4). This was in contrast with Hi-B, for which regression analysis indicated a 4.7-fold higher average microbial load in non-acute baseline samples compared to acute samples (p-value < 0.001) (Table 4). For Hi-non B and *S. pneumoniae*, there was a 7.7-fold or 19.4-fold increase in average microbial load in non-acute samples collected at the end of follow-up compared to acute samples collected during an URI episode, respectively (p-values ≤0.002).

Time to sample collection

There was no significant difference in delay between symptom onset and specimen collection in acute samples containing one (median delay: 2 days; interquartile range (IQR): 1–3) or more (median delay: 2 days; IQR: 1–3) organisms (p-value = 0.536). Six acute specimens were negative for all agents tested (median delay: 0.5 days; IQR: 0–1). Thus, sampling delay is unlikely to account for any observed differences in Ct-value distributions.

Discussion

Microbe frequencies

We analyzed the patterns of infection with common respiratory agents in a well-defined population of military recruits. The use of highly sensitive multiplex PCR diagnostics allowed an accurate characterization of the spectrum of organisms contained in non-acute and acute samples.

Table 3 Frequency of co-detections with selected organism pairs among acute samples. Acute specimens were collected from individuals who developed upper respiratory tract infection during follow-up (n = 145)

Microbe 1	%(n) detected[a]	Microbe 2	%(n) detected[a]	%(n) co-detected[b]	p-value[c]
H. influenzae B	64.8 (94)	*H. influenzae non-B*	56.6 (82)	32.4 (47)	0.031
H. influenzae B	64.8 (94)	Rhinovirus	26.9 (39)	22.1 (32)	0.008
Influenza B	9.7 (14)	*H. influenzae non-B*	56.6 (82)	8.3 (12)	0.024*
H. influenzae B	64.8 (94)	*S. pneumoniae*	15.2 (22)	4.1 (6)	< 0.001
S. aureus	6.2 (9)	Rhinovirus	26.9 (39)	4.1 (6)	0.012*
S. pneumoniae	15.2 (22)	Influenza B	9.7 (14)	3.4 (5)	0.04*
H. influenzae B	64.8 (94)	Influenza B	9.7 (14)	2.1 (3)	0.001*
S. pneumoniae	15.2 (22)	Parainfluenza 2	1.4 (2)	1.4 (2)	0.022*
S. aureus	6.2 (9)	Human adenovirus	2.8 (4)	1.4 (2)	0.019*

[a]Percentages indicate proportion of acute samples where each microbe was identified

[b]Percentages indicate proportion of acute samples where each microbe pair was co-detected

[c]p-value computed by χ^2- or Fisher's exact (*) test, indicating that co-detection of each of the listed microbe pairs occurred more frequently than expected by chance

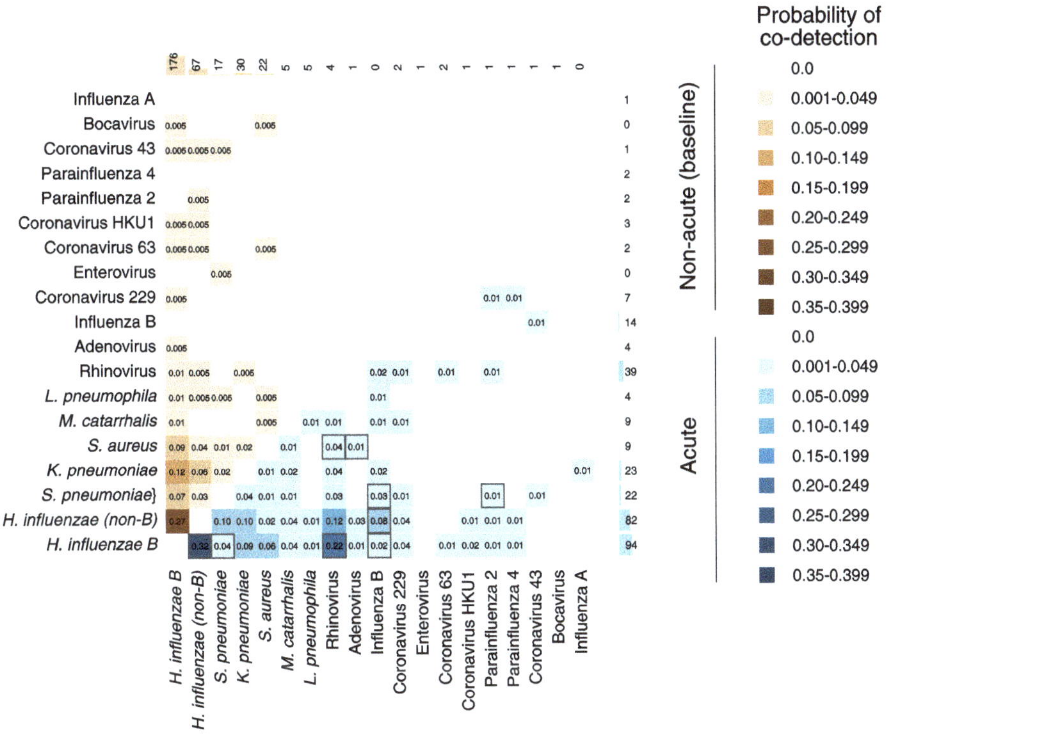

Fig. 1 Pairwise probabilities of co-detection of bacterial and viral agents. Probabilities indicate the percentage of non-acute baseline (orange shading; $n = 210$) or acute samples (blue shading; $n = 145$) positive with each microbe pair. Bar charts on the upper or right hand side indicate number of non-acute baseline or acute samples positive for each microbe, respectively. Dark box outlines indicate microbe pairs detected more frequently than expected by chance, as assessed by χ2- or Fisher's exact test (see also Table 3)

The data indicate co-circulation of several different viral agents, and high frequency of bacterial colonization in both non-acute and acute samples. Up to one third of respiratory illness cases among army personnel are reportedly caused by viral or bacterial infections [6]. The gathering of individuals from diverse geographic locations and the crowded living conditions increase the risk of microbe transmission in these settings [7]. Illnesses are usually self-limiting, although the emergence of highly virulent strains can lead to high morbidity and mortality [8]. *Streptococcus* bacteria, adenoviruses, coronaviruses and influenza are among the most widely distributed microbes in the military environment, and are implicated in > 50% of febrile illness cases reported at military medical facilities [6]. We identified each of these organisms in one or more samples. For most of these microbes, overall detection frequencies were comparable in non-acute and acute samples, although influenza B and coronavirus 229 were more commonly identified among acute specimens. Other infectious agents commonly circulating among military personnel include *H. influenzae*, rhinovirus, and, to a lesser extent, parainfluenza, RSV, and *L. pneumophila*, although their presence does not necessarily imply the occurrence of clinical symptoms [9–11]. *H. influenzae* and rhinoviruses were the most frequently detected organisms in our population in both non-acute and acute samples. We detected parainfluenza and *L. pneumophila*, but we did not find RSV in any of our samples.

Clinical relevance

For individuals developing URI during follow-up, illness etiology could not be unequivocally determined. Among acute samples, Hi-B was the most frequently detected organism. It was the sole agent identified in 12% of acute specimens, while it was co-detected with other microbes in > 50% of acute samples. However, colonisation with Hi-B was also common among non-acute baseline samples, where it was detected alone or in combination with other microbes in 40.5% and 43.3% of specimens, respectively.

For organisms rarely detected among asymptomatic individuals but frequently found in acute samples, a causal association may be more likely. For instance, influenza B was detected in none of the non-acute, but 9.7% of acute samples. Similarly, the proportion of both Hi-nonB- and rhinovirus-positive samples was significantly lower among non-acute specimens collected at baseline compared to acute samples. However, > 85% of acute samples positive for Hi-non B, rhinovirus or influenza B were also positive for one or more additional microbe, so that a causal

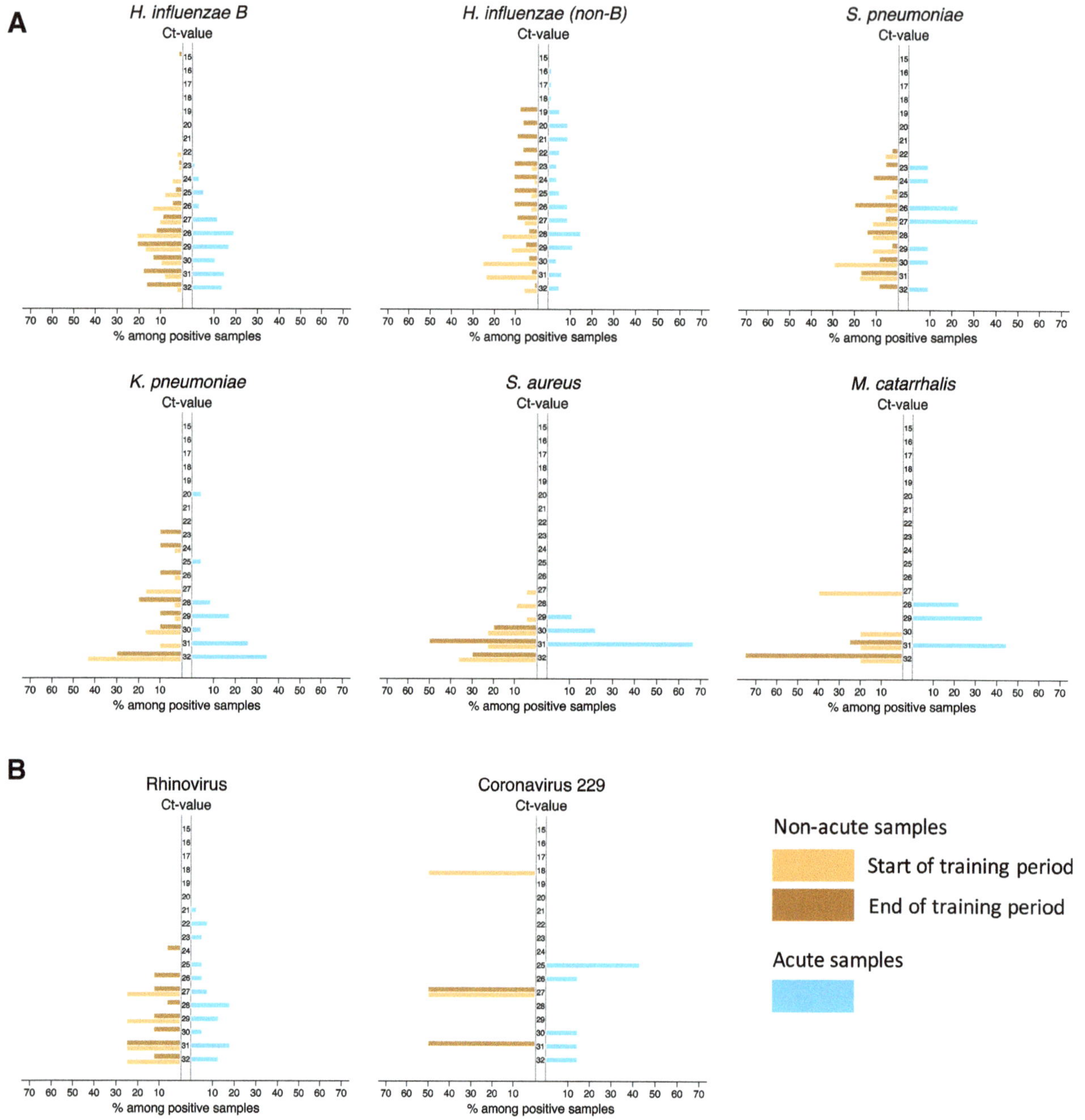

Fig. 2 Cycle threshold value distribution in non-acute and acute samples. Ct-value distribution for selected **a** bacteria and **b** viruses detected in non-acute samples collected at the start or end of the training period (orange bars) or acute samples from individuals experiencing an upper respiratory tract infection during follow-up (blue bars). A Ct-value of < 33 was considered a positive result

association could not be determined. Some agents, such as Hi-non B or adenovirus, were most frequently detected in non-acute samples collected at the end of follow-up, possibly indicating post-infectious shedding or persistent infection at sub-clinical levels.

In the clinical setting, overlapping clinical presentations and poor capabilities to determine the etiology of respiratory illnesses often lead to inappropriate treatment with broad-spectrum antibiotics [12]. This might occur even more frequently in the military setting, where molecular diagnostic tools are usually inaccessible [6]. Since a considerable fraction of respiratory illnesses is caused by viruses, the unsubstantiated use of antibiotics is particularly problematic, because it can lead to negative health outcomes and promote the development of antimicrobial resistance [3]. Studies evaluating the impact of multiplex diagnostic procedures on patient management report inconsistent results. In the outpatient setting, access to rapid molecular diagnostic tools for respiratory pathogens significantly reduced antibiotic

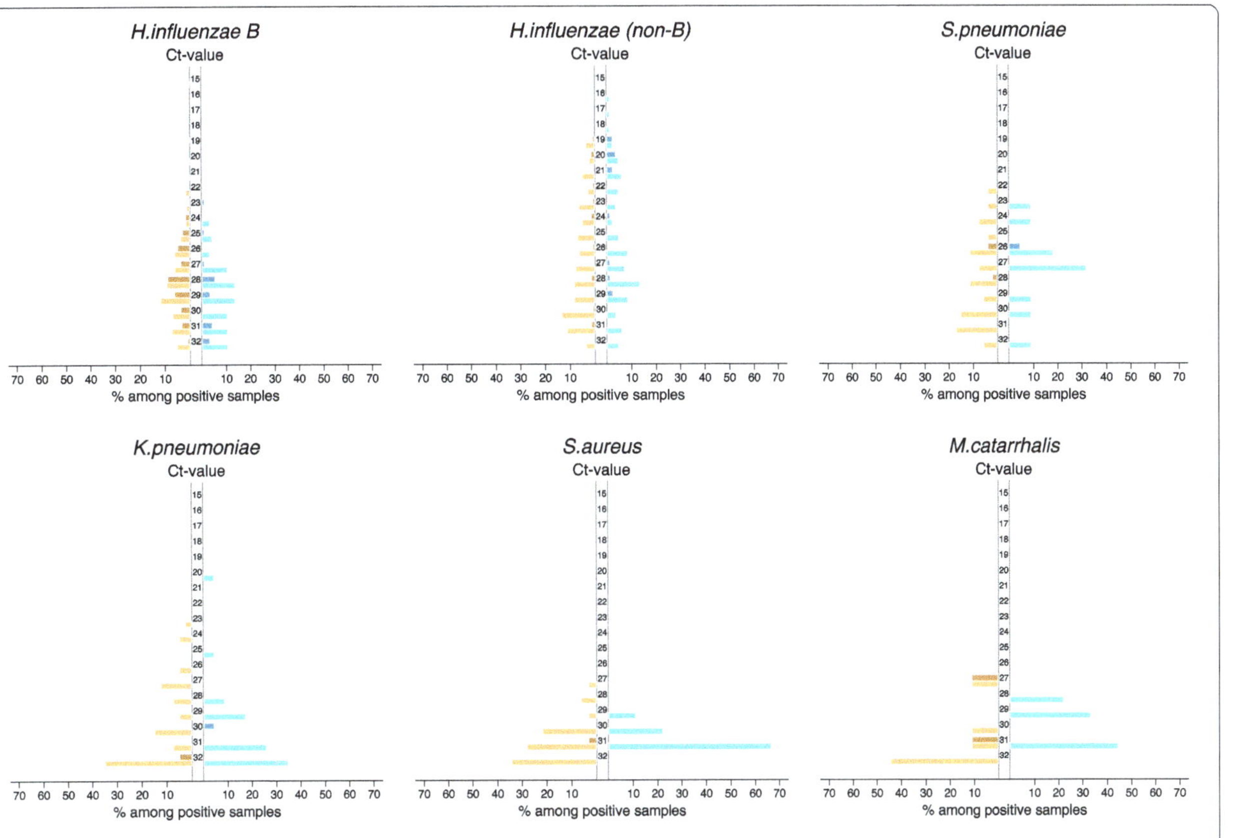

Fig. 3 Cycle threshold value distribution in samples containing one or multiple microbes. Ct-value distributions for selected bacteria detected in non-acute samples collected at the start or end of the training period (orange bars) and acute samples (blue bars) containing a single or multiple microbes. A Ct-value of < 33 was considered a positive result

Table 4 Tobit regression analysis. Tobit regression model assessing differences in Ct-value distributions in non-acute samples collected at the start (R0) or end (RF) of the training period and acute samples collected from symptomatic individuals during follow-up. Acute samples are used as a reference

Bacteria	Sample type	Coefficient	95%CI	*p*-value
H. influenzae B	R0	−2.22	−2.94; −1.49	< 0.001
	RF	0.11	−0.80; 1.02	0.809
H. influenza non-B	R0	5.56	4.05; 7.08	< 0.001
	RF	−2.95	−4.62; −1.27	0.001
S. pneumoniae	R0	3.04	0.41; 5.67	0.024
	RF	−4.28	−7.00; −1.56	0.002
K. pneumoniae	R0	0.52	−1.01; 2.05	0.506
	RF	1.45	−0.55; 3.45	0.155
S. aureus	R0	−0.98	−2.43; 0.47	0.186
	RF	−0.74	−2.47; 0.99	0.401
Viruses				
Rhinovirus	R0	10.04	6.49; 13.58	< 0.001
	RF	2.83	0.39; 5.27	0.023

prescription rates for patients presenting with respiratory illness [13]. However, these findings were not confirmed in the hospital setting. PCR-based testing failed to reduce hospital admissions and duration of hospital stay in patients with acute respiratory infection [14, 15]. Although molecular diagnostic tools may help to differentiate bacterial and viral respiratory agents, it is unlikely that antibacterial treatment would be terminated based on the mere presence of viral agents in an acute respiratory sample, especially considering the high rates of bacterial co-infection [16].

Microbial load

Quantitative or semi-quantitative diagnostic tools can potentially help define clinically significant pathogen densities, and have proven highly valuable to understand the dynamics of diarrheal disease [17] and to improve the management of gastrointestinal illnesses [18]. Among acute diarrhea patients, quantitative amplification of norovirus RNA from fecal samples can help determine pathogen load thresholds that effectively distinguish between causal association and sub-pathogenic carriage [19]. Similarly, rotavirus load correlates with disease severity among children with gastroenteritis [20]. Because of the crucial role of microbial replication in viral pathogenesis, the value of pathogen load quantitation could be most clearly established for gastrointestinal illnesses of viral etiology, although some evidence is available for bacterial infections as well. For instance, microbial load of enteropathogenic *E. coli* is significantly higher among children with diarrhea compared to control subjects, especially when enteropathogenic *E. coli* is the sole agent identified [21].

In this study, tobit regression indicated significantly lower microbial load in non-acute relative to acute samples for rhinovirus, HI-nonB, and *S. pneumoniae.* However, due to a substantial overlap in Ct-value distributions, it was not possible to identify a Ct-value threshold indicating causality for any of these organisms. Previous studies assessing the association of viral load with clinical symptoms of respiratory infections reported similar findings. Mean viral load for rhinovirus and six additional viruses was significantly higher in upper respiratory tract aspirates from children with pneumonia compared to healthy controls, but the overlap in viral load distribution was substantial [22]. In pediatric patients, high rhinovirus load was associated with the presence of lower respiratory tract symptoms [23, 24], but a threshold for clinical relevance could only be determined if rhinovirus was the sole agent identified [24]. Additional studies reported a correlation between microbial load and occurrence or severity of respiratory symptoms for RSV [25], bocavirus [26], and human metapneumovirus (HMPV) [27, 28], although these findings were inconsistent [29, 30] or conditional on the presence of the virus as a single microbe [31]. We did not detect any significant association between microbial load and clinical manifestations for viruses other than rhinovirus.

For both *H. influenzae* and *Streptococcus* species, previous studies reported a significant correlation of bacterial densities with clinical manifestations of disease [32]. In young patients with acute respiratory tract infection, *S. pneumoniae* load fluctuated with symptom incidence and resolution [33]. Among children hospitalized with pneumonia, median nasopharyngeal *S. pneumoniae* load was substantially higher compared to healthy controls [32]. Pneumococcal density was also associated with severity of symptoms [34] and increased duration of children's hospital stay [35]. Similar associations were observed in pneumonic adults, although the correlation was not significant in this population [36].

The association between microbial load and clinical manifestations may depend on specific pathogen-host interactions. If pathogenesis is primarily related to microbial replication, a stronger correlation between microbial load and illness magnitude may be observed [37]. If clinical manifestations are largely attributable to host immune defences or bacterial toxins, the correlation with microbial load may not be obvious [37]. Temporal variations in microbial load may also play an important role if the quantity of nucleic acid is significantly more abundant at the time and location of pathology [30, 33]. In acute respiratory illness patients, high bacterial colonization densities are often associated with the presence of viral co-infections [38], and clinical manifestations may vary depending on specific co-infection patterns [39].

The ecology of respiratory pathogens is also likely to be influenced by the living conditions in military settings. Mixing of individuals from diverse backgrounds living in close-quarters with high levels of inter-personal contact increases the potential for introduction and spread of multiple microbes in this population, which could account for the broad range of organisms and co-detections in this study.

Strengths and limitations

We analysed both non-acute and acute samples from a closely monitored population in a semi-closed, longitudinal setting. The study population was well-defined and relatively homogeneous with regards to demographics and living conditions. However, our findings may not be applicable to populations with different socio-demographic characteristics and populations outside the military environment, such as cohorts of children among whom the impact of respiratory infections may be greater.

The frequent co-detection of multiple respiratory agents and the failure to distinguish between viable and dead organisms, or microbes that colonize the host at sub-pathogenic levels, may prevent the unambiguous interpretation of test results [2]. A positive result may indicate illness aetiology, asymptomatic colonisation, post-infectious shedding, or an incipient infection. Therefore, Ct-values may not always be a reliable surrogate for infectious load.

Samples from only two out of six cohorts were tested by real-time PCR. Although there might be bias from seasonal effects, these are usually less pronounced in the tropics. Given the relatively low frequencies of viral detection, a larger sample size and a longer follow-up may have captured a more precise picture of infection patterns in this population. This study was also limited to the detection of organisms contained in the respiratory panel. We cannot exclude the presence of additional organisms in our specimens. In addition, the data were obtained from throat and nasal swab samples, but our findings may not apply to nasopharyngeal or sputum specimens. Finally, the quality and quantity of material obtained through nose and throat swabs may differ significantly among subjects, and the success of PCR-based methods also depends on the availability of intact genome sequences and the absence of random mutations.

Conclusions

Overall, the multiplex respiratory panel provided a comprehensive characterization of the microbe spectrum contained in non-acute and acute respiratory samples collected among recruits. However, semi-quantitative assessment of microbial load could not reliably distinguish between symptomatic and asymptomatic samples. More research is warranted to compare new multiplex diagnostic techniques with traditional methods and evaluate their potential with regards to diagnostic accuracy [40] and clinical utility [16, 40] in the context of respiratory infections.

Abbreviations

PCR: Polymerase chain reactionURIUpper respiratory illnessILIInfluenza-like illnessFTDFast Track DiagnosticsCtCycle thresholdHi-B*Haemophilus influenzae* type BHi-nonBnon-type B *Haemophilus influenzae*IQRInterquartile rangeHMPVHuman metapneumovirus

Acknowledgements

We are grateful to the participants of this study, the Royal Thai Army, and the clinical, laboratory and administrative personnel at AFRIMS. Material has been reviewed by the Walter Reed Army Institute of Research. There is no objection to its presentation and/or publication. The opinions or assertions contained herein are the private views of the authors, and are not to be construed as official, or as reflecting true views of the Department of the Army or the Department of Defense.

Funding

This work was supported by the United States Department of Defense - Global Emerging Infectious Disease Surveillance (DoD - GEIS), Protocol 989A.

Author's contributions

CCT conceived the idea for this paper, VO conducted the analysis and wrote the manuscript. KA, AW, LM, DE, RR, and SS participated in project oversight. SF, RG, RR, SS, and IY participated in the design of the study. All authors contributed to drafting the manuscript and approved the final submission.

Consent for publication

Not applicable.

Competing interests

CCT is associate editor for *BMC Infectious Diseases*, research area Viral Diseases. All other authors declare that they have no competing interests.

Author details

[1]Saw Swee Hock School of Public Health, National University of Singapore and National University Health System, Singapore 117549, Singapore. [2]London School of Hygiene & Tropical Medicine, WC1E7HT, London, UK. [3]University of Minnesota, Minneapolis 55455, USA. [4]Armed Forces Research Institute of Medical Sciences, Bangkok 10400, Thailand. [5]Phramongkutklao College of Medicine, Bangkok 10400, Thailand. [6]University of Texas at San Antonio, San Antonio 78249, USA. [7]International Vaccine Institute, Seoul 08826, South Korea. [8]Phramongkutklao Hospital, Bangkok 10400, Thailand.

References

1. Reddington K, Tuite N, Barry T, O'Grady J, Zumla A. Advances in multiparametric molecular diagnostics technologies for respiratory tract infections. Curr Opin Pulm Med. 2013;19:298–304. https://doi.org/10.1097/MCP.0b013e32835f1b32.
2. Gray J, Coupland LJ. The increasing application of multiplex nucleic acid detection tests to the diagnosis of syndromic infections. Epidemiol Infect. 2014;142:1–11. https://doi.org/10.1017/S0950268813002367.
3. Infectious Diseases Society of A. An unmet medical need: rapid molecular diagnostics tests for respiratory tract infections. Clin Infect Dis. 2011;52 Suppl 4:S384–95. https://doi.org/10.1093/cid/cir055.
4. Jansen RR, Wieringa J, Koekkoek SM, Visser CE, Pajkrt D, Molenkamp R, et al. Frequent detection of respiratory viruses without symptoms: toward defining clinically relevant cutoff values. J Clin Microbiol. 2011;49:2631–6. https://doi.org/10.1128/JCM.02094-10.
5. Levy JW, Bhoomiboonchoo P, Simasathien S, Salje H, Huang A, Rangsin R, et al. Elevated transmission of upper respiratory illness among new recruits in military barracks in Thailand. Influenza Other Respir Viruses. 2015;9:308–14. https://doi.org/10.1111/irv.12345.
6. Korzeniewski K, Nitsch-Osuch A, Konior M, Lass A. Respiratory tract infections in the military environment. Respir Physiol Neurobiol. 2015;209:76–80. https://doi.org/10.1016/j.resp.2014.09.016.
7. Korzeniewski K, Nitsch-Osuch A, Chciałowski A, Korsak J. Environmental factors, immune changes and respiratory diseases in troops during military activities. Respir Physiol Neurobiol. 2013;187:118–22. https://doi.org/10.1016/j.resp.2013.02.003.
8. Aligne CA. Overcrowding and mortality during the influenza pandemic of 1918. Am J Public Health. 2016;106:642–4. https://doi.org/10.2105/AJPH.2015.303018.
9. Wang Z, Malanoski AP, Lin B, Long NC, Leski TA, Blaney KM, et al. Broad spectrum respiratory pathogen analysis of throat swabs from military recruits reveals interference between rhinoviruses and adenoviruses. Microb Ecol. 2010;59:623–34. https://doi.org/10.1007/s00248-010-9636-3.
10. Gray GC, Callahan JD, Hawksworth AW, Fisher CA, Gaydos JC. Respiratory diseases among U.S. military personnel: countering emerging threats. Emerg Infect Dis. 1999;5:379–85. https://doi.org/10.3201/eid0503.990308.
11. Eick AA, Faix DJ, Tobler SK, Nevin RL, Lindler LE, Hu Z, et al. Serosurvey of bacterial and viral respiratory pathogens among deployed U.S. service members. Am J Prev Med. 2011;41:573–80. https://doi.org/10.1016/j.amepre.2011.08.006.
12. McGeer A, Green KA, Plevneshi A, Shigayeva A, Siddiqi N, Raboud J, et al. Antiviral therapy and outcomes of influenza requiring hospitalization in Ontario. Canada Clin Infect Dis. 2007;45:1568–75. https://doi.org/10.1086/523584.
13. Brittain-Long R, Westin J, Olofsson S, Lindh M, Andersson L-M. Access to a polymerase chain reaction assay method targeting 13 respiratory viruses can reduce antibiotics: a randomised, controlled trial. BMC Med. 2011;9:44. https://doi.org/10.1186/1741-7015-9-44.
14. Oosterheert JJ, van Loon AM, Schuurman R, Hoepelman AI, Hak E, Thijsen S, et al. Impact of rapid detection of viral and atypical bacterial pathogens by real-time polymerase chain reaction for patients with lower respiratory tract infection. Clin Infect Dis. 2005;41:1438–44. https://doi.org/10.1086/497134.
15. Wishaupt JO, Russcher A, Smeets LC, Versteegh FGA, Hartwig NG. Clinical impact of RT-PCR for pediatric acute respiratory infections: a controlled clinical trial. Pediatrics. 2011;128:e1113–20. https://doi.org/10.1542/peds.2010-2779.
16. Murdoch DR. Impact of rapid microbiological testing on the Management of Lower Respiratory Tract Infection. Clin Infect Dis. 2005;41:1445–7. https://doi.org/10.1086/497145.
17. Binnicker MJ. Multiplex molecular panels for diagnosis of gastrointestinal infection: performance, result interpretation, and cost-effectiveness. J Clin Microbiol. 2015;53:3723–8. https://doi.org/10.1128/JCM.02103-15.

18. Rand KH, Tremblay EE, Hoidal M, Fisher LB, Grau KR, Karst SM. Multiplex gastrointestinal pathogen panels: implications for infection control. Diagn Microbiol Infect Dis. 2015;82:154–7. https://doi.org/10.1016/j.diagmicrobio.2015.01.007.
19. Phillips G, Lopman B, Tam CC, Iturriza-Gomara M, Brown D, Gray J. Diagnosing norovirus-associated infectious intestinal disease using viral load. BMC Infect Dis. 2009;9:63. https://doi.org/10.1186/1471-2334-9-63.
20. Kang G, Iturriza-Gomara M, Wheeler JG, Crystal P, Monica B, Ramani S, et al. Quantitation of group a rotavirus by real-time reverse-transcription-polymerase chain reaction: correlation with clinical severity in children in South India. J Med Virol. 2004;73:118–22. https://doi.org/10.1002/jmv.20053.
21. Barletta F, Ochoa TJ, Mercado E, Ruiz J, Ecker L, Lopez G, et al. Quantitative real-time polymerase chain reaction for enteropathogenic Escherichia coli: a tool for investigation of asymptomatic versus symptomatic infections. Clin Infect Dis. 2011;53:1223–9. https://doi.org/10.1093/cid/cir730.
22. Feikin DR, Fu W, Park DE, Shi Q, Higdon MM, Baggett HC, et al. Is Higher Viral Load in the Upper Respiratory Tract Associated With Severe Pneumonia? Findings From the PERCH Study. Clin Infect Dis. 2017;64 suppl_3:S337–S346. doi:https://doi.org/10.1093/cid/cix148.
23. Utokaparch S, Marchant D, Gosselink JV, McDonough JE, Thomas EE, Hogg JC, et al. The relationship between respiratory viral loads and diagnosis in children presenting to a pediatric hospital emergency department. Pediatr Infect Dis J. 2011;30:e18–23. https://doi.org/10.1097/INF.0b013e3181ff2fac.
24. Gerna G, Piralla A, Rovida F, Rognoni V, Marchi A, Locatelli F, et al. Correlation of rhinovirus load in the respiratory tract and clinical symptoms in hospitalized immunocompetent and immunocompromised patients. J Med Virol. 2009;81:1498–507. https://doi.org/10.1002/jmv.21548.
25. Gerna G, Campanini G, Rognoni V, Marchi A, Rovida F, Piralla A, et al. Correlation of viral load as determined by real-time RT-PCR and clinical characteristics of respiratory syncytial virus lower respiratory tract infections in early infancy. J Clin Virol. 2008;41:45–8. https://doi.org/10.1016/j.jcv.2007.10.018.
26. Jiang W, Yin F, Zhou W, Yan Y, Ji W. Clinical significance of different virus load of human bocavirus in patients with lower respiratory tract infection. Sci Rep. 2016;6:20246. https://doi.org/10.1038/srep20246.
27. Bosis S, Esposito S, Osterhaus ADME, Tremolati E, Begliatti E, Tagliabue C, et al. Association between high nasopharyngeal viral load and disease severity in children with human metapneumovirus infection. J Clin Virol. 2008;42:286–90. https://doi.org/10.1016/j.jcv.2008.03.029.
28. Martin ET, Kuypers J, Heugel J, Englund JA. Clinical disease and viral load in children infected with respiratory syncytial virus or human metapneumovirus. Diagn Microbiol Infect Dis. 2008;62:382–8. https://doi.org/10.1016/j.diagmicrobio.2008.08.002.
29. Yan X-L, Li Y-N, Tang Y-J, Xie Z-P, Gao H-C, Yang X-M, et al. Clinical characteristics and viral load of respiratory syncytial virus and human metapneumovirus in children hospitaled for acute lower respiratory tract infection. J Med Virol. 2017;89:589–97. https://doi.org/10.1002/jmv.24687.
30. Peng D, Zhao X, Liu E, Huang Y, Yang X, Zhao Y, et al. Analysis of viral load in children infected with human metapneumovirus. Iran J Pediatr. 2010;20:393–400. http://www.ncbi.nlm.nih.gov/pubmed/23056737. Accessed 4 Aug 2017
31. Christensen A, Nordbo SA, Krokstad S, Rognlien AG, Dollner H. Human bocavirus in children: mono-detection, high viral load and viraemia are associated with respiratory tract infection. J Clin Virol. 2010;49:158–62. https://doi.org/10.1016/j.jcv.2010.07.016.
32. Vu HTT, Yoshida LM, Suzuki M, Nguyen HAT, Nguyen CDL, Nguyen ATT, et al. Association between nasopharyngeal load of Streptococcus pneumoniae, viral coinfection, and radiologically confirmed pneumonia in Vietnamese children. Pediatr Infect Dis J. 2011;30:11–8. https://doi.org/10.1097/INF.0b013e3181f111a2.
33. Fan RR, Howard LM, Griffin MR, Edwards KM, Zhu Y, Williams JV, et al. Nasopharyngeal pneumococcal density and evolution of acute respiratory illnesses in young children, Peru, 2009-2011. Emerg Infect Dis. 2016;22:1996–9. https://doi.org/10.3201/eid2211.160902.
34. Esposito S, Marchese A, Tozzi AE, Rossi GA, Da Dalt L, Bona G, et al. DNA bacterial load in children with bacteremic pneumococcal community-acquired pneumonia. Eur J Clin Microbiol Infect Dis. 2013;32:877–81. https://doi.org/10.1007/s10096-013-1821-0.
35. Muñoz-Almagro C, Gala S, Selva L, Jordan I, Tarragó D, Pallares R. DNA bacterial load in children and adolescents with pneumococcal pneumonia and empyema. Eur J Clin Microbiol Infect Dis. 2011;30:327–35. https://doi.org/10.1007/s10096-010-1086-9.
36. Gadsby NJ, Russell CD, McHugh MP, Mark H, Conway Morris A, Laurenson IF, et al. Comprehensive molecular testing for respiratory pathogens in community-acquired pneumonia. Clin Infect Dis. 2016;62:817–23. https://doi.org/10.1093/cid/civ1214.
37. Platts-Mills JA, Liu J, Houpt ER. New concepts in diagnostics for infectious diarrhea. Mucosal Immunol. 2013;6:876–85. https://doi.org/10.1038/mi.2013.50.
38. Wolter N, Tempia S, Cohen C, Madhi SA, Venter M, Moyes J, et al. High nasopharyngeal pneumococcal density, increased by viral coinfection, is associated with invasive pneumococcal pneumonia. J Infect Dis. 2014;210:1649–57. https://doi.org/10.1093/infdis/jiu326.
39. Tenenbaum T, Franz A, Neuhausen N, Willems R, Brade J, Schweitzer-Krantz S, et al. Clinical characteristics of children with lower respiratory tract infections are dependent on the carriage of specific pathogens in the nasopharynx. Eur J Clin Microbiol Infect Dis. 2012;31:3173–82. https://doi.org/10.1007/s10096-012-1682-y.
40. Gadsby NJ, McHugh MP, Russell CD, Mark H, Conway Morris A, Laurenson IF, et al. Development of two real-time multiplex PCR assays for the detection and quantification of eight key bacterial pathogens in lower respiratory tract infections. Clin Microbiol Infect. 2015;21:788.e1–788.e13. https://doi.org/10.1016/j.cmi.2015.05.004.

Complications of miliary tuberculosis: low mortality and predictive biomarkers from a UK cohort

Jonathan Underwood[1*], Fiona Cresswell[2], Alex P Salam[3], Alex J Keeley[4], Charles Cleland[5], Laurence John[6] and Robert N Davidson[6]

Abstract

Background: Untreated, miliary tuberculosis (TB) has a mortality approaching 100%. As it is uncommon there is little specific data to guide its management. We report detailed data from a UK cohort of patients with miliary tuberculosis and the associations and predictive ability of admission blood tests with clinical outcomes.

Methods: Routinely collected demographic, clinical, blood, imaging, histopathological and microbiological data were assessed for all patients with miliary TB identified from the London TB register from 2008 to 2012 from Northwest London Hospitals NHS Trust. Multivariable logistic regression was used to assess factors independently associated with the need for critical care intervention. Receiver operator characteristics (ROC) were calculated to assess the discriminatory ability of admission blood tests to predict clinical outcomes.

Results: Fifty-two patients were identified with miliary tuberculosis, of whom 29% had confirmed central nervous system (CNS) involvement. Magnetic resonance imaging (MRI) was more sensitive than computed tomography (CT) or lumbar puncture for detecting CNS disease. Severe complications were frequent, with 15% requiring critical care intervention with mechanical ventilation. This was independently associated with admission hyponatraemia and elevated alanine aminotransferase (ALT). Having an admission sodium ≥125 mmol/L and an ALT <180 IU/L had 82% sensitivity and 100% specificity for predicting a favourable outcome with an area under the ROC curve (AUC) of 0.91. Despite the frequency of severe complications, one-year mortality was low at 2%.

Conclusions: Although severe complications of miliary tuberculosis were frequent, mortality was low with timely access to critical care intervention, anti-tuberculous therapy and possibly corticosteroid use. Clinical outcomes could accurately be predicted using routinely collected biochemistry data.

Keywords: Tuberculosis, Miliary tuberculosis, Central nervous system infection, Mortality, Biomarkers

Background

Tuberculosis is one of the leading causes of death from infectious diseases worldwide [1]. Miliary tuberculosis results from widespread haematogenous spread of the *Mycobacterium tuberculosis* bacilli (TB). Clinical presentations are protean and vary from vague constitutional upset in ambulatory patients to abrupt multi-organ failure [2]. Untreated, miliary TB has a mortality approaching 100% [3], reducing to 7.1-30% with treatment [2, 4–6].

Miliary TB is uncommon, comprising 1-2% of TB cases [2], thus specific data regarding its management, particularly the ability to identify patients at high risk of poor outcomes, are lacking [2]. Current treatment guidelines are largely extrapolated from randomised controlled trials of pulmonary TB rather than specific trials of patients with miliary TB. As such, insights provided by cohort studies are important in guiding best practice. However, most cohorts are small and from the developing world, with limited neuroimaging and microbiological data. We sought to characterise the clinical course, investigation findings, and outcomes of a cohort with miliary TB from an ethnically

* Correspondence: jonathan.underwood@imperial.ac.uk
[1]Division of Infectious Diseases, Imperial College London, London, UK
Full list of author information is available at the end of the article

diverse population with one of the highest TB incidences in the UK [7].

Methods

Participants

Patients with miliary TB were identified from the London TB register (LTBR) from 2008 to 2012 at Northwest London Hospitals NHS Trust. These records were cross-checked against the hospital database of all in-patient admissions.

Data collection

Diagnosis of miliary TB was confirmed by identification of the characteristic miliary pattern on chest radiograph or computed tomography (CT) along with one or more of the following features: clinical features compatible with TB and response to anti-tuberculous therapy (ATT); histopathological evidence of TB; microbiological evidence of TB (positive smear or culture). Demographic, clinical, biochemical, radiological, histopathological evidence of TB (caseating or non-caseating granulomas with or without acid-alcohol fast bacilli on Ziehl-Neelson staining), and microbiological data were obtained from the LTBR and the hospital electronic patient records.

Statistical analysis and biomarker selection

Univariate analysis of continuous data was performed using t-tests and the Mann-Whitney U tests as appropriate. For subsequent biomarker analysis, the primary outcome of interest, defined as an 'unfavourable outcome', was the need for critical care intervention with mechanical intervention. Whereas, a 'favourable outcome' was defined as not requiring critical care intervention with mechanical ventilation.

Multivariable logistic regression ($p < 0.1$ for entry from univariable logistic regression) was used to assess factors associated with the need for critical care intervention. Biomarkers that were independently associated with the need for critical care intervention (i.e. an 'unfavourable outcome') in the multivariable model were then assessed for their predictive performance by determining their receiver operator characteristics (ROC). Biomarker classification thresholds were determined by optimising the balance of sensitivity and specificity. Biomarker classification performance was assessed and thresholds determined using the area under the ROC curve (AUC). This is equivalent to the balanced accuracy of the classifier (i.e. accuracy taking account of differences in prevalence of the outcome between groups) for both 'favourable' (i.e. not requiring critical care intervention) and 'unfavourable' outcomes. Additionally, sensitivity, specificity, positive and negative predictive values were calculated. Confidence intervals were determined using bootstrapping with 1000 replicates.

Biomarkers were combined using an exhaustive grid across the range of all possible values and combinations to determine the optimum threshold for each biomarker in combination so that the AUC was maximised.

Biomarker validation

Given the relatively small size of the dataset, splitting the data into separate training and testing datasets would be subject to bias. Therefore, to validate the predictive rule in this dataset, a leave-one-out-cross-validation (LOOCV) scheme was used. This entailed leaving one subject out of the dataset, then performing an exhaustive grid search, as before, to determine the optimal thresholds for the biomarker(s) of interest. This threshold(s) was then applied to the case that was left out. These steps were then repeated and summary statistics across the range of folds were calculated. Accuracy was determined by the percentage of correct responses across all the cross-validation folds.

Results

Baseline characteristics

Table 1 summarises the demographic data, investigations and clinical outcomes of the cohort of 52 patients with miliary TB. Thirty-six (69%) had typical miliary changes on chest radiographs with the remainder having miliary appearances confirmed on chest CT. The majority of patients (90%) were not born in the UK, had no significant comorbidity, and were nearly all (94%) vitamin D deficient. Half (14/24) had tuberculin skin test anergy and 6% were HIV co-infected. All but one patient (98%) were admitted to hospital with a median length of stay of 11 days (range 1 – 233 days).

Neuroimaging

Nineteen patients (37%) had a CT brain scan performed on their initial admission. Of these, 6 (31%) had ring-enhancing lesions typical of tuberculomas. Eleven patients (21%) underwent magnetic resonance imaging (MRI) of their brain, of whom 10 (91%) demonstrated tuberculomas. Notably, 4 patients with normal/nonspecific admission CT had subsequent MRI because due to clinical concern of neurological disease, all of whom demonstrated tuberculomas. The overall prevalence of tuberculomas seen on MRI or CT was 12 of 23 (52%), but we may have missed lesions in the 29 patients who did not undergo neuroimaging, and in patients in whom tuberculomas developed subsequently.

Microbiology

Forty patients (77%) had positive cultures for *M. tuberculosis* (MTB) complex. Induced sputa lead to a positive culture in thirty (58%) patients. Only ten sputum samples (19%)

Table 1 Baseline characteristics, co-morbidities, admission blood tests, neurological tests and outcomes of a UK cohort of patients with miliary tuberculosis

Variable	n (%) or median (range)
Age (years)	41 (10-87)
Sex	
Male	31 (60%)
Ethnic Origin	
Asian	32 (62%)
Black-African	11 (21%)
White	5 (10%)
Other	4 (8%)
Previous diagnosis of TB	2 (4%)
Co-morbidities	
None	33 (63%)
Diabetes	6 (12%)
CKD	4 (8%)
Anti-TNF therapy	3 (6%)
Alcoholism	3 (6%)
Heart failure	2 (4%)
HIV positive	3/49 (6%)
Hepatitis B sAg positive	3/49 (6%)
Hepatitis C positive	1/47 (2%)
Vitamin D deficient	44/57 (94%)
Admission blood tests	
Sodium (mmol/L)	132 (106-141)
Creatinine (mmol/L)	68 (44-559)
Alanine aminotransferase (IU/L)	46 (5-453)
Alkaline phosphatase (iU/L)	121 (39-866)
Bilirubin (μmol/L)	12 (4-39)
Erythrocyte sedimentation rate (mm/h)	33 (1-127)
C-reactive protein (mg/L)	56 (3-433)
White cell count ($\times 10^9$/L)	7.1 (1.1-17.0)
Neutrophil count ($\times 10^9$/L)	5.3 (0.9-15.7)
Platelet count ($\times 10^9$/L)	238 (53-574)
Ferritin (μg/L)	522 (10-19,070)
Vitamin D (nmol/L)	16 (2-117)
Assessment for CNS involvement	
Number of patients assessed for CNS infection	29 (56%)
- CT head consistent with CNS infection	6/19 (32%)
- MRI brain consistent with CNS infection	10/11 (91%)
- Lumbar puncture consistent with CNS infection	4/17 (24%)
Total number with confirmed CNS infection	15 (29%)
Outcomes and adverse events	
Death (by one-year)	1 (2%)
Mechanical ventilation	8 (15%)
Drug-induced hepatitis	7 (13%)
Seizure	4 (8%)
Pneumothorax	3 (6%)
Haemophagocytic lymphohistiocytosis	2 (4%)
Pericardial effusion	2 (4%)

Data are presented as n (%), except for age and blood tests results which are presented as median (range)
Abbreviations: *TB* Tuberculosis, *CKD* chronic kidney disease, *TNF* tumour necrosis factor, *HIV* human immunodeficiency virus, *CNS* central nervous system, *CT* computer tomography; MRI: magnetic resonance imaging, *sAG* surface antigen

revealed acid-alcohol fast bacilli (AFB) on microscopy. Seventeen patients (33%) had cerebrospinal fluid (CSF) examination. Of these, four (24%) had findings compatible with TB meningitis, all of whom subsequently cultured MTB (two of four [50%] had tuberculomas). Aside from sputa and CSF, MTB was cultured from joint (n = 2), pericardial (n = 2) and pleural (n = 1) fluids (n = 1), transbronchial biopsy (n = 1) and bone marrow (n = 1). Four (10%) were resistant to isoniazid, three (6%) to pyrazinamide, three (6%) to streptomycin, one to rifampicin and isoniazid (i.e. multidrug resistant – MDR) and none to ethambutol.

Treatment

All patients were commenced on quadruple ATT with most receiving rifampicin, isoniazid, pyrazinamide and ethambutol. Median (range) duration of ATT was 12 (1.5 – 28) months. Ten (19%) patients stopped pyrazinamide due to drug-induced liver injury (15%) or intolerance (4%). 29 patients (56%) received corticosteroids during their ATT for a variety of indications including central nervous system (CNS) involvement, systemic inflammatory response syndrome and paradoxical reactions.

Complications

Follow-up to one-year was complete for 49 patients (94%). One 87-year-old patient with multiple co-morbidities, including chronic renal failure, died during treatment (after 1.5 months' therapy). One patient died subsequently from constrictive pericarditis secondary to pericardial involvement, two years after successfully completing 12 months of ATT.

Eight patients (15%) required critical care intervention with mechanical ventilation, seven with respiratory failure and one with neurologic deterioration. Other serious adverse events are shown in Table 1. Corticosteroid use was more frequent (88% vs. 50%, p = 0.11) in patients that required mechanical ventilation. In a univariate model, requirement for mechanical ventilation was associated with thrombocytopenia (median platelet count in those needing: 148×10^9/L vs. not needing mechanical ventilation: 266×10^9/L, $p = 0.04$), hyponatraemia (125 vs. 133 mmol/L, $p = 0.03$), hyperbilirubinaemia (17 vs. 11 μmol/L, $p < 0.01$), and increased alanine aminotransferase (ALT: 196 vs. 35 IU/L, $p < 0.001$). There were borderline associations with increased erythrocyte sedimentation rate (37 vs. 18 mm/h, $p = 0.08$) and c-reactive protein (97 vs 48 mg/L, $p = 0.06$) among those requiring mechanical ventilation. There was no significant association between requirement for mechanical ventilation and age ($p = 0.72$), admission vitamin D ($p = 0.39$), total white cell count ($p = 0.14$), neutrophil count ($p = 0.45$), creatinine ($p = 0.34$), alkaline phosphatase ($p = 0.53$) nor ferritin ($p = 0.54$ but data were only available for 23/52). Additionally, neither comorbidity nor ethnicity were associated with the need for critical care intervention ($p > 0.8$ for all). Whilst there was a trend for a difference in the distribution of ESR between those who did and did not require critical care intervention, in a univariable logistic regression model it was not predictive (odds ratio [95% confidence intervals]: 0.98 [0.94-1.01] per 100 mm/h; $p = 0.19$). Therefore, ESR was not included in the multivariable model. In a multivariable logistic regression model, only sodium (OR [95% CIs] 0.19 [0.02-0.93] per 10 mmol/L reduction, $p = 0.04$) and an ALT (1.33 [1.11-1.78] per 10 IU/L increase, $p < 0.0001$) were independently associated with the need for mechanical ventilation (Table 2).

Admission ALT and sodium were both independently associated with the need for critical care intervention with mechanical ventilation and therefore underwent further ROC analysis to determine predictive thresholds. For the independent prediction of an unfavourable outcome, the optimal threshold for admission ALT was ≥180 IU/L and for admission sodium was <132 mmol/L (Fig. 1 and Table 3). The addition of sodium to ALT did not alter classification performance, suggesting that using ALT ≥180 IU/L is sufficient to predict an unfavourable outcome with a positive likelihood ratio of 32.6. Conversely, for the prediction of a favourable outcome, a different threshold for sodium was evident and classification performance was improved by combining ALT <180 IU/L (individual AUC: 0.864) and sodium ≥125 mmol/L (individual AUC: 0.670) thresholds (combined AUC 0.909, Table 3). It should be noted that this is equivalent to using an ALT threshold ≥180 IU/L *or* sodium <125 mmol/L as criteria from predicting an unfavourable outcome. The relationship between admission sodium and ALT with outcomes is displayed graphically in Fig. 1.

Given the size of the dataset, biomarker prediction validity was assessed using LOOCV. For the prediction of an unfavourable outcome the median (range) ALT threshold was: ≥180 (180-191) IU/L with diagnostic accuracy of 92.3% across the cross-validation folds. For the prediction of a favourable outcome, the median (range) ALT threshold was <191 (180-200) IU/L; and for sodium was: ≥125 (106-126) mmol/L yielding a diagnostic accuracy of 76.9% across the cross-validation folds.

Discussion

We report the lowest one-year mortality from miliary TB (2%), despite significant rates of severe complications. Additionally, we demonstrate how routinely collected biochemical measures can be used to accurately predict clinical outcomes.

The mortality rate in our cohort compares favourably to previously reported rates of 10-30% from the developing world and 7.1%-21% from the developed world [2, 4–6]. Critical care intervention and mechanical ventilation, which was required in 15% of our cohort, are likely to be responsible for the low mortality we report as these patients would almost certainly have died if these facilities were not available. Additionally, extensive experience in the management of complicated tuberculosis at a high-volume centre are likely to have contributed to our low mortality. Due to the retrospective nature of data collection it was not possible to assess the impact of corticosteroid usage on outcome, and whilst corticosteroid usage was higher in patients requiring mechanical ventilation this may reflect increased rates of CNS involvement and systemic inflammatory response syndrome in patients requiring critical care support. The impact of corticosteroids on mortality in CNS TB infection has been demonstrated, particularly in non HIV-infected individuals [8]. Furthermore, meta-analysis of corticosteroid use in all forms of TB suggest a beneficial effect on mortality, however many of the 41 randomised controlled trials were identified as being

Table 2 Univariable and multivariable logistic regression model results for the outcome of requiring critical care intervention

Parameter	Univariable		Multivariable	
	Odds ratio (95% CI)	*p*-value	Odds ratio (95% CI)	*p*-value
ALT (per 10 IU/L)	1.29 (1.13-1.56)	<0.001	1.33 (1.11-1.78)	<0.001
Bilirubin (per 10 μmol/L)	2.99 (1.29-7.84)	0.01	0.69 (0.07-3.86)	0.68
CRP (per 10 mg/L)	1.14 (1.02-1.35)	0.02	1.13 (0.93-1.61)	0.27
Platelet count (per 100 cells/mm3)	0.39 (0.14-0.87)	0.02	0.75 (0.13-3.60)	0.71
Sodium (per 10 mmol/L)	0.40 (0.14-1.03)	0.06	0.19 (0.02-0.93)	0.04

Abbreviations: *ALT* alanine aminotransferase, *CI* confidence intervals; *CRP* c-reactive protein

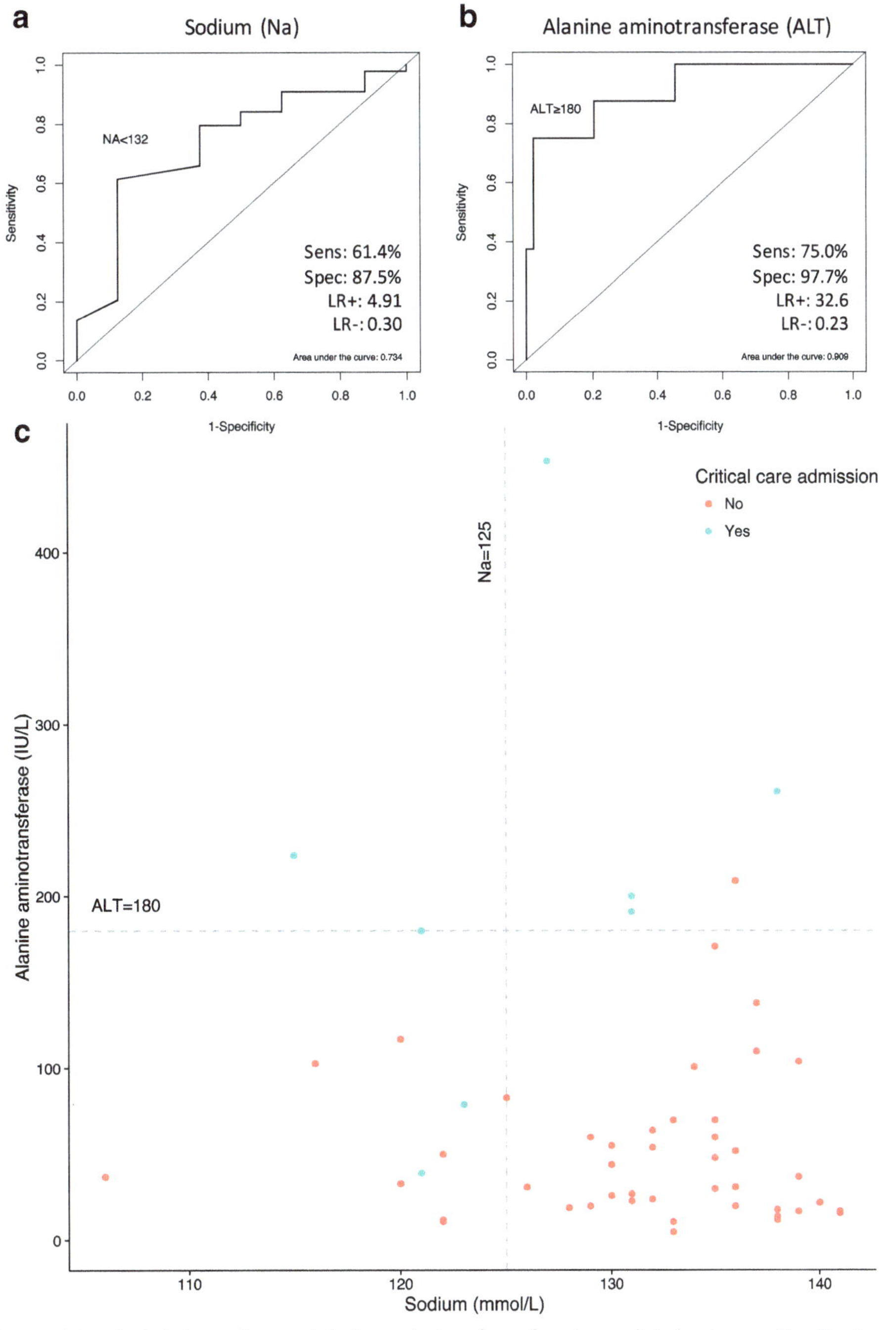

Fig. 1 Predictive characteristics of admission sodium and alanine aminotransferase for adverse clinical outcomes. Top: Receiver operator characteristics of admission sodium (**a**) and alanine aminotransferase (**b**) for predicting the need for critical care intervention with mechanical intervention with displayed statistics. Bottom: **c** graphically depicts patients by need for critical care intervention with cut-offs for admission sodium and alanine aminotransferase that identify a favourable outcome with 100% specificity. Abbreviations: ALT: alanine aminotransferase; Na: sodium; Sens: sensitivity; Spec: specificity; LR+: positive likelihood ratio; LR-: negative likelihood ratio

at high risk of bias, and none were performed to assess corticosteroid usage specifically in miliary TB [9]. Given the multisystem nature of miliary TB with frequent and potentially under-recognised CNS involvement, further research is warranted to clarify the role of corticosteroids.

Hyponatraemia and an elevated ALT on admission were associated with an unfavourable clinical course. The causes of hyponatraemia in those with miliary TB are numerous, but are likely to include brain injury as well as adrenal and pituitary dysfunction. Whereas, an increased ALT identifies those with significant liver injury and in this cohort a

Table 3 Classification performance of different biomarkers and their optimum threshold by outcome determined using bootstrapping

Predictor	Outcome	Sensitivity (%)	Specificity (%)	PPV (%)	NPV (%)	AUC
ALT ≥180 IU/L	Unfavourable	75.0 (41.7-100)	97.3 (92.5-100)	85.7 (50.0-100)	95.6 (88.6-100)	0.864 (0.692-1.00)
Sodium <132 mmol/L	Unfavourable	87.5 (57.1-100)	61.4 (46.5-76.1)	29.2 (11.1-48.3)	96.4 (88.9-100)	0.744 (0.583-0.869)
ALT <180 IU/L & sodium ≥125 mmol/L	Favourable	81.8 (69.8-92.5)	100 (100-100)	100 (100-100)	50.0 (25.0-76.9)	0.909 (0.849-0.963)

An unfavourable outcome was defined as the need for critical care intervention with mechanical ventilation, whereas a favourable outcome was defined as not requiring critical care intervention with mechanical ventilation. 95% confidence intervals determined by bootstrapping (1000 replicates) are in parentheses for each parameter. *Abbreviations*: *ALT* alanine aminotransferase, *AUC* area under the receiver operator curve (equivalent to the balanced accuracy), *PPV* positive predictive value, *NPV* negative predictive value

threshold of ≥180 IU/L was strongly predictive of an unfavourable outcome. Both factors are likely surrogates of disease burden, hence their association with clinical outcomes. Our data suggests these routinely collected biochemical measures could be used to identify patients with severe disease at risk of deterioration. However, these thresholds need verifying in an independent dataset. Pending further study, they should be interpreted with caution given the relatively low number of patients in our study. Furthermore, the influence of co-morbidity, in particular HIV-infection and type 2 diabetes given their increasing prevalence in regions with the highest burden of tuberculosis, on the relationship between predictive biomarkers and outcomes needs to be determined.

UK National Institute for Health and Care Excellence (NICE) guidelines [10] currently recommend neuroimaging only for miliary TB patients with CNS signs or symptoms. Given that miliary TB is caused by the widespread haematogenous dissemination of *MTB*, it is unsurprising that CNS involvement was proven in 29% of our cohort. However, as not all our patients underwent systematic neuroimaging or CSF sampling, this represents the lower bound of the true prevalence of CNS disease and confirms historical autopsy data documenting high rates of CNS disease [11]. In keeping with other studies, MRI was more sensitive than CT in detecting tuberculomas [4]. CSF examination demonstrated TB meningitis in a minority, suggesting that meningitis may be a late manifestation of disease, however, normal CSF biochemistry and microscopy did not exclude CNS involvement. In addition, CNS tubercles may initially be below the size of detection by CT or MRI, and may paradoxically appear during treatment.

There are no randomised trials to provide guidance on duration of therapy for miliary TB. A 6-month course is currently recommended for miliary TB without CNS involvement in UK, USA, Europe and WHO international guidelines [10, 12–14]. However, as we suspect CNS involvement in miliary TB is often under-recognised, a 6-month course of ATT may risk later relapse and complications. Generally, patients in our cohort were treated for 12-months. Whether this contributed to our low mortality is unclear. Given the ubiquity of CNS involvement, we advocate performing contrast-enhanced neuroimaging (ideally MRI) in all patients and CSF examination in those with symptoms or signs of meningitis. Ideally, this should be at the time of diagnosis and possibly repeated 6-12 weeks later to detect tuberculomas which appear during treatment [15]. In settings where this is not possible, 9-12 months' treatment to cover CNS disease may be prudent. Given the high *a priori* probability of CNS disease, we advocate consideration for longer empirical duration of therapy (9-12 months) if contrast-enhanced MRI and CSF examination cannot be undertaken, such as in the developing world.

The limitations of this case series include the retrospective and non-systematic nature of initial data collection and incomplete post-treatment follow-up. However, most mortality attributed to miliary TB occurs in the early stages of disease so it is unlikely that longer follow-up would significantly change our conclusions [16, 17]. Additionally, due to the low mortality in our cohort, where there was only one death, we lacked power to detect associations with this important outcome.

Conclusions

CNS involvement in miliary TB is common and is likely to be under-recognised and under-treated. Although severe complications occur frequently, they can be predicted by admission hyponatraemia and increased ALT. A low one-year mortality is achievable in a high resource setting with critical care support and mechanical ventilation. Further research is required to establish the role of corticosteroids and prolonged ATT in the management of miliary TB.

Abbreviations

ALT: Alanine aminotransferase; ATT: Anti-tuberculous therapy; CNS: Central nervous system; CSF: Cerebrospinal fluid; CT: Computer tomography; HIV: Human immunodeficiency virus; MRI: Magnetic resonance imaging; MTB: *Mycobacterium tuberculosis*; TB: Tuberculosis

Acknowledgements

We gratefully acknowledge the assistance of the TB nurses at Northwest London Hospitals NHS Trust for their assistance with this study.

Funding

No specific funding for this study was received.

Authors' contributions
JU, FC, APS, LJ and RND conceived of and designed the study. JU, FC, APS and CC collected data from participating sites. JU conducted statistical analyses. JU, FC and AJK compiled the first draft of the study manuscript and all authors contributed to subsequent revisions. All authors read and approved the final manuscript.

Competing interests
The authors declare that they have no competing interests.

Consent for publication
Not applicable.

Author details
[1]Division of Infectious Diseases, Imperial College London, London, UK. [2]Lawson Unit, Brighton and Sussex University Hospitals NHS Trust, Brighton, UK. [3]King's College London, London, UK. [4]Department of Medicine, Western Sussex Hospitals Trust, Worthing, UK. [5]Royal Free Hospital, London, UK. [6]Department of Infectious Diseases, Northwick Park Hospital, Northwest London Teaching Hospitals NHS Trust, London, UK.

References

1. Murray CJ, Lopez AD. Global mortality, disability, and the contribution of risk factors: global burden of disease study. Lancet. 1997;349:1436–42.
2. Sharma SK, Mohan A, Sharma A, Mitra DK. Miliary tuberculosis: new insights into an old disease. Lancet Infect Dis. 2005;5:415–30.
3. Falk A. U. S. veterans administration-armed forces cooperative study on the chemotherapy of tuberculosis. Tuberculous meningitis in adults, with special reference to survival, neurologic residuals, and work status. Am Rev Respir Dis. 1965;91:823–31.
4. Venkatraman N, King T, Bell D, Woltmann G, Wiselka M, Abubakar I, et al. High levels of neurological involvement but low mortality in miliary tuberculosis: a 6-year case-series from the UK. Eur Respir J. 2016;47:1578–81.
5. Ormerod LP, Horsfield N. Miliary tuberculosis in a high prevalence area of the U.K.: Blackburn 1978-1993. Respir Med. 1995;89:555–7.
6. Touré NO, Cissé MF, Dia Kane Y, Diatta A, Bouker Bakioui B, Ndiaye EHM, et al. Miliary tuberculosis: a report of 49 cases. Rev Mal Respir. 2011;28:312–6.
7. Tuberculosis in the UK, 2014 report. Public Health England (https://www.gov.uk/government/uploads/system/uploads/attachment_data/file/360335/TB_Annual_report__4_0_300914.pdf); 2014.
8. Prasad K, Singh MB, Ryan H. Corticosteroids for managing tuberculous meningitis. Cochrane Database Syst Rev. 2016;4:CD002244.
9. Critchley JA, Young F, Orton L, Garner P. Corticosteroids for prevention of mortality in people with tuberculosis: a systematic review and meta-analysis. Lancet Infect Dis. 2013;13:223–37.
10. Tuberculosis. National Institute for Health and Care Excellence; 2016. (https://www.nice.org.uk/guidance/ng33/).
11. American College of Physicians. Tuberculoma of the brain. Ann Intern Med. 1934;7:1141–5.
12. American Thoracic Society - AJRCCM. American Thoracic Society/Centers for Disease Control and Prevention/Infectious Diseases Society of America. Am J Respir Crit Care Med. 2003;167:603–62.
13. Migliori GB, Zellweger JP, Abubakar I, Ibraim E, Caminero JA, De Vries G, et al. European union standards for tuberculosis care. Eur Respir J. 2012;39:807–19.
14. World Health Organization. Guidelines for treatment of tuberculosis. WHO. World Health Organization; 2010. (http://www.who.int/tb/publications/2010/9789241547833/en/).
15. Afghani B, Lieberman JM. Paradoxical enlargement or development of intracranial tuberculomas during therapy: case report and review. Clin Infect Dis. 1994;19:1092–9.
16. Lin C-H, Lin C-J, Kuo Y-W, Wang J-Y, Hsu C-L, Chen J-M, et al. Tuberculosis mortality: patient characteristics and causes. BMC Infect Dis BioMed Central. 2014;14:5.
17. Gelb AF, Leffler C, Brewin A, Mascatello V, Lyons HA. Miliary Tuberculosis. American Review of Respiratory Disease. Am Lung Assoc. 1973;108(6):1327–33.

12

Genomic sequencing is required for identification of tuberculosis transmission in Hawaii

Kent J. Koster[1], Angela Largen[2], Jeffrey T. Foster[3,6], Kevin P. Drees[3], Lishi Qian[1], Ed Desmond[4], Xuehua Wan[5], Shaobin Hou[5] and James T. Douglas[1,6*]

Abstract

Background: Tuberculosis (TB) caused an estimated 1.4 million deaths and 10.4 million new cases globally in 2015. TB rates in the United States continue to steadily decline, yet rates in the State of Hawaii are perennially among the highest in the nation due to a continuous influx of immigrants from the Western Pacific and Asia. TB in Hawaii is composed of a unique distribution of genetic lineages, with the Beijing and Manila families of *Mycobacterium tuberculosis* (*Mtb*) comprising over two-thirds of TB cases. Standard fingerprinting methods (spoligotyping plus 24-loci Mycobacterial Interspersed Repetitive Units-Variable Number Tandem Repeats [MIRU-VNTR] fingerprinting) perform poorly when used to identify actual transmission clusters composed of isolates from these two families. Those typing methods typically group isolates from these families into large clusters of non-linked isolates with identical fingerprints. Next-generation whole-genome sequencing (WGS) provides a new tool for molecular epidemiology that can resolve clusters of isolates with identical spoligotyping and MIRU-VNTR fingerprints.

Methods: We performed WGS and SNP analysis and evaluated epidemiological data to investigate 19 apparent TB transmission clusters in Hawaii from 2003 to 2017 in order to assess WGS' ability to resolve putative *Mtb* clusters from the Beijing and Manila families. This project additionally investigated MIRU-VNTR allele prevalence to determine why standard *Mtb* fingerprinting fails to usefully distinguish actual transmission clusters from these two *Mtb* families.

Results: WGS excluded transmission events in seven of these putative clusters, confirmed transmission in eight, and identified both transmission-linked and non-linked isolates in four. For epidemiologically identified clusters, while the sensitivity of MIRU-VNTR fingerprinting for identifying actual transmission clusters was found to be 100%, its specificity was only 28.6% relative to WGS. We identified that the Beijing and Manila families' significantly lower Shannon evenness of MIRU-VNTR allele distributions than lineage 4 was the cause of standard fingerprinting's poor performance when identifying transmission in Beijing and Manila family clusters.

Conclusions: This study demonstrated that WGS is necessary for epidemiological investigation of TB in Hawaii and the Pacific.

Keywords: *Mycobacterium tuberculosis*, Hawaii, Spoligotyping, Genomic epidemiology

* Correspondence: jtd379@gmail.com
[1]University of Hawaii at Manoa, Honolulu, HI, USA
[6]Present Address: Pathogen and Microbiome Institute, Northern Arizona University, Flagstaff, AZ, USA
Full list of author information is available at the end of the article

Background

The World Health Organization has shown that the worldwide tuberculosis (TB) epidemic is larger than was previously estimated [1]. Tuberculosis caused an estimated 1.4 million deaths in 2015, with an estimated 10.4 million new cases. TB rates in the United States continue to steadily drop, yet TB rates in the State of Hawaii remain steady [2]. Hawaii experienced an average of 120 incident cases per year from 2006 to 2017, ranging from a low of 114 in 2006 to a high of 136 in 2014. Hawaii currently displays the highest incidence rate of TB in the US, at 8.1 per 100,000 in 2017. Comparing this rate to the median US state rate of 1.8 per 100,000 illustrates the public health burden of TB in Hawaii. Of the 119 incident TB cases in Hawaii in 2016, 100 (84%) were non-US born, well above the national average of 68.5%. Furthermore, of those 100 cases, 69 were in persons born in the Philippines.

Thus, it is not surprising that Hawaii perennially experiences among the highest rates of TB cases in the United States due to a continuous influx of immigrants from the Western Pacific and Asian regions. As a result of this immigration pattern, TB in Hawaii is composed of a unique distribution of genetic lineages relative to the continental United States or Europe, but similar to the United States Affiliated Pacific Islands [3–5]. The Beijing and Manila families of *Mycobacterium tuberculosis* (*Mtb*) comprise over two-thirds of the TB cases in Hawaii [6, 7]. These families are defined by spoligotyping (reverse-line hybridization of 43 sequences complementary to CRISPR spacers), mycobacterial interspersed repetitive units–variable number of tandem repeats (MIRU-VNTR) patterns, and whole-genome single nucleotide polymorphism (SNP) phylogenies [6–10]. The Manila family has been shown to comprise the majority of *Mtb* lineage 1 and has spread into the Pacific islands with Filipino migration, while the Beijing family comprises the majority of lineage 2 and is the dominant family in East Asia [10]. In contrast, lineage 4, whose members are the most commonly found among TB cases in Europe and North America, contains a larger set of spoligotyping clades [4].

Potentially long latency periods in tuberculosis cases make molecular epidemiological tools an essential part of its control. IS*6110* restriction fragment length polymorphism (RFLP) typing historically represented the "gold standard" for *Mtb* genotyping [11]. However, IS*6110* typing is time consuming and labor intensive, and provides limited resolving power for clusters composed of isolates with low IS*6110* copy numbers [12, 13]. Two other methods, spoligotyping and MIRU-VNTR fingerprinting, are currently the standard employed by the Centers for Disease Control and Prevention (CDC) in the United States [8, 12, 14]. However, these fingerprinting methods still perform poorly when used to identify actual transmission. One study conducted in the English Midlands found that the positive predictive value (PPV) that two isolates with identical MIRU-VNTR fingerprints represent actual recent transmission between those cases was only 18.6% [15]. Furthermore, they found that this PPV varied by lineage, with lineage 4 displaying a PPV of 30.6%, while lineage 1 displayed a PPV of only 8.0% and lineage 2 only 13.8%. Even more previous work has demonstrated that these genetic fingerprinting methods perform poorly for identifying actual transmission of Beijing family isolates, showing that MIRU-VNTR fingerprinting is superior to IS*6110* when only lineage 4 isolates are being typed, but performs poorly when Beijing family isolates are being typed [16]. Multiple other studies have also indicated that 12-loci MIRU-VNTR is insufficient to resolve suspected Beijing family clusters, and that 24-loci MIRU-VNTR is similarly ineffective when Beijing family isolates are present [17–19]. However, similar studies are not available for the Manila family.

Attempts to optimize VNTR typing for the Beijing family have been proposed and implemented with the switch from 12-loci to 24-loci typing, but as we further demonstrate in this study, have failed to result in a comprehensively effective solution [12, 20]. The need for effective epidemiological tracking for the Beijing family is highlighted by this family's association with drug resistance. The population structure of TB in areas of high drug resistance has been shown to be rapidly shifting towards the Beijing family, which specifically has a significantly higher rate of developing rifampin resistance [21]. Alarmingly, the Beijing family has been shown to manifest increased transmission fitness relative to a non-Beijing lineage while streptomycin resistant [22]. However, limited research has been performed on the Manila family, despite its dominance in Hawaii and the Philippines, and despite the prediction that rates of multiple drug resistant (MDR) TB in the Philippines will continue to increase [23].

As a result of the predominance of these two *Mtb* families in Hawaii and the Pacific, identifying autochthonous *Mtb* transmission is especially difficult both in Hawaii and throughout the Western Pacific Region. Although extensive TB screening is implemented in Hawaii (including requiring tuberculin skin tests prior to enrolment in education or prior to employment as a food-handler), frequent travel of Hawaii residents to visit family in high-incidence areas throughout the Pacific, combined with insufficient existing molecular fingerprinting methods, prevents TB controllers in Hawaii from developing a comprehensive understanding of local TB transmission. In this study, we examined the ability of CDC-standard genetic fingerprinting (spoligotyping plus 24-loci MIRU-VNTR fingerprinting) for *Mtb* to identify Beijing and Manila family transmission clusters, and attempted to identify the cause of its reduction in genotyping resolution compared to when applied to lineage 4. We previously observed that the Beijing and Manila families demonstrated lower allelic Shannon evenness at most MIRU-VNTR loci [J.T. Douglas unpublished data]. The Shannon diversity index is a measurement of diversity in a community that considers both the richness (total number of alleles at each MIRU-VNTR locus, in our case) present in the community and evenness (relative abundance) of each of those alleles. Our study utilizes this measurement to determine if certain *Mtb* genetic lineages possess a dominance of specific alleles (indicated by reduced Shannon evenness values) at any MIRU-VNTR loci that may explain why MIRU-VNTR performs poorly when utilized for molecular epidemiology on these lineages. Here, we utilized a dataset of all fully fingerprinted *Mtb* isolates recorded in Hawaii from 2002 through 2016 to further investigate this apparent cause for MIRU-VNTR's poor ability to resolve apparent lineage 1 and 2 clusters relative to its considerably greater ability for lineage 4 clusters.

Our previous cooperation with the State of Hawaii Department of Health Tuberculosis Control Branch revealed that the CDC's standard *Mtb* fingerprinting methodology was of limited epidemiological use for Hawaii's TB clinicians. Large numbers of epidemiologically unrelated Beijing and Manila family isolates frequently shared identical fingerprints, and nearly all suspected transmission clusters also fingerprinted identically within those suspected clusters, preventing fingerprinting results from being a useful tool for confirming or disproving suspected transmission events.

Whole genome sequencing (WGS) has been shown to be able to identify specific transmission chains within fingerprinting clusters [24]. Advances in next-generation sequencing have resulted in the cost of WGS decreasing to the point where it is feasible for many laboratories to sequence most or all clustered isolates [25]. WGS is increasingly being employed for tuberculosis epidemiology, including identifying the transmission chains of a TB outbreak in British Columbia, Canada, verifying contact investigation-based links in an outbreak in San Francisco, California, and use in a large, retrospective observational study in the UK Midlands [26–28]. For this study, we selected 19 apparent TB transmission clusters that were identified by fingerprinting or epidemiological data in Hawaii from 2003 to 2017 and conducted Illumina whole genome sequencing to determine if WGS could be used to further resolve these clusters and identify the transmission connections among isolates.

Making full use of the resulting WGS dataset, we further examined isolates from clusters that WGS identified to represent actual transmission events and investigated which genes or regions were developing mutations that differentiated individual isolates in a cluster. Our previous work has identified virulence factor mutations in the Beijing and Manila families that may be involved in virulence or latency, and this work seeks to help us further characterize these historically under-studied families [29, 30].

Methods

Identification of clusters for WGS

Records of all genotyped tuberculosis cases processed by the Hawaii State Department of Health Tuberculosis Control Program from 2004 to 2016—as well as partial data from 2002, 2003, and 2017—were analyzed to identify fingerprinting clusters that possibly represented actual transmission clusters. One thousand sixty-one isolate records were available for analysis. Names were assigned to spoligotypes using the SpolDB4 database [31]. Genetic fingerprints, dates and locations, patient histories, and nursing contact investigation records were all considered in the selection of these clusters. Four large historic *Mtb* fingerprinting clusters in Hawaii were selected for investigation (Table 1).

As we hypothesized that these large fingerprinting clusters did not represent actual transmission clusters due to their relatively high number of cases, geographic distribution throughout the state, and chronological diversity, we further selected five clusters with spoligotypes that were less common in Hawaii, including two clusters with "Manila-like" patterns, one cluster with an uncommon Beijing family pattern (000000000003751 versus the common 000000000003771), one cluster with no spoligotype match in SpolDB4, and one H3 cluster (which is common globally, but uncommon in Hawaii) in order to analyze clusters with greater suspected likelihood of being transmission-derived. Nineteen isolates were selected for WGS from those clusters in order to maximize chronological diversity for the largest clusters and to fully sequence the smaller clusters.

We further worked with staff at the State of Hawaii Tuberculosis Control Program's Lanakila Tuberculosis Clinic, including doctors, nurses, and Tuberculosis Epidemiological Studies Consortium (TBESC) staff, to identify 17 epidemiologically-derived possible transmission clusters, of which ten had two or more isolates sent to CDC-contracted laboratories for genetic fingerprinting (Table 1). Twenty-one isolates from these clusters were selected for sequencing.

Recall of state of Hawaii *Mtb* isolates

Twenty isolates were requested from the Michigan Department of Community Health, where they had been previously sent by the State of Hawaii for contracted fingerprinting, and where they had been archived. We received extracted DNA from those isolates. Sixty-one

Table 1 Sequenced *Mtb* Fingerprinting or Epidemiological Clusters

Cluster Name	Cluster Family	# of Isolates	# of WGS Isolates	# of SNP Loci in Cluster	SNP Range	Transmission Linked?
Large Clusters Identified by Identical Genetic Fingerprints						
Manila Cluster 1	Manila	23	3	178	73–148	No
Manila Cluster 2	Manila	24	2	161	–	No
Beijing Cluster 1	Beijing	11	4	63	0–52	Partial
Beijing Cluster 2	Beijing	7	7	0	–	Yes
Clusters Identified by Shared Uncommon Spoligotypes						
Manila-like Cluster 1	Manila	2	2	3	–	Yes
Manila-like Cluster 2	Manila	2	2	4	–	Yes
Beijing Cluster 5	Beijing	2	2	1	–	Yes
Manila-like Cluster 3	Manila-like	3	3	3	1–3	Yes
H3 Cluster 1	H3	3 (1)	3	1230	3–1230	Partial
Epidemiologically Identified Putative Clusters						
Manila Cluster 3	Manila	2	2	90	–	No
Manila Cluster 4	Manila	2	2	0	–	Yes
Manila Cluster 5	Manila	2	2	192	–	No
Manila Cluster 6	Manila	2	2	229	–	No
Beijing Cluster 3	Beijing	2	2	3	–	Yes
Mixed Cluster 2	U/Beijing	2	2	1153	–	No
U Cluster 1	U	4	4	131	1–117	Partial
Mixed Cluster 1	Beijing/Manila	3	3	1762	1–1762	Partial
Manila Cluster 7	Manila	2	2	142	–	No
Beijing Cluster 4	Beijing	2	2	0	–	Yes

# of WGS Isolates is the number of isolates from each cluster that were sequenced with Illumina whole genome sequencing. # of SNP Loci in Cluster is the total number of SNP loci possessing alleles that differentiate isolates within the cluster. SNP Range lists the smallest and largest numbers of SNPs between any two isolates in the cluster. Transmission Linked is marked as "No" if all isolates in the cluster differ by 12 SNPs or more, "Yes" if they differ by 5 SNPs or fewer, or "Partial" if some, but not all, isolates within the cluster differ by 5 SNPs or fewer. H3 Cluster 1 includes a fourth isolate that was not available for sequencing. Clusters are listed in the order in which they are discussed in the text

isolates were sent from the California Department of Public Health State Laboratory as "double-killed" sample preps using a treatment of immersion in 70% ethanol followed by heating at 80 °C for 1 h.

DNA extraction and whole genome sequencing

DNA extraction was performed as previously described by the National Institute of Public Health and Environmental Protection (RIVM), Bilthoven, The Netherlands (Isolation of Genomic DNA from Mycobacteria Protocol), or according to the source state laboratory's standard protocol. In brief, *Mtb* cultures were harvested and lysed with lysozyme followed by a SDS/proteinase K mix. Non-nucleic acid cell debris was precipitated using a CTAB/NaCl solution and removed using a chloroform/isoamyl alcohol extraction. Finally, DNA was precipitated using isopropanol. DNA was quantified with the Qubit 2.0 dsDNA Broad Range Assay. Isolate libraries were prepared using the Illumina Nextera XT DNA Library Kit using manual normalization and sequenced on the Illumina MiSeq Platform with v3 Chemistry for 300 bp paired-end reads.

Data analysis

SNP matrices were produced using a modification of the NASP pipeline [32], with Bowtie2 used for alignment [33], and GATK used for SNP-calling [34], and SNPs being filtered for ten-fold read coverage and 75% read consensus as previously described [28]. Repetitive regions were removed by the NASP pipeline utilizing MUMmer to perform a self-self comparison with a minimum match length of 20. When two compared isolates presented with 30 SNPs or fewer between them during analysis of the pipeline output, those differentiating SNP loci were compared against their alignment's annotated scaffold genomes in NCBI GenBank (https://www.ncbi.nlm.nih.gov/nuccore/) to identify and discard any SNPs in repetitive regions that were not automatically excluded by the NASP pipeline. Relatedness of isolates was determined by the method developed by Walker et al. [28], with the stepwise 95% prediction interval from the mean rate of change between their paired isolates being used as our baseline. Identification of SNPs among members of clusters, or between isolate pairs, was performed by importing the SNP matrices produced by the NASP pipeline into a database and performing custom SQL queries. Minimum spanning trees were produced for selected clusters with PHYLOViZ 2.0 using goeBURST Full MST [35, 36].

Analysis of the resolving capability of CDC-standard *Mtb* fingerprinting (spoligotyping plus 24 loci MIRU-VNTR typing) was conducted on all 562 fully fingerprinted *Mtb* isolates recorded in the State of Hawaii from 2002 through 2016. Only isolates with the "EAI2_MANILLA" designation in SpolDB4 were utilized as "lineage 1" isolates, as we have previously shown that other spoligotypes with "EAI" designations can span diverse evolutionary lineages [37]. All isolates with "BEIJING" or "BEIJING-LIKE" spoligotypes were placed in "lineage 2." All isolates with LAM, H, S, T, U, and X spoligotypes were grouped into "lineage 4." MIRU-VNTR loci were individually analyzed using the Shannon diversity index. Evenness of allelic distribution at each locus was calculated by dividing the Shannon diversity index by the maximum possible Shannon diversity index for that locus, assuming that all alleles could possibly be observed at each locus. Statistical significance of the means of diversity indices for all 24 MIRU-VNTR loci was calculated in Microsoft Excel using the t-Test: Two-Sample Assuming Unequal Variances, with p-values < 0.05 being considered significant. Sensitivity and specificity for genetic fingerprinting were calculated using VassarStats Clinical Calculator 1 [38].

Isolates discussed in this paper are identified by their one or two-digit University of Hawaii DNA extraction number. Gene names are presented as annotated in their respective genomes hosted in GenBank (see accession numbers below).

Results

Resolution of *Mtb* fingerprinting clusters in Hawaii through whole genome sequencing

Nineteen *Mtb* fingerprinting clusters were either fully (n = 15) or partially (n = 4) sequenced, with two or more isolates selected for initial sequencing to evaluate the possibility that the fingerprinting cluster represents a direct or recent transmission cluster. Eight of the fingerprinting clusters were determined to represent actual transmission clusters due to isolates in those clusters being separated by fewer than six SNPs. Four clusters were determined to partially represent direct transmission, meaning that while some isolates in the fingerprinting cluster were separated by five or fewer SNPs, other isolates within the fingerprinting cluster were separated by 12 or more SNPs. All sequenced fingerprinting clusters are summarized in Table 1.

Results of each investigated fingerprinting or epidemiological cluster

The following sections present background information, epidemiological details, and whole genome SNP numbers for each *Mtb* fingerprinting or epidemiological cluster investigated in this study. The clusters are divided into three groups: 1.) Large Clusters Identified by Identical Genetic Fingerprints, 2.) Clusters Identified by Shared Uncommon Spoligotypes, and 3.) Epidemiologically Identified Putative Clusters. Epidemiological details were primarily derived from the chart reviews and reviews of Lanakila TB Clinic Nursing Contact Investigation records that were conducted for a more detailed understanding of transmission. These reviews reinforced several cases where clusters were determined to represent or not represent transmission based on SNP count.

Large clusters identified by identical genetic fingerprints

These large clusters were identified through CDC-standard genetic fingerprinting (spoligotyping plus 24-loci MIRU-VNTR) of all isolates in Hawaii from 2004 to 2016, plus a selection from 2002, 2003, and 2017. All clusters are detailed in Additional file 1, and their SNP matrices are presented in Table 2.

Manila cluster 1

This cluster was composed of 23 isolates spanning 2004–2013. The oldest and newest isolates, plus an intermediate isolate from 2009, were selected for WGS to determine if this fingerprinting cluster might represent an actual transmission cluster. All isolates shared the 677,777,477,413,731 spoligotype and a 254,326,223,432 14A943263217 24-loci MIRU-VNTR fingerprint. The large number of SNPs among isolates in this fingerprinting cluster indicates that it does not

Table 2 SNPs between Sequenced Isolates from Clusters Identified by Identical Genetic Fingerprints

Manila Cluster 1				
	2	**9**	**46**	
2	X	–	–	
9	73	X	–	
46	148	135	X	
Beijing Cluster 1				
	10	**28**	**29**	**40**
10	X	–	–	–
28	49	X	–	–
29	49	0	X	–
40	52	25	25	X

Matrix displaying the number of SNPs between each pair of isolates from Manila Cluster 1 and Beijing Cluster 1

represent an actual transmission cluster (Table 2, Fig. 1a). Isolates in this cluster had no epidemiological linkages, reinforcing the WGS-based determination of no comprehensive direct transmission.

Manila cluster 2

This cluster was composed of 24 isolates spanning 2004–2013. The oldest and newest isolates (3 and 45, respectively) were selected for WGS to determine if this fingerprinting cluster represents an actual transmission cluster. All isolates shared the 677,777,477,413,771 spoligotype and a 254,326,223,432 14A943263217 24-loci MIRU-VNTR fingerprint. We identified 161 SNPs between the two sequenced isolates, thus allowing us to exclude the possibility that all isolates in this cluster belong to an actual transmission cluster. That result illustrates the need for further WGS fingerprinting to investigate the remaining isolates in the cluster after demonstrating that MIRU-VNTR based clustering is insufficient to conclude that all identically fingerprinting isolates here are actually transmission-linked. Similar to Manila Cluster 1, isolates in this cluster had no epidemiological linkages, reinforcing the WGS-based determination of no comprehensive direct transmission.

Beijing cluster 1

This cluster was composed of 11 isolates spanning 2009–2012. The oldest and newest isolates were selected for WGS to determine if this fingerprinting cluster represents an actual transmission cluster. Two intermediate isolates were also sequenced, both to represent possible intermediate transmission isolates and also due to the fact that both patients were originally from the Democratic People's Republic of Korea (North Korea), and both cases were counted on the same date. All isolates shared the 000000000003771 spoligotype and a 222,325,173,533 445,644,423,328 24-loci MIRU-VNTR fingerprint. The > 20 SNPs displayed by all isolates other than 28 and 29 (which were identical) indicates that this fingerprinting cluster contains both transmission-linked and non-linked isolates (Table 2, Fig. 1b). This fingerprinting cluster revealed no epidemiological linkages, but it is notable that the two isolates that were linked by WGS (separated by no SNPs) were from two retirement-aged, North Korean women.

Beijing cluster 2

This cluster was composed of seven Beijing family isolates from 2010 to 2012. All isolates in the cluster were

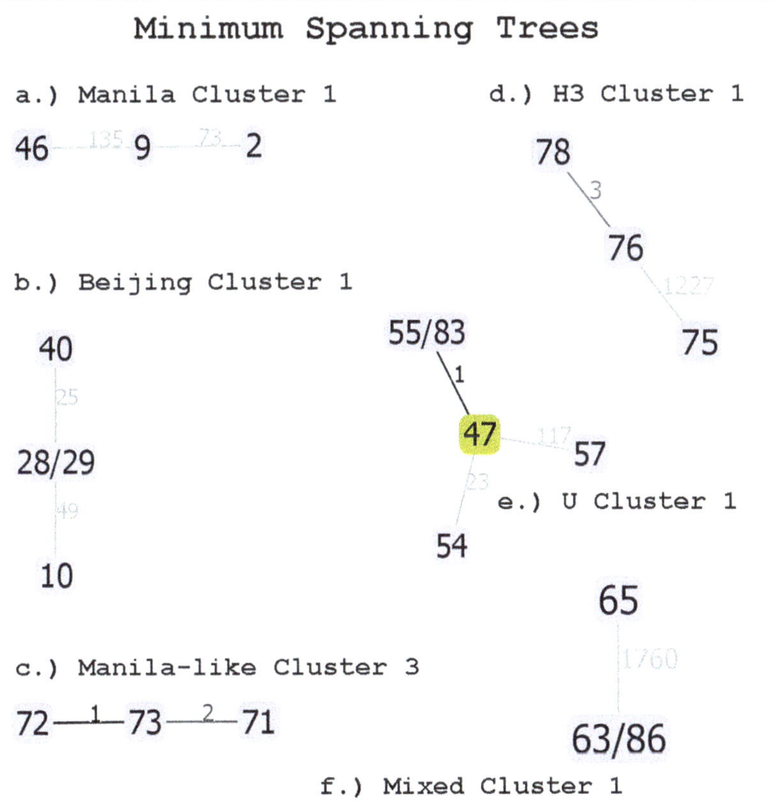

Fig. 1 Minimum Spanning Trees for Selected Clusters. Plates a-f present minimum spanning trees for selected putative clusters that contain more than two sequenced isolates. These clusters are discussed individually in following sections. Isolates are identified by their University of Hawaii DNA extraction numbers. The number of SNPs separating each isolate or group of isolates is shown next to each connecting line. Trees shown were determined by PHYLOViZ 2.0 using goeBURST Full MST.

sequenced. All isolates shared the 000000000003771 spoligotype and a 222,325,173,533 445,644,423,326 24-loci MIRU-VNTR fingerprint. All isolates are separated by no SNPs at the 75% read consensus level, indicating that this fingerprinting cluster represents an actual transmission cluster. However, Isolate 35 was distinguished from all other isolates in the cluster by a single SNP in a ~ 100 bp region between a hypothetical protein and a glycosyl hydrolase, which had a read depth of 27x and a 74.4% read consensus (20 reads supporting the SNP and 7 reads supporting the reference), though this SNP was discarded here with a strict read consensus cut-off of 75%. In this fingerprinting cluster (where all isolates were determined to be transmission-linked by WGS) one patient was originally evaluated as a link to another (though he was asymptomatic at the time), and possibly linked to a third case. Of the two possibly linked cases, both were young men from Chuuk (in the Federated States of Micronesia) who entered Hawaii within 5 months of each other.

Clusters identified by shared uncommon Spoligotypes

All clusters are detailed in Additional file 2, and their SNP matrices are presented in Table 3.

Manila-like cluster 1

This cluster was composed of two isolates from 2011 (21) and 2013 (44) with the Manila-like spoligotype of 600,777,477,413,771 with no SpolDB4 match. Three SNPs were found between the two isolates, indicating that direct or recent transmission is likely. Neither of the cases comprising this fingerprinting cluster were epidemiologically connected to each other.

Table 3 SNPs between Isolates from Clusters Identified by Shared Uncommon Spoligotypes

Manila-like Cluster 3				
	71	**72**	**73**	
71	X			
72	3	X		
73	1	2	X	
H3 Cluster 1				
	75	**76**	**78**	**XX**
75	X	–	–	–
76	1227	X	–	–
78	1230	3	X	–
XX	NA	NA	NA	X

Matrix displaying the number of SNPs between each pair of isolates from Manila-like Cluster 3 and H3 Cluster 1. With all isolates in Manila-like Cluster 3 separated by only one to three SNPs, this fingerprinting cluster was determined to represent an actual transmission cluster. For H3 Cluster 1, with only three SNPs between isolates 76 and 78, transmission is indicated between them, but not between them and 75. One final isolate has not been sequenced for this project as it was unavailable, and its DNA extraction number has been notated here as "XX"

Manila-like cluster 2

This cluster was composed of two isolates from 2011 (30) and 2012 (37) with the Manila-like spoligotype of 677,777,402,003,771 with no SpolDB4 match. Isolate 30 was from the island of Kauai, while 37 was from the island of Hawaii. Four SNPs were found between the two isolates, indicating that transmission is likely, possibly with an intermediate host, or extended incubation period between transmission events. Both patients were from Micronesia, where transmission might have occurred.

Beijing cluster 5

This cluster was composed of two isolates from 2008 (74) and 2009 (77), both sharing an uncommon Beijing family spoligotype (000000000003751). Only a single SNP was found between the two isolates, indicating that this fingerprinting cluster likely represents an actual transmission cluster. The two patients in this cluster were niece and uncle.

Manila-like cluster 3

This cluster was composed of three isolates from 2002 (71) and 2006 (72 and 73), all sharing a spoligotype with no SpolDB4 match (737777377413771). One to three SNPs were found among the isolates, indicating that this fingerprinting cluster represents an actual transmission cluster (Table 3, Fig. 1c). Two of the isolates belonged to a mother and her son, and both were isoniazid and streptomycin resistant. The third case was caught by an abnormal chest X-ray on entry to the US in 2006, was originally from the Philippines (unlike the mother, who was from Vietnam), and had no drug susceptibility testing results available.

H3 cluster 1

This cluster was composed of four isolates with an H3 spoligotype (777777770020771). Isolate 76 was from 2009, and Isolate 78 was from 2010. Isolate 75's full records were not available in Hawaii, and one additional isolate was not available for sequencing. With only three SNPs between 76 and 78, but over 1000 SNPs among those and the other isolate, this cluster includes both transmission-linked and non-linked isolates (Table 3, Fig. 1d). All four persons in this fingerprinting/epidemiological cluster were from the Republic of the Marshall Islands, though no epidemiological linkage between them could be found. However, multiple members of this cluster reported that they traveled back and forth between Hawaii and the Marshall Islands. Interestingly, a mother in this cluster (76) had a son (75) who also had TB, but the son's isolate was in the Beijing family instead of H3 and as expected, was separated from the mother's isolate by over 1000 SNPs.

Epidemiologically identified putative clusters

These clusters were initially identified as possible transmission clusters by epidemiological investigations instead of by fingerprinting. All clusters are detailed in Additional file 3, and their SNP matrices are presented in Table 4.

Manila cluster 3

This cluster was composed of two Manila family isolates from patients from the Philippines (53 from 2015 and 61 from 2016). We identified 90 SNPs between the two isolates, allowing direct transmission to be ruled out. Initially (prior to WGS analysis), this fingerprinting cluster appeared to represent a transmission cluster due to being composed of an uncle and nephew, though WGS later disproved that possibility.

Manila cluster 4

This cluster was composed of two Manila family isolates from a husband and wife, both originally from the Philippines (51 and 59). Zero SNPs separated the two isolates, indicating direct transmission.

Table 4 SNPs between Isolates from Epidemiologically Identified Clusters

U Cluster 1					
	47	**54**	**57**	**83**	***55***
47	X	–	–	–	–
54	23	X	–	–	–
57	117	120	X	–	–
83	1	24	118	X	–
55	*1*	*24*	*118*	*0*	*X*
Mixed Cluster 1					
	63	**65**	**86**		
63	X				
65	1761	X			
86	0	1762	X		

Matrix displaying the number of SNPs between each pair of isolates from two epidemiologically identified clusters. Isolate 55 (italicized) from Mixed Cluster 2 was added to U Cluster 1 for comparison due to having an identical spoligotype and MIRU-VNTR fingerprint. With only a single SNP separating isolates 55 and 83 from isolate 47, but a larger number of SNPs separating those isolates from isolates 54 and 57, this cluster includes both direct transmission and non-linked isolates. The presence of zero SNPs between isolates 63 and 86 from Mixed Cluster 1 indicates direct transmission. The presence of more than 12 SNPs between isolates 63 and 65 or 65 and 86 indicates that direct transmission between them can be ruled out. This confirms the expected result indicated by their different spoligotyping lineages

Manila cluster 5

This cluster was composed of two Manila family isolates from two siblings living in the same city, both originally from the Philippines, who were diagnosed 2 years apart (50 and 62). One isolate was multiple drug resistant (MDR), while the other isolate was pan-susceptible to antibiotics, initially suggesting to TB controllers that these two isolates were not transmission-linked. The 192 SNPs found between the two isolates further excluded the possibility of direct transmission.

Manila cluster 6

This cluster was composed of two Manila family isolates from an aunt and nephew, both originally from the Philippines (84 and 60). One isolate was isoniazid and pyrazinamide resistant while the other was pan-susceptible. The 229 SNPs identified between the two isolates allowed direct transmission to be further ruled out.

Beijing cluster 3

This cluster was composed of two Beijing family isolates from a husband and wife, one of whom was US-born and the other (the index patient) was from the Republic of the Marshall Islands (RMI) (58 and 85). The three SNPs identified between the two isolates supported the epidemiological assessment that direct or recent transmission had occurred.

Mixed cluster 2

This cluster was included in this study prior to CDC fingerprinting being conducted. Isolate 56 was from a retirement-aged man from the RMI who had entered the US 1 month prior to his case being documented. Isolate 55 came from a young woman, also from the RMI, who entered the US roughly 15 years prior, and had a suspicious chest X-ray (but negative follow-up X-ray) 2 years prior to her diagnosis, and then was determined to have TB when examined as a contact to the patient providing isolate 56. However, the two isolates had different spoligotypes (Beijing for 56 and U for 55), and the 1153 SNPs between them further confirmed that transmission of these strains had not occurred between these two patients.

U cluster 1

U Cluster 1 is perhaps the most interesting epidemiologically identified cluster for multiple reasons (Fig. 1e). It was identified not by contact-investigation in Hawaii, but by the US Centers for Disease Control and

Prevention (CDC), who notified the State of Hawaii TB Control Program of it. The TB Control Program reviewed the cases, but was unable to find any epidemiological linkages among them. All isolates shared the same uncommon, unclassified "U" SpolDB4 spoligotype designation (777777760000000) and the same 24-loci MIRU-VNTR fingerprint (223,325,143,322 242,324,223,422). All cases were young men from either the Federated States of Micronesia or the Marshall Islands (Additional file 4). We further noted that isolate 55 from Mixed Cluster 2 shared the same spoligotype and MIRU-VNTR fingerprint as the isolates in this cluster, and thus we included it in our comparison. WGS identified likely direct transmission between two patients in this fingerprinting/outbreak notification cluster (isolates 47 and 83), with only one SNPs between them, and 0–1 SNPs between them and the addition from Mixed Cluster 2, isolate 55 (Fig. 1). However, the SNP numbers between those three isolates and the remaining two isolates in the fingerprinting cluster (54 and 57) are considerably higher, indicating that some isolates in this cluster are linked by direct transmission, while others are not. Thus, while this outbreak notification cluster does contain transmission-linked isolates, the linkage does not extend to all isolates in the notification. Furthermore, it appears that one additional isolate (55) is linked to this cluster, despite not being included in the notification.

Mixed cluster 1

This putative cluster is composed of three isolates from the island of Maui, two of which are in the Beijing family (63 and 86) and one of which is in the Manila family (65). The two Manila family isolates represent direct transmission with zero SNPs separating them, while the Beijing family isolate is not related, with 1700+ SNPs separating it from the Manila family isolates (Table 4, Fig. 1f). Although detailed epidemiological information was not available for this cluster, the two Manila family isolates being separated by only a single SNP indicates that this epidemiologically identified cluster represents a partial transmission cluster.

Manila cluster 7

This cluster was composed of two Manila family isolates from a grandfather and grandson, both originally from the Philippines and who both lived together in Hawaii (48 and 49). Both cases were counted by the State of Hawaii on the same month, but the grandfather's isolate was MDR, while the grandson's isolate was pan-susceptible. The 142 SNPs between the two isolates confirmed that the two cases were not the result of direct transmission.

Beijing cluster 4

This cluster was composed of two Beijing family isolates from a juvenile male and a middle-aged man from the Marshall Islands (whose relationship with the juvenile is unclear, but may have served as his guardian at some point) (52 and 64). The older man previously had TB and was treated in the Marshall Islands, but his tuberculin skin test (TST) showed a negative reaction upon entering Hawaii. Later, the juvenile, living in a shelter at the time, was treated for TB and the man was identified as a contact, at which time the man produced a suspicious chest X-ray and a positive T-SPOT.TB interferon gamma release assay (IGRA) test. However, his TST and QuantiFERON-TB IGRA test were negative, in addition to no acid-fast bacilli being found in his sputum and his sputum culture growing no bacteria, so he was not treated at that time. Regardless, he produced a culture-positive sputum sample 16 months later, at which time the juvenile was also re-identified as a contact. Despite this complexity, zero SNPs were found between the two isolates, unambiguously indicating direct transmission.

Sensitivity and specificity of standard *Mtb* fingerprinting

Comparing the ability of WGS and standard *Mtb* fingerprinting to resolve the ten epidemiologically identified *Mtb* clusters in this study showed that fingerprinting indicated that eight of the ten epidemiological clusters were genetic clusters, while WGS indicated that only three of the ten epidemiological clusters were genetic clusters (Additional file 5). Standard fingerprinting was unable to resolve any of the clusters indicated by WGS. If WGS is designated as the "gold standard" for *Mtb* typing, then the sensitivity *Mtb* fingerprinting for identifying actual transmission clusters was found to be 100% (95% CI, 31.0–100%), while its specificity was only 28.6% (95% CI, 5.1–69.7%).

MIRU-VNTR resolution of Beijing and Manila family clusters

Of the 562 isolates in this study that were fully fingerprinted with 24-loci MIRU-VNTR and that had no loci that failed to sequence, 369 were in the Manila family (lineage 1), 150 were in the Beijing family (lineage 2), and 43 were in the various spoligotyping clades of lineage 4. (All of Hawaii's *Mtb* isolates were typed with 24 loci MIRU-VNTR fingerprinting from 2009 onwards, but most isolates prior to 2009 were only typed with 12-loci MIRU-VNTR typing and thus were not included in this analysis.) Analysis of MIRU-VNTR allele distribution over the full set of 24 loci indicated reduced Shannon diversity indices and Shannon evenness values of MIRU-VNTR allele distribution in the Beijing and Manila families (lineages 2 and 1) compared to lineage 4 (Additional file 6).

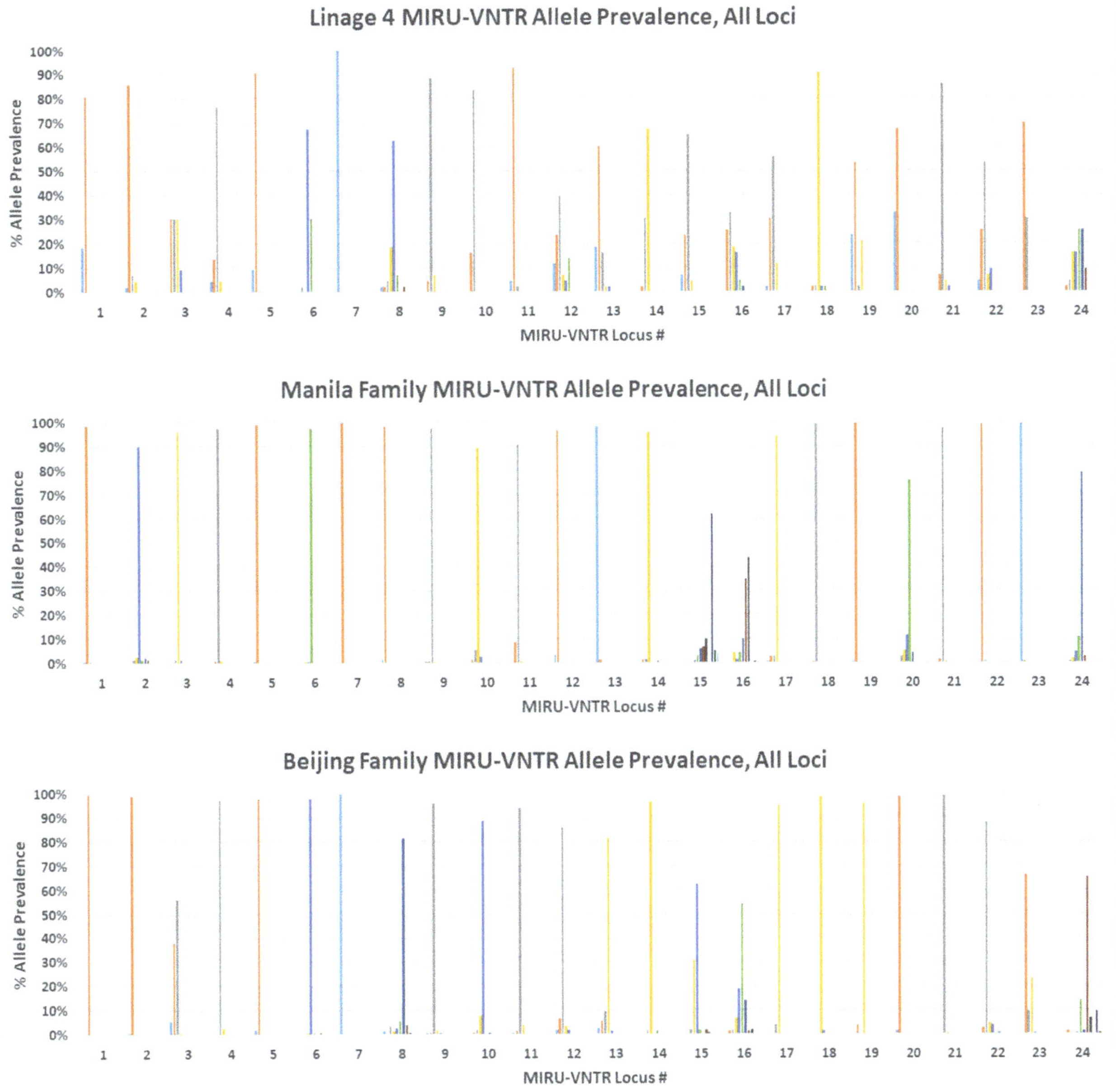

Fig. 2 Comparison of MIRU-VNTR Allele Prevalence by Lineage and Family. Each numbered group of bars represents one locus used in 24 loci MIRU-VNTR typing of *Mtb*. Vertical bars represent the percentage of all alleles at each locus that each allele comprises. The reduced allelic evenness demonstrated by the Beijing and Manila families relative to lineage 4 at most loci is readily observed

This reduced evenness is readily apparent from the histogram of allele distributions presented in Fig. 2. The Beijing family displayed significantly lower average Shannon diversity indices ($p \leq 0.002$) and Shannon evenness values ($p \leq 0.002$) over the full set of 24 loci than lineage 4 (Fig. 3). Likewise, the Manila family displayed significantly lower average Shannon diversity indices ($p \leq 0.001$) and Shannon evenness values ($p \leq 0.001$) over the full set of 24 loci than lineage 4. However, the Beijing and Manila families were not significantly different from each other by that index ($p = 0.4$).

Genes containing intra-cluster SNPs

Every putative cluster that was determined to represent an actual transmission cluster and whose isolates were separated by at least one SNP was examined to determine which genes hosted the intra-cluster mutations. Additional file 7 displays these genes, their mutations, and their TubercuList annotations and descriptions. SNPs from repetitive PPE and PE-PGRS family genes were discarded as questionable SNPs (possibly resulting from alignment errors) in this study because we did not confirm individual SNPs with PCR assays or Sanger sequencing.

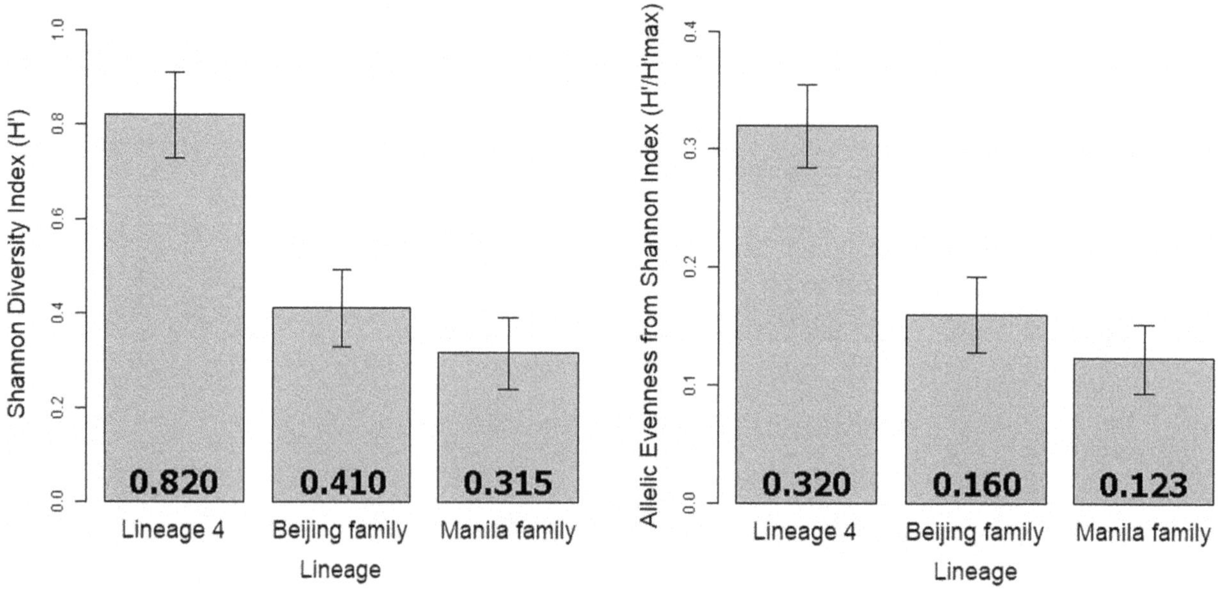

Fig. 3 Mean Shannon Diversity Index and Evenness Values for 24 MIRU-VNTR Loci, by Lineage. The Shannon diversity index and evenness values of the Beijing and Manila families are statistcally significantly lower than lineage 4 for both metrics at the $p = 0.005$ level, but the Beijing and Manila families are not significantly different from each other at the $p = 0.05$ level for either metric. Error bars represent 95% confidence intervals

Discussion

This work demonstrated that established standard molecular fingerprinting methods for *Mtb* (spoligotyping plus 24-loci MIRU-VNTR typing) are insufficient for epidemiological investigation of TB in Hawaii. Our study is not alone in such findings. One study that utilized 1999 consecutive *MTb* isolates processed by a laboratory in the English Midlands from 2012 to 2015 identified that the performance of MIRU-VNTR profiles for identifying genomic relatedness in *Mtb* differed by lineage [15]. Notably, when they modeled the number of SNPs between paired isolates assuming a linear relationship over 1–3 MIRU-VNTR locus differences, they found that while paired lineage 4 isolates with identical MIRU-VNTR profiles displayed a median of 10 SNPs, lineages 1 and 2 displayed 122 and 159 SNPs, respectively. However, this study also showed that the number of pairwise SNPs between isolates was significantly higher when one or both isolates were from a recent immigrant, suggesting that the study's specific conclusions partially represented trends in domestic versus foreign transmission associated with different lineages. Regardless, it further illustrates the necessity of WGS over MIRU-VNTR for investigation of Mtb transmission.

With WGS serving as our "gold standard," we demonstrated the specificity of CDC-standard fingerprinting (spoligotyping plus MIRU-VNTR) in our geographic region with high levels of Beijing and Manila family *Mtb* to be only 28.6% (Additional file 5). Such a low level provides clinicians and epidemiologists with very low confidence that a purported transmission cluster identified by standard fingerprinting represents an actual transmission cluster. Note that these data are not intended to propose that WGS be considered the gold standard for *Mtb* epidemiological analysis; rather, they are intended to illustrate how high prevalence of certain *Mtb* families exposes shortcomings in presently-employed *Mtb* genetic fingerprinting methods. However, although IS*6110* has previously been considered the "gold standard" for *Mtb* molecular epidemiology, isolates with as many as 130 SNPs between them have been shown to have identical IS*6110* fingerprints, adding support that WGS has become the de-facto "gold standard" for *Mtb* molecular epidemiology [39, 40].

Our previous work illustrated that even with the full set of 24 MIRU-VNTR loci, potential Beijing and Manila family transmission clusters are poorly resolved by this method of fingerprinting [29]. Here, we identified that MIRU-VNTR's lack of resolving ability results from the Beijing and Manila families both being characterized by a greater number of loci that are dominated by either one allele or a small set of alleles than lineage 4. While the Shannon diversity index itself does not indicate how much of its diversity is derived from allelic richness versus allelic evenness, evenness can be easily calculated using values from the Shannon diversity index. Figure 3 shows that most of the reduction in Shannon diversity demonstrated by the Beijing and

Manila families is due to a decrease in allelic evenness instead of a decrease in allelic diversity. However, it should be noted that lineage 4 contains multiple major clades, compared to one clade each for lineages 1 and 2, and thus higher allelic evenness should generally be expected from lineage 4 overall. Regardless, this work illustrates why MIRU-VNTR fingerprinting is less effective at identifying actual transmission when applied to Beijing and Manila family isolates.

These data help demonstrate why CDC-standard molecular fingerprinting of *Mtb* is insufficient for areas of the world where the Beijing and Manila families are dominant. Thus, this study investigated in detail the ability of whole genome sequencing-based analysis to compensate for MIRU-VNTR's shortcoming by resolving fingerprinting-derived clusters from those two families in order to identify actual transmission.

Combining epidemiology with whole genome sequencing for cluster resolution

Of the 19 possible transmission clusters we investigated, definitive verdicts of recent transmission, partial transmission, or non-transmission were reached for all clusters. Epidemiological investigation was used to further strengthen or disprove the determinations of transmission or non-transmission. Although WGS analysis was able to disprove the apparent transmission that was initially suspected based on epidemiological connections for several apparent clusters, there were no cases where epidemiological information was sufficient to call WGS-derived transmission determinations into question.

Genes containing cluster-informative SNPs

In order to explore which genes could be experiencing rapid mutation and producing the SNPs that distinguished isolates within individual transmission clusters, isolates from those clusters were aligned against GenBank genome CP003248.2, which was selected due to its manually-curated annotation at TubercuList. These informative SNPs that distinguished isolates in actual transmission clusters are contained in a broad range of genes (Additional file 7). The genes identified in this study differ from those identified by a previous study examining an outbreak in San Francisco with the H1 spoligotype [27]. The genes where intra-cluster SNPs were located did not appear to demonstrate any lineage association, and included an ATPase, an ABC transporter membrane protein, a PHOH-like protein PhoH2 phosphate starvation-inducible protein, a PSIH-like sequence-specific RNA helicase, an RNAse, and several hypothetical proteins, among others [41, 42].

Determining isolate relatedness through whole genome sequencing

The selection of cut-off points for a SNP's required read coverage and read consensus (allele frequency) are of interest for developing a system for applied WGS epidemiology. Previous studies have required 75% read consensus or 10x read coverage and 80% read consensus, and found a mutation rate of ~ 0.5 SNPs per genome per year and 0.4 SNPs per genome per year [16, 28]. At the extreme ends of range proposed by Walker et al. for identifying transmission-linked or possibly linked isolates (0–1 SNPs and 6–12 SNPS), this information may suggest to tuberculosis controllers whether two isolates were likely the result of recent, direct transmission, or whether the transmission occurred in the more distant past (allowing time for divergent accumulation of SNPs in each infection) or through an intermediate host [28]. However, with several transmission clusters investigated in this work displaying 3–4 SNPs distinguishing their isolates, we cannot propose whether they represent direct transmission or not – only recent transmission.

Conclusion

This project demonstrated use of whole genome sequencing to successfully overcome the Beijing and Manila families' current fingerprinting difficulties, which have been a persistent problem for State of Hawaii tuberculosis control efforts. We identified why even 24-loci MIRU-VNTR fingerprinting fails to effectively resolve Beijing and Manila family clusters, and illustrated the advantage and necessity of utilizing WGS for molecular epidemiology in this region. As we continue to characterize the epidemiology of tuberculosis in Hawaii, more isolates from the largest Beijing and Manila family fingerprinting clusters will be sequenced to provide a more complete picture of their transmission.

Additional files

Additional file 1: Isolates Selected for WGS from Clusters Identified by Identical Genetic Fingerprints. This table summarizes the isolates that were selected for WGS from clusters that were initially identified by their shared genetic fingerprints.

Additional file 2: Clusters Identified by Shared Uncommon Spoligotypes. This table summarizes the isolates that were selected for WGS from clusters that were initially identified by their shared uncommon spoligotypes.

Additional file 3: Epidemiologically Identified Clusters. This table summarizes the isolates that were selected for WGS from clusters that were initially identified by epidemiology.

Additional file 4: U Cluster 1 Demographics. This table displays the demographics of the patients providing isolates from U Cluster 1.

Additional file 5: Comparison of the Sensitivity and Specificity of Standard *Mtb* Fingerprinting against Whole Genome Sequencing (WGS). This "2 x 2 Table" illustrates how the sensitivity and specificity of standard

Mtb fingerprinting for the epidemiologically-identified clusters in this study were calculated.

Additional file 6: Comparison of Individual MIRU-VNTR Loci through the Shannon Diversity Index and Shannon Evenness. This table contains the Diversity Shannon Diversity Index and Shannon Evenness values for each of the 24 standard MIRU-VNTR loci.

Additional file 7: Genes Containing Intra-cluster SNPs. This table displays the genes and mutation sites where SNPs that distinguished isolates within clusters were found.

Abbreviations

CDC: Centers for Disease Control and Prevention; MIRU-VNTR: Mycobacterial Interspersed Repetitive Units-Variable Number Tandem Repeats; *Mtb*: *Mycobacterium tuberculosis*; PE-PGRS: Proline-glutamic Acid - Polymorphic GC-Rich Sequence; PPE: Proline-Proline-glutamic Acid; PPV: Positive Predictive Value; SNP: Single Nucleotide Polymorphism; TB: Tuberculosis; WGS: Whole Genome Sequencing; WHO: World Health Organization

Acknowledgements

We thank Dr. Richard Brostrom for his conversations and insights that proved invaluable to this project. We thank Dr. Steven Seifried for his contributions to our analysis.

Funding

This research was partially supported by the University of Hawaii College of Natural Sciences and the Office of the Vice Chancellor for Research. This funding was provided to support general laboratory operations, and the funders had no role in the design of this study, the collection, analysis, and interpretation of data, or in writing the manuscript. No additional external funding supported this work.

Authors' contributions

Study conception and design: KJK, JTD, LQ. Data acquisition, analysis, and interpretation: KJK, JTD, AL, JTF, KPD, ED, XW, SH. Manuscript writing: KJK, JTD, JTF. All authors read and approved the final manuscript.

Consent for publication

Not applicable – all details relating to patients were de-identified pursuant to State of Hawaii HIPAA guidelines prior to inclusion in this study.

Competing interests

The authors declare that they have no competing interests.

Author details

[1]University of Hawaii at Manoa, Honolulu, HI, USA. [2]Hawaii State Department of Health, Honolulu, HI, USA. [3]University of New Hampshire, Durham, NH, USA. [4]California Department of Public Health, Richmond, CA, USA. [5]Advanced Studies in Genomics, Proteomics and Bioinformatics, Honolulu, HI, USA. [6]Present Address: Pathogen and Microbiome Institute, Northern Arizona University, Flagstaff, AZ, USA.

References

1. Global Tuberculosis Report 2016. http://apps.who.int/medicinedocs/documents/s23098en/s23098en.pdf. Accessed 5 Dec 2017.
2. Stewart RJ, Tsang CA, Pratt RH, Price SF, Langer AJ. Tuberculosis — United States, 2017. Morb Mortal Wkly Rep. 2018;67:317–23.
3. Gagneux S. Ecology and evolution of Mycobacterium tuberculosis. Nat Rev Microbiol. 2018;16(4):202–13.
4. Comas I, Gagneux S. The past and future of tuberculosis research. PLoS Pathog. 2009;5(10):e1000600.
5. Bamrah S, Desmond E, Ghosh S, France AM, Kammerer JS, Cowan LS, et al. Molecular epidemiology of Mycobacterium tuberculosis in the United States–affiliated Pacific Islands. Asia Pac J Public Health. 2014;26(1):77–84.
6. Douglas JT, Qian L, Montoya J, Musser J, Van Embden J, Van Soolingen D, et al. Characterization of the Manila family of Mycobacterium tuberculosis. J Clin Microbiol. 2003;41:2723–6.
7. van Soolingen D, Qian L, de Haas PE, Douglas JT, Traore H, Portaels F, et al. Predominance of a single genotype of Mycobacterium tuberculosis in countries of East Asia. J Clin Microbiol. 1995;33:3234–8.
8. Kamerbeek J, Schouls L, Kolk A, van Agterveld M, van Soolingen D, et al. Simultaneous detection and strain differentiation of Mycobacterium tuberculosis for diagnosis and epidemiology. J Clin Microbiol. 1997;35:907–14.
9. Gagneux S, DeRiemer K, Van T, Kato-Maeda M, de Jong BC, Narayanan S, et al. Variable host–pathogen compatibility in Mycobacterium tuberculosis. Proc Natl Acad Sci U S A. 2006;103(8):2869–73.
10. Comas I, Homolka S, Niemann S, Gagneux S. Genotyping of Genetically Monomorphic Bacteria: DNA Sequencing in Mycobacterium tuberculosis Highlights the Limitations of Current Methodologies. PLoS One. 2009;4(11):e7815.
11. van Embden J, Cave M, Crawford J, Dale J, Eisenach K, Gicquel B, et al. Strain identification of Mycobacterium tuberculosis by DNA fingerprinting: recommendations for a standardized methodology. J Clin Microbiol. 1993;31:406–9.
12. Supply P, Allix C, Lesjean S, Cardoso-Oelemann M, Rusch-Gerdes S, Willery E, et al. Proposal for standardization of optimized mycobacterial interspersed repetitive unit–variable-number tandem repeat typing of Mycobacterium tuberculosis. J Clin Microbiol. 2006;44:4498–510.
13. Cowan L, Diem L, Monson T, Wand P, Temporado D, Oemig T, Crawford J. Evaluation of a two-step approach for large-scale, prospective genotyping of Mycobacterium tuberculosis isolates in the United States. J Clin Microbiol. 2005;43:688–95.
14. Tuberculosis (TB) Laboratory Information. https://www.cdc.gov/tb/topic/laboratory/default.htm. Accessed 5 Dec 2017.
15. Wyllie DH, Davidson JA, Grace Smith E, Rathod P, Crook DW, Peto TEA, Robinson E, Walker T, Campbell C. A quantitative evaluation of MIRU-VNTR typing against whole-genome sequencing for identifying Mycobacterium tuberculosis transmission: a prospective observational cohort study. EBioMedicine. 2018;34:122–30.
16. Roetzer A, Schuback S, Diel R, Gasau F, Ubben T, di Nauta A, et al. Evaluation of Mycobacterium tuberculosis typing methods in a 4-year study in Schleswig-Holstein, Northern Germany. J Clin Microbiol. 2011;49:4173–8.
17. Guo YL, Liu Y, Wang SM, Li CY, Jiang GL, Shi GL, et al. Genotyping and drug resistance patterns of Mycobacterium tuberculosis strains in five provinces of China. Int J Tuberc Lung Dis. 2011;15:789–94.
18. Hanekom M, van der Spuy GD, Gey van Pittius NC, CR ME, Hoek KG, Ndabambi SL, et al. Discordance between mycobacterial interspersed repetitive-unit-variable-number tandem-repeat typing and IS6110 restriction fragment length polymorphism genotyping for analysis of Mycobacterium tuberculosis Beijing strains in a setting of high incidence of tuberculosis. J Clin Microbiol. 2008;46:3338–45.
19. Kam KM, Yip CW, Tse LW, Wong KL, Lam TK, Kremer K, et al. Utility of mycobacterial interspersed repetitive unit typing for differentiating multidrug-resistant Mycobacterium tuberculosis isolates of the Beijing family. J Clin Microbiol. 2005;43:306–13.
20. Kam K, Yip C, Tse L, Leung K, Wong K, Ko W, et al. Optimization of variable number tandem repeat typing set for differentiating Mycobacterium tuberculosis strains in the Beijing family. FEMS Microbiol Lett. 2006;256:258–65.
21. de Steenwinkel J, ten Kate M, de Knegt G, Kremer K, Aarnoutse R, Boeree M, et al. Drug susceptibility of Mycobacterium tuberculosis Beijing genotype and association with MDR TB. Emerg Infect Dis. 2012;18(4):660–3.

22. Buu T, van Soolingen D, Huyen M, Lan N, Quy H, Tiemersma E, et al. Increased transmission of Mycobacterium tuberculosis Beijing genotype strains associated with resistance to streptomycin: a population-based study. PLoS One. 2012;7(8):e42323.
23. Sharma A, Hill A, Kurbatova E, van der Walt M, Kvasnovsky C, Tupasi TE, et al. Estimating the future burden of multidrug-resistant and extensively drug-resistant tuberculosis in India, the Philippines, Russia, and South Africa: a mathematical modelling study. Lancet Infect Dis. 2017. https://doi.org/10.1016/S1473-3099(17)30247-5.
24. Schürch A, Kremer K, Daviena O, Kiers A, Boeree MJ, Siezen RJ, et al. High-resolution typing by integration of genome sequencing data in a large tuberculosis cluster. J Clin Microbiol. 2010;48(9):3403–6.
25. Mokrousov I, Chernyaeva E, Vyazovaya A, Sinkov V, Zhuravlev V, Narvskaya O. Next-generation sequencing of Mycobacterium tuberculosis. Emerg Infect Dis. 2016;22(6):1127–9.
26. Gardy J, Johnston JC, Ho Sui S, Cook VJ, Shah L, Brodkin E, et al. Whole-genome sequencing and social-network analysis of a tuberculosis outbreak. N Engl J Med. 2011;364:730–9.
27. Kato-Maeda M, Ho C, Passarelli B, Banaei N, Grinsdale J, Flores L, et al. Use of whole genome sequencing to determine the microevolution of Mycobacterium tuberculosis during an outbreak. PLoS One. 2013;8(3):e58235.
28. Walker TM, Ip CL, Harrell RH, Evans JT, Kapatai G, Dedicoat MJ, et al. Whole-genome sequencing to delineate Mycobacterium tuberculosis outbreaks: a retrospective observational study. Lancet Infect Dis. 2013;13:137–46.
29. Wan X, Koster K, Qian L, Desmond E, Brostrom R, et al. Genomic analyses of the ancestral Manila family of Mycobacterium tuberculosis. PLoS One. 2017;12(4):e0175330.
30. Koster K, Largen A, Foster JT, Drees KP, Qian L, Desmond EP, Wan X, Hou S, Douglas JT. Whole genome SNP analysis suggests unique virulence factor differences of the Beijing and Manila families of Mycobacterium tuberculosis found in Hawaii. PLoS One. 2018;13(7):e0201146. https://doi.org/10.1371/journal.pone.0201146.
31. Brudey K, Driscoll JR, Rigouts L, Prodinger WM, Gori A, Al-Hajoj SA, et al. Mycobacterium tuberculosis complex genetic diversity: mining the fourth international spoligotyping database (SpolDB4) for classification, population genetics and epidemiology. BMC Microbiol. 2006;6:23.
32. Sahl JW, Lemmer D, Travis J, Schupp JM, Gillece JD, Aziz M, et al. NASP: an accurate, rapid method for the identification of SNPs in WGS datasets that supports flexible input and output formats. Microbial Genomics. 2016;2:e000074.
33. Langmead B, Salzberg SL. Fast gapped-read alignment with bowtie 2. Nat Methods. 2012;9(4):357–9.
34. McKenna A, Hanna M, Banks E, Sivachenko A, Cibulskis K, Kernytsky A, et al. The genome analysis toolkit: a MapReduce framework for analyzing next-generation DNA sequencing data. Genome Res. 2010;20:1297–303.
35. Nascimento M, Sousa A, Francisco AP, Carriço JA, Vaz C. PHYLOViZ 2.0: providing scalable data integration and visualization for multiple phylogenetic inference methods. Bioinformatics. 2017;33(1):128–9.
36. Francisco AP, Bugalho M, Ramirez M, Carriço JA. Global optimal eBURST analysis of multilocus typing data using a graphic matroid approach. BMC Bioinformatics. 2009;10:152.
37. Koster K, Qian L, Flores C, Desmond E, Brostrom R, Foster J, et al. Cluster identification and analysis of clinical Mycobacterium tuberculosis isolates in the state of Hawaii. Washington, DC: Abstr 115th gen meet am Soc Microbiol. American Society for Microbiology; 2015.
38. Clinical Calculator 1. http://vassarstats.net/clin1.html. Accessed 5 Dec 2017.
39. Roetzer A, Diel R, Kohl TA, Rückert C, Nübel U, Blom J, et al. Whole genome sequencing versus traditional genotyping for investigation of a Mycobacterium tuberculosis outbreak: a longitudinal molecular epidemiological study. PLoS Med. 2013;10(2):e1001387.
40. Lee RS, Behr MA. Does choice matter? Reference-based alignment for molecular epidemiology of tuberculosis. J Clin Microbiol. 2016;54(7):1891–5.
41. TubercuList. http://tuberculist.epfl.ch/. Accessed 8 Nov 2017.
42. Andrews ES, Arcus VL. The mycobacterial PhoH2 proteins are type II toxin antitoxins coupled to RNA helicase domains. Tuberculosis (Edinb). 2015;95(4):385–94.

13

Upper respiratory infections in a rural area with reduced malaria transmission in Senegal

Roger C. Tine[1*†], Léon A. Ndiaye[1†], Mbayame N. Niang[2], Davy E. Kiori[2], Ndongo Dia[2], Oumar Gaye[1] and Hélène Broutin[1,3]

Abstract

Background: Acute Respiratory Infections (ARI) are common causes of febrile illnesses in many settings in Senegal. These infections are usually managed presumptively due to lack of appropriate diagnostic tools. This situation, can lead to poor management of febrile illness or antibiotic misuse. In addition, there are limited data on the spectrum of pathogens commonly responsible for these ARI. This study was conducted to explore the pathogens community among patients with acute respiratory infection in a rural area in Senegal.

Methods: A cross sectional study was conducted from August to December 2015. Children and adult patients attending Keur Socé health post for signs suggestive of acute respiratory infection were enrolled after providing inform consent. Eligible participants were recruited using a consecutive sampling method. Paired nose and throat swabs were collected for pathogen detection. Samples were processed using a multiplex PCR designed to identify 21 pathogens including both virus and bacteria.

Results: Two hundred and fifty patients participated in the study. Samples positivity rate was evaluated at 95.2% (238/250). *Streptococcus pneumoniae* was the predominant pathogen (74%) and was present in all months and all age-groups, followed by *Staphylococcus aureus* (28,8%) and rhinovirus (28,4%). Respiratory syncytial virus (RSV) was detected only among children under 5 years old in August and September while coronavirus was present in all age groups, during the months of October and December.

Conclusion: This pilot study revealed a diversity of pathogens over the time and across all age groups, highlighting the need for further exploration. A pathogen community approach including both virus and bacteria at a larger scale becomes crucial for a better understanding of transmission dynamics at population level in order to help shape ARI control strategies.

Keywords: ARI, Senegal, Pathogen community, *Streptococcus pneumoniae*, RSV, Influenza

Background

Progress in the fight against malaria achieved through increased deployment of insecticide-treated bed-nets and artemisinin combination therapy (ACTs) has led to significant reduction of the disease burden in many malaria-endemic countries [1–3]. In Senegal, malaria has been a major disease for many years, accounting for 35% of all outpatients consultations in health care services [4]. The introduction of rapid diagnostic tests (RDT) in the country, has contributed to a better documentation of malaria cases and has resulted in a reduction of anti-malarial consumption [5]. While RDTs can improve targeting of anti-malarial drugs, there is no comparable test for bacterial or viral diseases and these pathogens are known to be leading causes of febrile illnesses [6]. Thus, patients with negative malaria RDT are being managed presumptively in many settings [7] and many febrile patients may be prescribed broad spectrum of antibiotics. In the context of declining of malaria reported in many

* Correspondence: roger.tine@ucad.edu.sn
†Roger C. Tine and Léon A. Ndiaye contributed equally to this work.
1Service de Parasitologie, Faculté de Médecine, Université Cheikh Anta Diop de Dakar (UCAD), BP5005 Dakar-Fann, Senegal
Full list of author information is available at the end of the article

African countries [8], this situation can lead to the occurrence and the spread of antibiotic resistance as well as poor management of febrile illnesses [9]. Thus, appropriate treatment guidelines are needed [10]. To achieve this, a better understanding in the epidemiology of non-malaria febrile illnesses is required. A prospective study conducted by the department of medical parasitology in Keur Socé rural area, a malaria sentinel site in the central part of Senegal, revealed that 75% of febrile illnesses among outpatients with negative malaria RDT were caused by acute respiratory infections (Tine et al. unpublished). However, the study was mainly a syndromic-based disease surveillance approach with limited biological investigations for pathogens identification. A better understanding of pathogens distribution and frequency during acute respiratory tract infections will improve current treatment guidelines and help shape preventive strategies related to these diseases.

Studies conducted in Africa, identified respiratory tract infections due to *Streptococcus pneumoniae* as a main cause of non-malaria febrile illnesses among other causes such as typhoid fever, urinary tract infection and other parasitic infections other than malaria [11–13].

Although several studies showed the importance of Acute Respiratory Infections (ARI) on febrile illness occurrence [11–13], few of them were conducted among adult patients [14, 15]. However, understanding ARI transmission dynamic may require additional investigations among higher age group population. Indeed the route transmission of these ARI is still unclear and looking at pathogens distribution across all age-groups has become crucial for a better understanding of pathogens reservoir, especially in rural settings with high burden of ARI such as the central part of Senegal. In the meantime, most of the previous studies focused on bacterial ARI and did not include assessment of viral causes like influenza, which is known to be present in all age-groups [16–18].

To provide first insights on these important gaps, we conducted a pilot study in Senegal, to explore the pathogens community in the nasopharyngeal tract among individuals with ARI in a rural primary health care unit, including all age groups and targeting both bacteria and viruses.

Methods

Study settings

The study was carried out at the rural area of Keur Socé, a malaria sentinel site located in the central part of Senegal, at 200 km from the capital city of Dakar. The area of "Keur Socé" covers 73 villages with 2 health posts providing mainly primary care (Keur Socé health post and Lamarame health post), headed by nurses. A demographic surveillance system (DSS) is going on within the 73 villages with a total population size at 35000 inhabitants.

Study design and participants

A cross sectional study was carried out from August to December 2015. Children and adults attending the Keur Socé Health post for symptoms suggestive of acute respiratory infection according to IMCI guideline [10] were screened by the health post staff for eligibility. Eligible participants were then sent to the research team for enrolment in the study if they consented to participate. Participants, who were previously screened for respiratory tract infection within the same study period and patients with severe illness, were excluded. Eligible participants were recruited using a consecutive sampling method.

Data collection methods

A code was given to each enrolled participant and a physician examined each participant prior to the biological assessments, which included naso-pharyngeal swab collection for PCR analysis. The patient was interviewed directly to determine socio-demographic characteristics, patient's medical history and vaccination status, using a standard questionnaire. For children, these information were obtained from their mothers or care takers. For each enrolled study participant, paired nose and throat swabs were collected for pathogens detection. Symptoms presented by each participant on the day of survey, as well as data obtained from interviews and biological investigations were assigned on a case report form (CRF).

Laboratory methods

Samples were collected by the study physician using a sterile nylon flocked swab and placed in viral transport medium *("BD Universal Viral")*, labelled and transported on ice at Pasteur Institute Dakar for further processing and storage of the samples. Nucleic acids were extracted using the Qiamp viral Kit according to manufacturer's instructions. Pathogens detection was performed using the Fast track Diagnostic Kit (FTD Respiratory pathogens 21 kit Luxembourg) which is a multiplex PCR essay designed to detect 21 pathogens. The kit presents 6 tubes multiplex PCR for the detection of different pathogens: (i) First tube: influenza A, influenza B, influenza A H1N1, human rhinovirus; (ii) second tube: coronavirus NL63, coronavirus 229E, coronavirus OC43, coronavirus (HKU1); (iii) third tube: parainfluenza 2, parainfluenza 3, parainfluenza 4, Internal Control; [19] fourth tube: parainfluenza 1, human metapneumovirus A/B, bocavirus, *Mycoplasma pneumoniae*; (v) fifth tube (respiratory syncytial viruses A/B, adenovirus, enterovirus, parechovirus; (vi) sixth tube: *Chlamydia pneumoniae*, *Streptococcus pneumoniae*, *Haemophilus influenzae* type B,

Table 1 Number of samples done by month and by age group from August to December 2015

Month	< 1 year	1–5 years	6–15 years	> 15 years	Total
August	15	29	1	5	50
September	11	28	4	7	50
October	12	23	4	11	50
November	16	20	1	13	50
December	17	23	4	6	50
Screened at health post for eligibility	160	223	49	130	565
Enrolled in the study	71	123	14	42	250

Staphylococcus aureus. The multiplex real-time PCR FTD assay was performed on an ABI 7500 Fast instrument (Life Technologies, USA) as described elsewere [20] and PCR programme was as follow: 50 °C for 15 min, 95 °C for 10 min, 40 cycles of 95 °C for 8 s, 60 °C for 34 s.

Statistical methods

Sample size assumption: with 250 participants sampled, the study was powered at 80% to provide an estimate for each pathogen with a 10% precision, assuming a 75% morbidity related to acute respiratory infection among febrile outpatients (temperature > 37 °C) seen at the health post (Tine et al. unpublished) with alpha at 0.05 (two sided).

Data were entered in Excel software and all analyses were conducted using Stata package (StataCorp, Texas). For categorical data, percentage was used to assess the frequency of each outcome with a 95% confidence interval. For continuous data, mean and standard deviation were used to describe normally distributed variables, median and range for other data. Characteristics of all participants included in the study were tabulated. Proportions were compared using chi square test or Fisher exact test where appropriated (univariate analysis). To assess the effect of age on pathogens distribution, a multivariate logistic regression was done with adjustment on covariates such as study period. From the final model, adjusted odds ratios were derived with their 95% confidence interval. Model validity was tested using the Hosmer-Lemeshow goodness of fit test. The performance of the final model was assessed by the area under the curve and Akaike and Bayesian information criterion; in addition a test for multicolinearity between variables was done using the variance inflation factor. Significance level of the different tests was 0.05, two sided.

Ethical considerations

Participation to the study was strictly voluntary and patients who refused to be enrolled were not included in the study. A signed informed consent was obtained from each eligible participant prior to any investigation. For minor participants (age < 18 years) informed consent was obtained from parents or children's legal representative prior to their enrollement. To ensure confidentiality, information collected during the study were analysed using participant's identification code. The study protocol and other study related documents (CRF, Inform consent Form) were approved by the Senegalese national ethics committee (*Conseil National d'Ethique et de Recherche en Santé – N°0166 MSAS/DPRS/CNERS du 10 Mai 2014).*

Results

Participant's characteristics at enrollment

Among the 565 patients who consulted at the health post for signs suggestive of respiratory infections, 250 of

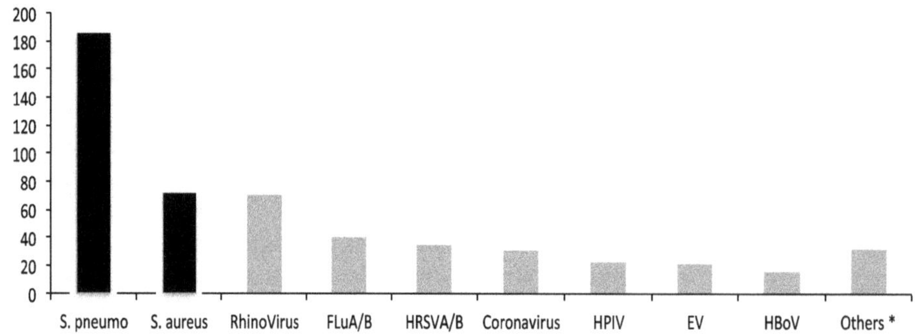

Fig. 1 Pathogens distribution among the 250 analysed samples

Table 2 Overall distribution of sample positivity and pathogens association ($N = 250$)

Type of pathogenes	Number	Percentage	(95%CI)
Virus			
Absence	75	30	24.4–36.1
patients with viral species	124	49.6	43.2–55.9
patients carrying 2 viral species	44	17.6	13.1–22.9
patients with 3 viral species	07	02.8	1.1–5.7
Combined (at least 1 viral pathogen)	175	70	63.9–75.6
Bacteria			
Absence	43	17.2	12.7–22.5
patients with 1 bacterial species	139	55.6	49.2–61.8
Patients with 2 bacterial species	68	27.2	21.8–33.2
Combined (at least 1 bacterial pathogen)[a]	207	82.8	77.5–87.3
Association of virus and bacteria			
Absence	12	4.8	2.5–8.2
Patients with at least 1 virus and 1 bacterial species	238	95.2	91.8–97.5

[a]Comparison between proportion of patients with at least one viral pathogen versus patients with bacterial pathogen: difference = 12.8% (95%CI (5.4–20.2) $p = 0.001$)

them fulfilled all defined inclusion criteria and were enrolled in the study. The majority of the samples were collected among the 1 to 5 years age-group which also represents the most affected age-group. Due to a very low number of samples in the 6–10 years (8 samples) and 11–15 years (6 samples), we aggregated both age groups in an unique age-group (6–15 years) for subsequent analyses (Table 1).

Frequency and spectrum of identified pathogens

Among the 250 samples, at least one pathogen was identified in 238 samples (95,2%) and the most frequent pathogen identified was *Streptococcus pneumoniae* (185/250, 74%), followed by *Staphylococcus aureus* (72/250, 28,8%) and *rhinovirus* (71/250, 28,4%) (Fig. 1).

Overall, 124 participants (49.6%) were found with one viral species while 44 patients (17.6%) were infected by at least 2 viruses; a proportion of 2.8% (7 patients) were co-infected with 3 viruses. Patients with one bacterial species represented 55.6% while that was at 27.2% for patients with 2 bacterial species. In total, 238 patients were found with at least 1 bacteria and 1 virus at the same time (Table 2).

The highest number of pathogens was detected among the under 5 years age group; these pathogens were mainly represented by *Streptococcus pneumoniae*, rhinovirus (in < 1 year) and *Staphylococcus aureus* (1-5 years). Among patients with age above 15 years, the main pathogens detected at the nasopharyngeal level were rhinovirus (31%) and *Staphylococcus aureus* (28,6%). *Streptococcus pneumoniae* was found in all age groups, with a higher frequency among infants and children (i.e. > 70%); it was also identified among patients above the age of 15 years with a frequency of 23.8%. Similarly, rhinovirus was detected in all age groups with lower proportion among the above 15 years old age-group (13/71, 18%). These 2 pathogens are thus circulating in all age groups. In contrast, human respiratory syncytial virus was detected only among the less than 5 years old age-group. The majority of influenza A/B (27/40, 67,5%) and coronavirus (14/31, 45.1%) were detected in 1–5 years old age group. The rest of the pathogens were detected at low levels in all age-groups. The

Table 3 Spectrum of the identified pathogens from naso-pharyngeal swabs by age-groups

Age-group	*S. pneumo* (*n* = 185)	*S. aureus* (*n* = 72)	*RhinoVirus* (*n* = 71)	*FLu A/B* (*n* = 40)	*HRSV A/B* (*n* = 35)	*Corona-virus* (*n* = 31)	*HPIV* (*n* = 22)	*EV* (*n* = 21)	*HBoV* (*n* = 16)	*Others*[a] (*n* = 32)	*Total number of pathogens identified*
< 1 year (n = 71)	**61 (*85,9*)**	16 (*22,5*)	**29 (*40,8*)**	6 (*8,5*)	14 (*19,7*)	10 (*14,1*)	7 (*9,9*)	5 (*7*)	4 (*5,6*)	9 (*12,7*)	***161***
1–5 years (*n* = 123)	**104 (*84,6*)**	**37 (*30,1*)**	27 (*22,0*)	27 (*22,0*)	20 (*16,3*)	14 (*11,4*)	11 (*8,9*)	8 (*6,5*)	6 (*4,9*)	16 (*13,0*)	***270***
6–15 years (*n* = 14)	**10 (*71,4*)**	**7 (*50,0*)**	2 (*14,3*)	4 (*28,6*)	0	2 (*14,3*)	2 (*14,3*)	3 (*21,4*)	2 (*14,3*)	2 (*14,3*)	***34***
> 15 years (*n* = 42)	10 (*23,8*)	**12 (*28,6*)**	**13 (*31,0*)**	3 (*7,1*)	1 (*2,4*)	5 (*11,9*)	2 (*4,8*)	5 (*11,9*)	4 (*9,5*)	5 (*11,9*)	***60***

The number in italic corresponds to percentage (%) among the age-groups. Bold numbers represent the 2 main pathogens identified in the considered age-group. S. pneumo: Streptococcus pneumoniae; H. Saureus: Staphylococcus aureus; Flu A/B: Influenza A/B; HRSV A/B: Human Respiratory Syncytial viruses, HPIV Human ParaInfluenza Virus, EV Enterovirus, BoV Bocavirus

[a]Others: Human metapneumovirus (HMPV) A/B, H1N1, Mycoplasma pneumoniae, Human Parechovirus (HPeV), Human Adenovirus (HAdv), Chlamydia pneumoniae, Haemophilus influenzae type B

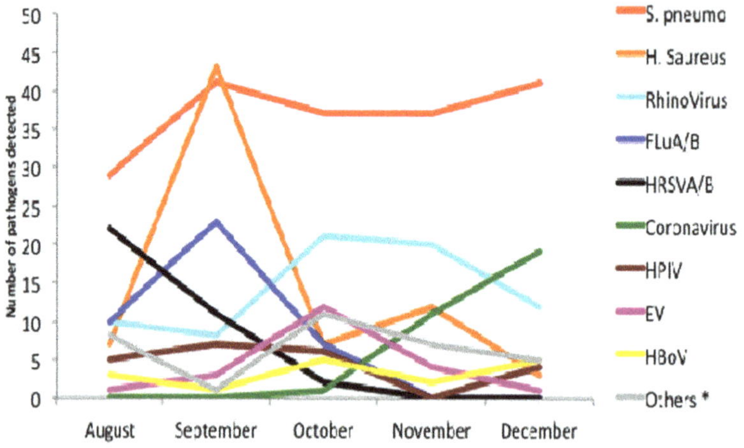

Fig. 2 Monthly Distribution of pathogens (2015)

distribution of the identified pathogens by age group is described in Table 3.

Pathogens distribution by age group and period

The 5 months sampling provided new insights about the temporal dynamics of pathogens. *Streptococcus pneumoniae* was detected in similar proportion during the 5 months and remained the major pathogen detected (Fig. 2). The majority of human respiratory syncytial virus (22/35, 63%) was detected in august, then it decreased in september and October; no respiratory syncytial virus was found during the months of november and december. *Staphylococcus aureus* and influenza virus A/B increased in september then decreased during the rest of the year. Rhinoviruses were detected at a low level in august and September; its frequency increased in october and november and then decreased in december. Finally, coronavirus were only detected from october and increased continuously up to december. All this temporal distribution shows a trend of successive pathogens over time within the population.

Overall, bacterial pathogens were more common among children compared to viral pathogens with significant statistical differences among children less than 1 year (prevalence difference: 34.1%; $p = 0.001$), and 1 to 5 years (prevalence difference: 19.5%; $p = 0.0002$); no significant difference was noted when comparing the frequency of bacterial versus viral pathogens both in the 6 to 15 years (prevalence difference: 28.8%; $p = 0.06$) and in the > 15 years (prevalence difference: 9.5%; $p = 0.38$) (Table 4).

A higher frequency of viral pathogens compared to bacterial pathogens was noted during the month of august (prevalence difference: 22%; $p = 0.009$). During the months of september, november, and december, bacterial pathogens were predominantly isolated compared to virus (all *p values* for these periods are < 0.05) (Table 5). Adjusted on age group, patients were less likely to carry viral infections during the months of september (adjusted Odds ratio:0.19, 95%CI(0.07–0.55)), november

Table 4 Pathogens distribution by age group and study period

	Viral pathogenes			Bacterial pathogenes			p value
	Number examined	Positive	Prevalence (95%CI)	Positive	Prevalence (95%CI)	Prevalence difference (95%CI)	
Age categories							
< 1 year	71	56	78.9 (67.5–87.7)	64	90.1 (80.7–95.9)	34.1 (20.6–47.6)	0.0001
1–5 years	123	85	69.1 (60.1–77.1)	109	88.6 (81.6 - 93.6)	19.5 (9.6–29.4)	0.0002
6–15 years	14	09	64.2 (35.1–87.2)	13	92.8 (66.1–99.8)	28.6 (0.06–57.1)	0.06
> 15 years	42	25	59.5 (43.3–74.4)	21	50.0 (34.2–65.8)	9.5 (11.7–30.7)	0.38
Study period							
August	50	44	88.0 (75.7–95.5)	33	66.0 (51.2–78.8)	22 (6.1–39.9)	0.009
September	50	29	58.0 (43.2–71.8)	49	98 (89.3–99.9)	40 (25.8–54.2)	< 0.001
October	50	41	82.0 (68.6–91.4)	40	80 (66.3–89.9)	02 (13.4–17.4)	0.79
November	50	30	60.0 (45.2–73.6)	42	84 (70.9–92.8)	24 (7.1–40.9)	0.007
December	50	31	62.0 (47.2–75.3)	43	86 (73.2–94.2)	24 (7.5–40.5)	0.006

Table 5 Adjusted effect of age and period on pathogens carriage among the study participants

Presence of virus				
	Frequency (95%CI)	OR (95%CI)	aOR (95%CI)	*p* value
Age categories				
< 1 year	78.9 (67.5–87.7)	*Reference*	*Reference*	
1–5 years	69.1 (60.1–77.1)	0.60 (0.30–1.19)	0.58 (0.28–1.19)	0.13
6–15 years	64.2 (35.1–87.2)	0.48 (0.14–1.65)	0.52 (0.14–1.87)	0.32
> 15 years	59.5 (43.3–74.4)	0.39 (0.17–0.97)	0.39 (0.16–0.94)	0.04
Study period				
August	88.0 (75.7–95.5)	*Reference*	*Reference*	
September	58.0 (43.2–71.8)	0.19 (0.07–0.52)	0.19 (0.07–0.55)	0.002
October	82.0 (68.6–91.4)	0.56 (0.19–1.68)	0.61 (0.20–1.85)	0.38
November	60.0 (45.2–73.6)	0.21 (0.08–0.60)	0.22 (0.08–0.64)	0.005
December	62.0 (47.2–75.3)	0.22 (0.08–0.62)	0.22 (0.08–0.63)	0.005
Presence of bacteria				
	Frequency (95%CI)	OR (95%CI)	aOR (95%CI)	*p* value
Age categories				
< 1 year	90.1 (80.7–95.9)	*Reference*	*Reference*	–
1–5 years	88.6 (81.6 - 93.6)	0.85 (0.33–2.22)	0.82 (0.30–2.24)	0.69
6–15 years	92.8 (66.1–99.8)	1.42 (0.16–12.56)	0.95 (0.09–9.25)	0.97
> 15 years	50.0 (34.2–65.8)	0.11 (0.04–0.29)	0.05 (0.02–0.18)	< 0.001
Study period				
August	66.0 (51.2–78.8)	*Reference*	*Reference*	–
September	98 (89.3–99.9)	25.2 (3.5–45.8)	56.5 (6.19–60.8)	< 0.001
October	80 (66.3–89.9)	1.87 (0.77–4.55)	3.55 (1.21–10.39)	0.02
November	84 (70.9–92.8)	3.09 (1.15–8.33)	8.66 (2.47–30.44)	0.001
December	86 (73.2–94.2)	3.16 (1.17–8.52)	4.51 (1.45–14.02)	0.009

Goodness of fit: chi (8df) = 3.74; p = 0.88. Area under the curve: 83.4%. Akaike information criterion (AIC) = 298.26; Bayesian information criterion = 326.43. Variance inflation factor (VIF) = 1.48

(adjusted Odds ratio: 0.22, 95%CI(0.08 - 0.64)) and december (adjusted Odds ratio: 0.22, 95%CI(0.08–0.63)) (Table 5).

Discussion

Acute Respiratory Infections are usually a clinical diagnosis in many primary health care units in Senegal. The diagnosis approach is often based on IMCI guidelines [10]. This pilot study was conducted to assess the spectrum and frequency of pathogens responsible of ARI using a highly sensitive multiplex RT-PCR technique. The study revealed a high positivity rate both for viral and bacterial pathogens and a broad spectrum of pathogens were detected in all age groups over the 5 months period of data collection, providing an original pathogens community study in the global population.

Streptococcus pneumoniae was the main pathogen detected and it remained constantly highly present over the 5 months of study, mainly among children but also among adults, suggesting a non-negligible and permanent reservoir of this pathogen among older age-groups. This observation deserves further investigation since it suggests that adults represent an important fraction of *Streptococcus pneumoniae* reservoir. The potential contribution of these adults in the transmission of *Streptococcus pneumoniae* to younger children needs to be investigated to determine whether they also need protection or not. Unfortunately, the study could not assess the diversity of the different pneumococcal serotypes in order to determine serotype variability across age-groups. In the context of recent introduction of pneumococcal conjugated vaccine-13 (PCV-13) in the Senegalese immunization program, it is now crucial to document the circulating serotypes, compared to the vaccine-serotypes, in all age-groups. This will help to generate evidence on the impact of vaccination on pneumococcal serotypes.

The highest diversity of pathogens detected from nasopharyngeal swab among patients with signs suggestive of ARI was observed among children under 5 years old. Indeed, under five children remained the most vulnerable group with regard to ARI as describe in other studies [14, 21]. *Streptococcus pneumoniae, Staphylococcus aureus* and *rhinovirus* were the major pathogens detected in all age-groups. In contrast, *respiratory syncytial virus* has been detected only in < 5 years old (except in 1 adult) children, suggesting a transmission route of the pathogen among this specific population group.

The 5 months study has also suggested a temporal dynamics of the pathogens with different seasonal patterns. For instance *respiratory syncytial virus* was only observed in august and september, while coronavirus was detected from october to december. That temporal dynamic of pathogens needs to be further investigated throughout a continuous surveillance system over several years, to look at potential seasonality of these pathogens. Establishing a clear temporal dynamic of pathogen could help shape treatment practices and preventive interventions.

This study presents some caveats. The first limit consists in the length of the study, which is not large enough to clearly establish a seasonally. Nevertheless, this pilot study revealed relevant trends to explore further, considering the specific pattern of pathogens (e.g. human respiratory syncytial virus, coronavirus) or the age-groups distribution of pathogens (e.g. *Streptococcus pneumoniae* vs human respiratory syncytial virus) to better understand the transmission dynamics.

The study used a highly sensitive multiplex RT-PCR to detect pathogens among patients with signs suggestive of ARI. However, it was not possible to clearly establish which of the identified pathogen was responsible of the observed symptoms, but still all these pathogens are circulating within the whole population.

Streptococcus pneumoniae remains the major pathogen circulating in all age groups over the 5 months of study. The next step consists in determining the serotypes that are circulating and responsible for ARI in the context of the recent introduction of the Pneumococcal vaccines in Africa, in the immunization programs. Only infants receive vaccines and the seroconversion is quick. It is perfectly timely to follow on the evolution of the pneumococcal serotypes under vaccine pressure in the whole population. *Streptococcus pneumoniae* carriage among adults is not negligible in our study highlighting the need for further investigations on adult's role in *Streptococcus pneumoniae* transmission to infants.

Conclusion

This first pilot study of 5 months surveillance at the community level, including both virus and bacteria deserves to be routinely implemented to assess the spatial and temporal dynamics of the pathogens community at the nasopharyngeal level. Such a surveillance system will allow improvement of current treatment practices and may contribute to reduce antibiotic consumption. Public health programs need a community pathogens overview to better control respiratory infections among high-risk groups. Co-infections are crucial to explore further to better understand the link between symptoms and pathogens and be able to provide appropriate treatment guidelines.

Acknowledgments

Authors are grateful to the population of Keur Socé health post for their diligent help during this study. We also thank the population for their participation and cooperation.

Funding

This work was funded by IRD (Projet PEERS-THERANGA) with additional funding support from the Department of Medical Parasitology, University Cheikh Anta Diop of Dakar, and Institut Pasteur of Dakar.

Authors' contributions

RCT, HB, OG conceived and designed the study. LAN, HB and RCT performed the data collection. LAN, MN, ND, DEK performed the laboratory essays. HB, RCT and LAN analysed the data. HB and RCT were responsible of the first draft of the manuscript. All authors participated to the writing of the paper and approved the final manuscript.

Ethics approval and consent to participate

Participation to the study was strictly voluntary and patients who refused to be enrolled were not included in the study. A signed informed consent was obtained from each eligible participant prior to any investigation. For minor participants (age < 18 years) informed consent was obtained from parents or children's legal representative prior to their enrollement. To ensure confidentiality, information collected during the study was analysed using participant's identification code. The study protocol and other study related documents (CRF, Inform consent Form) were approved by the Senegalese national ethics committee (Conseil National d'Ethique et de Recherche en Santé – N°0166 MSAS/DPRS/CNERS du 10 Mai 2014.

Consent for publication

Not applicable.

Competing interests

The authors declare that they have no competing interests.

Author details

[1]Service de Parasitologie, Faculté de Médecine, Université Cheikh Anta Diop de Dakar (UCAD), BP5005 Dakar-Fann, Senegal. [2]Laboratoire des Virus respiratoires, Institut Pasteur de Dakar, Dakar, Senegal. [3]MIVEGEC, UMR CNRS -IRD -University of Montpellier - 911, Avenue Agropolis BP 64501, Cédex 5 34394 Montpellier, France.

References

1. Cotter C, Sturrock HJ, Hsiang MS, Liu J, Phillips AA, Hwang J, Gueye CS, Fullman N, Gosling RD, Feachem RG. The changing epidemiology of malaria elimination: new strategies for new challenges. Lancet. 2013;382(9895):900–11.
2. Tatem AJ, Smith DL, Gething PW, Kabaria CW, Snow RW, Hay SI. Ranking of elimination feasibility between malaria-endemic countries. Lancet. 2010; 376(9752):1579–91.
3. WHO. World malaria report 2016. Geneva: World Health Organization 2016; 2016.
4. Etard JF, Le Hesran JY, Diallo A, Diallo JP, Ndiaye JL, Delaunay V. Childhood mortality and probable causes of death using verbal autopsy in Niakhar, Senegal, 1989-2000. Int J Epidemiol. 2004;33(6):1286–92.
5. Thiam S, Thior M, Faye B, Ndiop M, Diouf ML, Diouf MB, Diallo I, Fall FB, Ndiaye JL, Albertini A, et al. Major reduction in anti-malarial drug consumption in Senegal after nation-wide introduction of malaria rapid diagnostic tests. PLoS One. 2011;6(4):e18419.
6. Mtove G, Hendriksen IC, Amos B, Mrema H, Mandia V, Manjurano A, Muro F, Sykes A, Hildenwall H, Whitty CJ, et al. Treatment guided by rapid diagnostic tests for malaria in Tanzanian children: safety and alternative bacterial diagnoses. Malar J. 2011;10:290.
7. Punjabi NH, Taylor WR, Murphy GS, Purwaningsih S, Picarima H, Sisson J, Olson JG, Baso S, Wangsasaputra F, Lesmana M, et al. Etiology of acute, non-malaria, febrile illnesses in Jayapura, northeastern Papua, Indonesia. Am J Trop Med Hyg. 2012;86(1):46–51.
8. O'Meara WP, Mangeni JN, Steketee R, Greenwood B. Changes in the burden of malaria in sub-Saharan Africa. Lancet Infect Dis. 2010;10(8):545–55.
9. Kasper MR, Blair PJ, Touch S, Sokhal B, Yasuda CY, Williams M, Richards AL, Burgess TH, Wierzba TF, Putnam SD. Infectious etiologies of acute febrile illness among patients seeking health care in south-Central Cambodia. Am J Trop Med Hyg. 2012;86(2):246–53.
10. WHO: Technical updates of the guidelines on the integrated Management of Childhood Illness (IMCI): evidence and recommendations for further adaptations. World Health Organization. 2005, ISBN 92 4 159348 2 (NLM classification: WS 366). avalaible at: http://www.who.int/iris/handle/10665/43303.
11. Berkley JA, Lowe BS, Mwangi I, Williams T, Bauni E, Mwarumba S, Ngetsa C, Slack MP, Njenga S, Hart CA, et al. Bacteremia among children admitted to a rural hospital in Kenya. N Engl J Med. 2005;352(1):39–47.
12. D'Acremont V, Kilowoko M, Kyungu E, Philipina S, Sangu W, Kahama-Maro J, Lengeler C, Cherpillod P, Kaiser L, Genton B. Beyond malaria--causes of fever in outpatient Tanzanian children. N Engl J Med. 2014;370(9):809–17.
13. Mahende C, Ngasala B, Lusingu J, Butichi A, Lushino P, Lemnge M, Premji Z. Aetiology of acute febrile episodes in children attending Korogwe District hospital in North-Eastern Tanzania. PLoS One. 2014;9(8):e104197.
14. Hildenwall H, Amos B, Mtove G, Muro F, Cederlund K, Reyburn H. Causes of non-malarial febrile illness in outpatients in Tanzania. Trop Med Int Health. 2016;21(1):149–56.
15. Crump JA, Morrissey AB, Nicholson WL, Massung RF, Stoddard RA, Galloway RL, Ooi EE, Maro VP, Saganda W, Kinabo GD, et al. Etiology of severe non-malaria febrile illness in northern Tanzania: a prospective cohort study. PLoS Negl Trop Dis. 2013;7(7):e2324.

16. Liu L, Johnson HL, Cousens S, Perin J, Scott S, Lawn JE, Rudan I, Campbell H, Cibulskis R, Li M, et al. Global, regional, and national causes of child mortality: an updated systematic analysis for 2010 with time trends since 2000. Lancet. 2012;379(9832):2151–61.
17. Mayxay M, Castonguay-Vanier J, Chansamouth V, Dubot-Peres A, Paris DH, Phetsouvanh R, Tangkhabuanbutra J, Douangdala P, Inthalath S, Souvannasing P, et al. Causes of non-malarial fever in Laos: a prospective study. Lancet Glob Health. 2013;1(1):e46–54.
18. Pondei K, Kunle-Olowu O, Peterside O. The aetiology of non-malarial febrile illness in children in the malaria-endemic Niger Delta region of Nigeria. Asian Pac J Trop Dis. 2013;3(1):56–60.
19. Oliver-Williams C, Brown E, Devereux S, Fairhead C, Holeman I. Using mobile phones to improve vaccination uptake in 21 low- and middle-income countries: systematic review. JMIR Mhealth Uhealth. 2017;5(10):e148.
20. Malhotra B, Swamy MA, Reddy PV, Kumar N, Tiwari JK. Evaluation of custom multiplex real - time RT - PCR in comparison to fast - track diagnostics respiratory 21 pathogens kit for detection of multiple respiratory viruses. Virol J. 2016;13:91.
21. Niang MN, Diop NS, Fall A, Kiori DE, Sarr FD, Sy S, Goudiaby D, Barry MA, Fall M, Dia N. Respiratory viruses in patients with influenza-like illness in Senegal: focus on human respiratory adenoviruses. PLoS One. 2017;12(3): e0174287.

14

Bordetella bronchiseptica pneumonia in a patient with lung cancer

Manlio Monti[1*], Danila Diano[2], Francesco Allegrini[3], Angelo Delmonte[1], Valentina Fausti[1], Paola Cravero[1], Giulia Marcantognini[1] and Giovanni Luca Frassineti[1]

Abstract

Background: *Bordetella bronchiseptica* (*B.bronchiseptica*) is a frequent cause of respiratory infections in animals but rarely causes serious infection in humans. We present a rare case of *B. bronchiseptica* pneumonia in a patient with lung cancer.

Case presentation: A 52-year-old white male with non small cell lung cancer developed fever during treatment with nivolumab. A persistent productive cough and a deterioration in his clinical condition led to his hospitalization for evaluation. Bronchoscopy was performed and a diagnosis of *B. bronchiseptica* pneumonia was made. The infection was successfully managed by antiobiotic therapy.

Conclusions: *B. bronchiseptica* is a pathogen that can cause serious infection in humans, especially in immunocompromised or immunoincompetent individuals. In our patient it showed unusual resistance to cephalosporins and poor sensitivity to amikacin. To our knowledge this is the first case of such an infection in a lung cancer patient undergoing treatment with nivolumab. When B. *bronchiseptica* is identified, the possibility of a nosocomial transmission must be considered.

Keywords: *Bordetella bronchiseptica*, Cavitary lung lesion, Rare infection, Nivolumab, Nosocomial infection

Background

Of the 9 species of *Bordetella* (*B.*) identified to date, *B. bronchiseptica*, *B. parapertussis* and *B. holmesii* are associated with respiratory infections in humans and other mammals. Whooping cough (pertussis) is a highly contagious, acute respiratory illness of humans caused by the gram-negative bacterial pathogen *B. pertussis, which has* no known animal or environmental reservoir [1]. *B. avium* is a bird pathogen that causes coryza and rhinotracheitis in poultry. *B. ansorpii*, *B. hinzii*, *B. holmesii*, *B. petrii* and *B. trematum* are mainly associated with infections in immunocompromised patients [2, 3].

B. bronchiseptica is a gram-negative coccobacillus frequently isolated in the upper respiratory tract of domestic animals and wild animals, e.g. voles, seals, rodents and captive koalas. The infection is believed to be transmitted from animals with tracheobronchitis. Despite potentially frequent exposure to zoonotic sources of this opportunistic pathogen, human infections are rare. However, it is known to be an etiologic agent of upper respiratory tract infections, pneumonitis, endocarditis, peritonitis, meningitis, sepsis and recurrent bacteremia in immunocompromised or immunoincompetent patients [4]. *B. bronchiseptica* does not express pertussis toxin, which is one of the characteristic virulence factors of *B. pertussis*, but has the genes to do so, indicating the close evolutionary relationship between the two species. We report a rare case of *B.bronchiseptica* pneumonia in a patient with lung cancer.

Case presentation

In April 2014, a 52-year-old Caucasian male with a history of cigarette smoking was diagnosed with cavitating squamous cell lung carcinoma (SCC) cT4N2M0 of the inferior left lung lobe. Between August 2015 and January

* Correspondence: manlio.monti@irst.emr.it
[1]Department of Medical Oncology, Istituto Scientifico Romagnolo per lo Studio e la Cura dei Tumori (IRST) IRCCS, Meldola, Italy
Full list of author information is available at the end of the article

2016, he underwent 10 cycles of second-line treatment with nivolumab (3 mg/kg every 14 days) at our institute. Fourteen days after the end of the last treatment the patient developed low-grade fever (38.3 °C). A chest X ray excluded the hypothesis of pneumonia. Levofloxacin 500 mg/day was prescribed for 7 days and the patient initially responded. Two further cycles of nivolumab were administered. At a follow-up appointment in February 2016, the patient reported having had low-grade fever (38 °C) for about a month and complained of pain in his chest wall over the area of the lung cancer. He also had a productive cough and had lost around 7 kg over a period of 6 months. Performance status was poor. The patient was urgently admitted to our inpatient oncology ward; initial vital signs were blood pressure 110/60, heart rate125 beats/min and oxygen saturation 92% in room air. Auscultation of the patient's lungs revealed decreased breath sounds over the whole lung field. The abdomen was soft, without organomegaly. Laboratory exams showed a white blood cell count of 22.10 × 10^9/L with 84.5% neutrophils, 4.7% lymphocytes and 10.5% monocytes. Hemoglobin was 10 g/dl and platelets 690 × 10^9/L. Electrolytes, renal and liver function tests and coagulation studies were all normal apart from C-reactive protein (320 mg/L) and albumin (28 g/L). Urine analysis showed protein 25 mg/dl. A chest X ray confirmed the presence of the cavitary lesion of the primary tumor and pleural effusion. A blood culture was performed and empirical treatment was started with amikacin 20 mg/kg on day 1 (15 mg/kg/day thereafter) plus ceftazidime 2 g 3 times/day. The patient also started oxygen therapy (oxygen therapy eyeglasses) 5 L/min and became apyretic after 3 days of the dual antibiotic treatment. Bronchoscopy was performed to investigate the continuous productive cough and foul-smelling pus was removed, mainly from the left lower lobe. The patient's clinical conditions worsened after 7 days of the dual therapy, with a reappearance of fever and chills. A chest computerized tomography (CT) scan revealed the presence of multiple bilateral parenchymal accumulations mainly in the left lower lobe, leading to a first hypothesis of inflammatory phenomena (Fig. 1a). Minimal left pleural effusion was also noted, together with an increase in the size of the cavitary lesion in the inferior left lobe and increased lytic rib disease in the adjacent vertebral structures. Treatment with amikacin was maintained but ceftazidime was replaced by teicoplanin 6 mg/kg twice on the first day and once a day thereafter. Blood culture remained negative. Tests for human immunodeficiency virus (HIV) and quantitative cytomegalovirus DNA (< 233 UI/ml) were negative. Bronchoscopic alveolar lavage (BAL) revealed the presence of *B. bronchiseptica* 10,000 CFU (colon-forming units) which was resistant to cefepime (minimal inhibitory concentration [MIC] ≥ 64), cefotaxime (MIC ≥64) and ceftazidime (MIC 16), but sensitive to amikacin (MIC 8), gentamicin (MIC 2), imipenem (MIC 0.5), meropenem (MIC ≤0.25), piperacillin/tazobactam (MIC ≤4) and ciprofloxacin (MIC 1). The bronchoalveolar material was negative for *Mycobacterium tuberculosis* complex DNA. After several days of apyrexia the fever returned and the patient's clinical conditions deteriorated. A blood culture

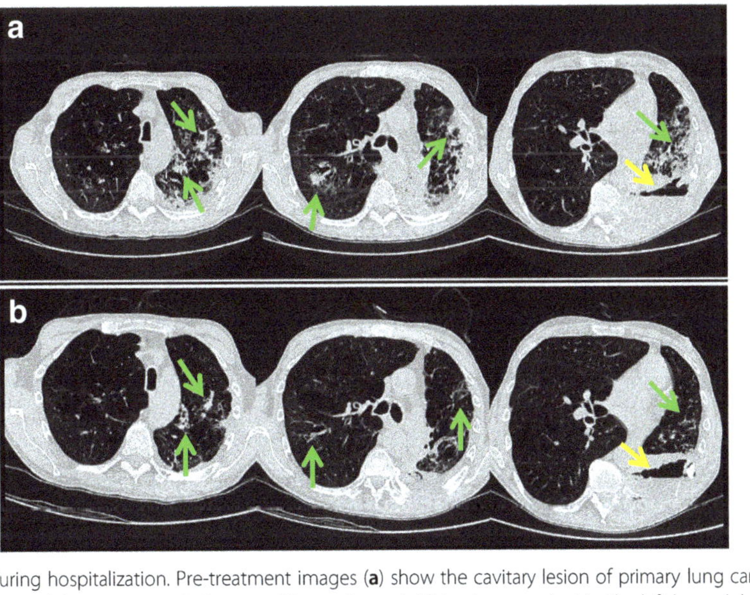

Fig. 1 Axial chest CT scans during hospitalization. Pre-treatment images (**a**) show the cavitary lesion of primary lung cancer (yellow arrow) and multiple bilateral pulmonary consolidations, ground glass opacities and septal thickening prevalent in the left lower lobe relating to inflammatory phenomena (green arrows). Images after 2 weeks of piperacillin/tazobactam therapy (**b**) reveal a stabilization of the cavitary lesion (yellow arrow) and a reduction in the inflammatory phenomena (green arrows)

was repeated and amikacin and teicolplanin were replaced by piperacillin 4 g plus tazobactam 500 mg three times/day. After 2 weeks' therapy, the chest CT scan (Fig. 1b) showed an improvement in the bilateral parenchymal inflammatory areas and a slight reduction in the pleural effusion. Blood culture remained negative. Antimicrobial treatment was continued for a total of 17 days after which, given the improvement in the pneumonia, clinical conditions and performance status, the patient was discharged. Levofloxacin 500 mg twice a day was prescribed for the first 6 days at home. The patient died 3 months later due to disease progression.

Discussion

Of the nine species of *Bordetella, B. bronchiseptica* is primarily a zoonotic pathogen associated with a wide spectrum of illnesses ranging in severity from mild respiratory symptoms to sepsis and death in humans [5]. In a review of the literature, the majority of patients infected with *B. bronchiseptica* had at least one predisposing disease such as acute lymphatic leukemia [6], chronic lymphocytic leukemia, lymphopenia associated with temozolomide treatment for glioblastoma, cystic fibrosis [7] and cancer (malignant thymoma, brain metastases of unknown origin, lung cancer and supraglottic cancer with no evidence of recurrence) [8], or had undergone hematopietic stem cell transplantation [9–11] or a lung transplant [12]. *B. bronchiseptica* has been reported in individuals with HIV [13], Down's syndrome, branchial cleft cyst [14], Crohn's disease, thoracic trauma, endocarditis, diabetes with "healed" pulmonary tuberculosis, post-traumatic meningitis, rheumatoid arthritis [15], and bronchitis [16].

Although little is known about the route of transmission of *B. bronchiseptica* infection, airborne human to human transmission has been reported in hospital settings [8, 10]. Our patient thus required droplet precautions and was placed in a single room.

B. bronchiseptica infects a wide range of mammals, causing tracheobronchitis (also known as 'kennel cough') in dogs and cats and atrophic rhinitis in pigs. Kennel cough vaccines containing live, attenuated *B. bronchiseptica* are commonly used in veterinary clinics. Transmission of vaccine strains to humans is a theoretical possibility [17]. When infections due to *B. bronchiseptica* occur in humans, they typically involve immunocompromised or immunoincompetent patients and are often acquired through contact with animals. The pathogen can survive intracellularly for several days after uptake by phagocytes, which may, in part, explain the persistence of infection in immunoincompetent individuals. Our patient had been a frequent visitor to a cat shelter a few years previously and his infection may thus have originated from an animal.

Lung cancer is the leading cause of cancer death in the world. In 2008, more than 1.6 million people were diagnosed with the disease, representing 13% of all new cancer diagnoses, and 1.4 million died, representing 18% of all cancer deaths [18]. Lung cancer is divided into two major classes based on its biology, therapy and prognosis, i.e. non small cell lung cancer (NSCLC) and small cell lung cancer (SCLC). The former accounts for more than 80% of all lung cancer cases and includes 2 major subtypes: non-squamous carcinoma of the lung (including adenocarcinoma, large-cell carcinoma, and other types) and squamous cell carcinoma (SCC). SCC accounts for 20%–30% of all lung cancers, representing a significant health burden [19]. The last 5–10 years have seen substantial advances in the development of molecular targeted therapies for advanced-stage lung adenocarcinoma, improving the outlook for patients with this disease. However, until recently, treatment for patients with advanced SCC was limited [20] and based on histologic type and performance status. Median overall survival for stage III B SCC is currently around 18 months. Our patient showed a slightly better overall survival and the *Bordetella* infection probably did not modify prognosis [21].

Advances in our understanding of the interaction between the immune system and tumors have led to the development of programmed death-1 (PD-1)/programmed death ligand-1 (PD-L1) inhibitors targeting the immune checkpoint pathway. The monoclonal antibody nivolumab was the first immune checkpoint inhibitor approved by the U.S. Food and Drug Administration for the treatment of advanced SCC and NSCLC following progression during or after platinum-based chemotherapy. Nivolumab binds the receptor PD-1, expressed in tumor-infiltrating lymphocytes, with high affinity. Its ligand, PD-L1, is expressed in different cancer types, including NSCLC, and PD-1/PD-L1 binding results in the suppression of the immune response. Nivolumab acts as a competitive agent and a PD-L1 antagonist, permitting a correct functioning of the immune system. It is a well tolerated treatment. Pneumonia is a possible side-effect of immune checkpoint inhibitors and nivolumab-associated pneumonia has been observed in melanoma patients (around 2%) and in those with renal cancer or NSCLC (around 5%). However, the presence of any symptom requires the interruption of the drug and the initiation of steroid treatment. In the case of our patient, methylprednisolone 20 mg/day was started on the 5th day of hospitalization.

B. bronchiseptica rarely responds to macrolide antibiotics [1, 4] but is usually susceptible in vitro to aminoglycosides (amikacin, gentamicin), antipseudomonal penicillins (mezlociclin, piperacillin, ticarcillin), quinolones, tetracycline, third-generation cephalosporins (cefoperazone, cefatazidime) and trimethoprim-sulfamethoxazole [22]. Conversely, in our patient, *B. bronchiseptica* was resistant to cephalosporins. Of note, the clinical response to the above antibiotics is sometimes disappointing but the discrepancy between in vitro sensitivity and in vivo efficacy is not clearly understood. The first antibiotic we used was levofloxacin, a member of the fluoroquinolone family which is considered an effective treatment option for acquired pneumonia and acute exacerbations of chronic bronchitis [23]. We then tried amikacin plus ceftazidime as empirical antibiotic therapy because this combination has broad-spectrum antibacterial coverage and synergistic bactericidal activity [24]. When the infection did not resolve we administered teicoplanin as it covers gram-positive organisms, but then changed to piperacillin/tazobactam on the basis of BAL results. Treatment duration for *B. bronchiseptica* is a controversial issue and varies from 2 to 4 weeks for patients with a good response [14], and from 2 weeks to 6 months for patients with recurrent symptoms. Therapy with piperacillin/tazobactam was maintained for more 2 weeks in our patient. The route of infection in our patient remains unknown but was probably caused by an animal. He had no recurrence of fever but died 3 months after being discharged due to cancer progression.

Although there are no distinctive radiographic features associated with *B. bronchiseptica* pulmonary infection, the most frequent manifestations are multiple lobular infiltrations, interstitial pneumonia [13], and lobular pneumonia [6, 9, 13]. Cavitary lesions are rarely encountered [13, 25]. The case we describe is noteworthy for a number of reasons. First, *B. bronchiseptica* was resistant to ceftazidime (an unusual occurrence) and showed poor sensitivity to amikacin. Secondly, to our knowledge this is the first case of pneumonia caused by *B. bronchiseptica* in a lung cancer patient undergoing nivolumab treatment. The diagnosis of cavitary lung cancer was made in 2013, but by July 2015 the tumor had increased in size. Thus, we do not know whether *B. bronchiseptica* was present at the diagnosis of the lung cancer or whether the cavitary lesion increased the patient's susceptibility to infection.

In conclusion, although *B. bronchiseptica* is a zoonotic pathogen, it can cause serious infection in humans, especially immunocompromised or immunoincompetent individuals. When *B. bronchiseptica* is identified, the possibility of nosocomial transmission must be taken into consideration. Lung cancer, bronchiectasis, emphysema, cystic fibrosis and other lung diseases causing structural changes may also be associated with *B. bronchiseptica* infection.

Abbreviations

B: *Bordetella*; CFU: Colony-forming unit; CT: Computerized tomography; HIV: Human immunodeficiency virus; MIC: Minimal inhibitory concentration

Acknowledgements

The authors thank Gráinne Tierney for editorial assistance.

Funding

No funding was received.

Authors' contributions

All authors contributed equally to the manuscript. All authors read and approved the final manuscript.

Consent for publication

Written informed consent for the publication of the case report was obtained from a relative of the patient.

Competing interests

The authors declare that they have no competing interests.

Author details

[1]Department of Medical Oncology, Istituto Scientifico Romagnolo per lo Studio e la Cura dei Tumori (IRST) IRCCS, Meldola, Italy. [2]Radiology Unit, Istituto Scientifico Romagnolo per lo Studio e la Cura dei Tumori (IRST) IRCCS, Meldola, Italy. [3]Department of Infectious Diseases, Morgagni-Pierantoni Hospital, Forlì, Italy.

References

1. Mattoo S, Cherry JD. Molecular pathogenesis, epidemiology, and clinical manifestations of respiratory infections due to bordetella pertussis and other bordetella subspecies. Clin Microbiol Rev. 2005;18(2):326–82.
2. Almuzara M, Barberis C, Traglia G, Sly G, Procopio A, Vilches V, et al. Isolation of Bordetella species from unusual infection sites. JMM Case Reports. 2015; doi:10.1099/jmmcr.0.000029.
3. Wirsing von König C-H, Riffelmann M, Coenye T. Bordetella and related genera. In: Versalovic J, Carroll KC, Funke G, Jorgensen JH, Landry ML, Warnock DW, editors. Manual of clinical microbiology. 10th ed. Washington, DC: ASM Press; 2011. p. 739–50.
4. Woolfrey BF, Moody JA. Human infections associated with bordetella bronchiseptica. Clin Microbiol Rev. 1991;4(3):243–55.
5. Gisel JJ, Brumble LM, Johnson MM. Bordetella bronchiseptica pneumonia in a kidney-pancreas transplant patient after exposure to recently vaccinated dogs. Transpl Infect Dis. 2010;12(1):73–6.
6. Gomez L, Grazziutti M, Sumoza D, Beran M, Rolston K. Bacterial pneumonia due to bordetella bronchiseptica in a patient with acute leukemia. Clin Infect Dis. 1998;26(4):1002–3.
7. Brady C, Ackerman P, Johnson M, McNamara J. Bordetella bronchiseptica in a pediatric cystic fibrosis center. J Cyst Fibros. 2014;13(1):43–5.
8. Yacoub AT, Katayama M, Tran J, Zadikany R, Kandula M, Greene J. Bordetella bronchiseptica in the immunosuppressed population - a case series and review. Mediterr J Hematol Infect Dis. 2014;6(1):e2014031.
9. Huebner ES, Christman B, Dummer S, Tang YW, Goodman S. Hospital-acquired Bordetella bronchiseptica infection following hematopoietic stem cell transplantation. J Clin Microbiol. 2006;44(7):2581–3.
10. Bauwens JE, Spach DH, Schacker TW, Mustafa MM, Bowden RA. Bordetella bronchiseptica pneumonia and bacteremia following bone marrow transplantation. J Clin Microbiol. 1992;30(9):2474–5.
11. Goldberg JD, Kamboj M, Ford R, Kiehn TE, Gilhuley K, Perales MA. 'Kennel cough' in a patient following allogeneic hematopoietic stem cell transplant. Bone Marrow Transplant. 2009;44(6):381–2.
12. Ner Z, Ross LA, Horn MV, Keens TG, MacLaughlin EF, Starnes VA, et al. Bordetella bronchiseptica infection in pediatric lung transplant recipients. Pediatr Transplant. 2003;7(5):413–7.
13. Dworkin MS, Sullivan PS, Buskin SE, Harrington RD, Olliffe J, MacArthur RD, et al. Bordetella bronchiseptica infection in human immunodeficiency virus-infected patients. Clin Infect Dis. 1999;28(5):1095–9.
14. Lo Re V, Brennan PJ, Wadlin J, Weaver R, Nachamkin I. Infected branchial cleft cyst due to bordetella bronchiseptica in an immunocompetent patient. J Clin Microbiol. 2001;39(11):4210–2.
15. Berkowitz DM, Bechara RI, Wolfenden LL. An unusual cause of cough and dyspnea in an immunocompromised patient. Chest. 2007;131(5):1599–602.

16. Papasian CJ, Downs NJ, Talley RL, Romberger DJ, Hodges GR. Bordetella bronchiseptica bronchitis. J Clin Microbiol. 1987;25(3):575–7.
17. Berkelman RL. Human illness associated with use of veterinary vaccines. Clin Infect Dis. 2003;37(3):407–14.
18. Alberg AJ, Brock MV, Ford JG, Samet JM, Spivack SD. Epidemiology of lung cancer; diagnosis and management of lung cancer, 3rd ed: American College of Chest Physicians Evidence-Based Clinical Practice Guidelines. Chest. 2013;143(5 Suppl):e1S–e29S.
19. Dela Cruz CS, Tanoue LT, Matthay RA. Lung cancer: epidemiology, etiology, and prevention. Clin Chest Med. 2011;32(4):605–44.
20. Ang YL, Lim JS, Soo RA. Profile of nivolumab in the treatment of metastatic squamous non-small-cell lung cancer. Onco Targets Ther. 2016;9:3187–95.
21. Choi HS, Jeong BK, Jeong H, Lee YH, Ha IB, Song JH, et al. Application of the new 8th TNM staging system for non-small cell lung cancer: treated with curative concurrent chemoradiotherapy. Radiat Oncol. 2017;12(1):122.
22. Mortensen JE, Brumbach A, Shryock TR. Antimicrobial susceptibility of Bordetella avium and bordetella bronchiseptica isolates. Antimicrob Agents Chemother. 1989;33(5):771–2.
23. Cantón R, Lode H, Graninger W, Milkovich G. Respiratory tract infections: at-risk patients, who are they? Implications for their management with levofloxacin. Int J Antimicrob Agents. 2006;28(Suppl 2):S115–27.
24. Ariffin H, Arasu A, Mahfuzah M, Ariffin WA, Chan LL, Lin HP. Single-daily ceftriaxone plus amikacin versus thrice-daily ceftazidime plus amikacin as empirical treatment of febrile neutropenia in children with cancer. J Paediatr Child Health. 2001;37(1):38–43.
25. Lorenzo-Pajuelo B, Villanueva JL, Rodríguez-Cuesta J, Vergara-Irigaray N, Bernabeu-Wittel M, Garcia-Curiel A, et al. Cavitary pneumonia in an AIDS patient caused by an unusual bordetella bronchiseptica variant producing reduced amounts of pertactin and other major antigens. J Clin Microbiol. 2002;40(9):3146–54.

15

Rapid detection of respiratory organisms with the FilmArray respiratory panel in a large children's hospital in China

Jin Li[1†], Yue Tao[2†], Mingyu Tang[1†], Bailu Du[1], Yijun Xia[3], Xi Mo[2*] and Qing Cao[1*]

Abstract

Background: Respiratory tract infections (RTIs) are the most common illness in children, and rapid diagnosis is required for the optimal management of RTIs, especially severe infections.

Methods: Nasopharyngeal swab or sputum specimens were collected from children aged 19 days to 15 years who were admitted to a hospital in Shanghai and diagnosed with RTIs. The specimens were tested with the FilmArray Respiratory Panel, a multiplex PCR assay that detects 16 viruses, *Mycoplasma pneumoniae* (*M. pneumoniae*), *Bordetella pertussis* (*B. pertussis*) and *Chlamydophila pneumoniae* (*C. pneumoniae*).

Results: Among the 775 children studied, 626 (80.8%, 626/775) tested positive for at least one organism, and multiple organisms were detected in 198 (25.5%). Rhinoviruses/enteroviruses (25.5%, 198/775) were detected most often, followed by respiratory syncytial virus (19.5%, 151/775), parainfluenza virus 3 (14.8%, 115/775), influenza A or B (10.9%), adenovirus (10.8%), *M. pneumoniae* (10.6%) and *B. pertussis* (6.3%). The prevalence of organisms differed by age, and most of the viruses were more common in winter. Of the 140 children suspected of having pertussis, 35.0% (49/140) tested positive for *B. pertussis*.

Conclusions: FilmArray RP allows the rapid simultaneous detection of a wide number of respiratory organisms, with limited hands-on time, in Chinese pediatric patients with RTIs.

Keywords: Respiratory tract infections, FilmArray respiratory panel, Respiratory organisms, Children

Background

Acute respiratory tract infections (RTIs) are the leading causes of outpatient visits and hospitalizations in all age groups, especially during winter and spring. For children under 5 years of age, RTIs are the second leading cause of death [1]. Most acute RTIs in children are caused by respiratory viruses, such as respiratory syncytial virus (RSV), adenovirus (ADV), rhinovirus (RV) and influenza viruses. In addition to viruses, atypical pathogens are major causes of pediatric RTIs. One of the most common atypical pathogens is *Mycoplasma pneumoniae* (*M. pneumoniae*), accounting for 10–40% of hospitalized children with community-acquired pneumonia [2, 3]. In addition to *M. pneumoniae*, the incidence of pertussis in China has significantly increased since 2010. Nevertheless, multiple epidemiological studies have suggested that the incidence of pertussis in China has been significantly underestimated [4, 5]. The early diagnosis of the pathogen is beneficial for the precise selection of medication, which can largely avoid the overuse or even abuse of the antibiotics and improve the clinical care of patients. More importantly, the early diagnosis of contagious pathogens, such as *Bordetella pertussis* (*B. pertussis*) and influenza viruses, can enable early isolation of patients, thus reducing the spread of pathogens.

At present, the routine detection methods for respiratory pathogens in China are mostly based on immunological methods, which include the detection of *M. pneumoniae* and several major viruses, such as RSV,

* Correspondence: moxi@scmc.com.cn; caoqing@scmc.com.cn
†Jin Li, Yue Tao and Mingyu Tang contributed equally to this work.
[2]The Laboratory of Pediatric Infectious Diseases, Pediatric Translational Medicine Institute, Shanghai Children's Medical Center, Shanghai Jiaotong University School of Medicine, Shanghai, China
[1]Department of Infectious Diseases, Shanghai Children's Medical Center, Shanghai Jiaotong University School of Medicine, Shanghai, China
Full list of author information is available at the end of the article

ADV, RV, parainfluenza virus (Para), influenza A virus (FluA) and influenza B virus (FluB). Other respiratory viruses and atypical bacteria, such as *Chlamydophila pneumoniae* (*C. pneumoniae*) and *B. pertussis,* are typically not routinely detected. Given their poor sensitivity and long turn-around time (TAT), immunological methods usually lead to broad-spectrum therapy and have been gradually replaced by molecular-based methods, such as conventional and real-time polymerase chain reaction (PCR), in developed countries [6, 7]. However, most of these molecular tests are technically challenging and require independent spaces, such as pre-PCR and post-PCR rooms, to eliminate the potential risk of cross-contamination, and such requirement limits their applications in China. Therefore, faster, more sensitive and easy-to-use assays for multiplex respiratory pathogen detection are urgently needed.

FilmArray (BioFire Diagnostics, Utah, USA, owned by bioMérieux) is a small, desktop, fully automated multiplex PCR device. The molecular system includes automated nucleic acid extraction, an initial reverse transcription step and multiplex nested PCR, followed by a melting curve analysis [8]. The FilmArray Respiratory Panel (FilmArray RP) is both FDA-approved and CE IVD-marked. The current version of FilmArray RP (v1.7) is able to detect 16 viral and 3 atypical respiratory organisms. The test is performed in a closed system that requires 5 min of hands-on time and 65 min of instrumentation time. Several comparison studies between FilmArray and other tests for respiratory organisms showed comparable results [9–11].

The aim of this study was to evaluate the application of FilmArray RP for the detection of respiratory organisms, and to provide information about the seasonality and prevalence of these organisms in pediatric patients with RTIs in a large children's hospital in China.

Methods

Subjects and specimens

The study population was enrolled according to protocol definitions and inclusion criteria. Patients with respiratory infections, with or without fever (defined as body temperature ≥ 37.5 °C), were included if they had at least one of the following symptoms: (1) cough; (2) nasal obstruction; (3) tachypnoea; (4) nasal flaring; or (5) hypoxia. Patients admitted to the hospital had at least one of the following conditions: (1) unabating high fever; (2) dyspnea, tachypnea or hypoxemia; (3) anorexia or dehydration; (4) radiological confirmation of lung infection; or (5) respiratory infection with underlying diseases, such as congenital heart disease, bronchopulmonary dysplasia, airway malformations, severe malnutrition.

According to the Chinese Center for Disease Control and Prevention (CDC), patients suspected of having pertussis should have a cough for more than 2 weeks and have at least one of the following symptoms: (1) paroxysmal cough; (2) inspiratory whoop; or (3) post-tussive vomiting. In the present study, patients suspected of having pertussis were diagnosed with pertussis when *B. pertussis* was positive by FilmArray RP detection and were otherwise diagnosed with pertussis-like syndrome.

Nasopharyngeal swab (NPS) or sputum specimens were obtained from patients with symptoms of RTIs on the day of hospitalization at Shanghai Children's Medical Center (SCMC) from December 1, 2016 to November 30, 2017. Demographic data and clinical features, as well as laboratory test and imaging results, were obtained for each enrolled patient. The study was approved by the Institutional Review Board and the Ethics Committee of Shanghai Children's Medical Center (SCMCIRB-K2017044), and written informed consent was obtained from the parents of each patient.

FilmArray RP v1.7 testing

The FilmArray RP v1.7 targets 19 organisms, including ADV, influenza A viruses H1, 2009H1, H3 (FluA-H1, FluA-2009H1, FluA-H3) and FluB, parainfluenza virus types 1 to 4 (Para 1–4), coronaviruses 229E, HKU1, OC43, and NL63 (Cov-HKU1, NL63, 229E, OC43), human metapneumovirus (hMPV), RSV, human rhinovirus/enterovirus (Rhino/Entero), *C. pneumoniae, M. pneumoniae* and *B. pertussis.* The FilmArray RP assay was performed according to the manufacturer's instructions. The principle of the assay has been previously described [8, 12]. Each pouch included internal run controls for every step, and results for the assay were only provided by the software if the quality control reactions showed appropriate results.

Statistical analysis

SPSS software package v21.0 was used for all statistical analyses. Categorical variables were expressed as frequencies and percentages. The chi-square and Fisher's exact tests were used to compare groups. Continuous variables are expressed as the mean and standard deviation. Student's *t*-test was used to assess the statistical significance between groups. $p < 0.05$ was considered to be statistically significant.

Results

Clinical characteristics of patients

A total of 775 patients diagnosed with upper or lower respiratory tract infections, aged 19 days to 15 years, were enrolled in the present study between December 1, 2016, and November 30, 2017. Congenital heart disease, congenital biliary atresia, malignancy and congenital immunodeficiency were the most frequently observed underlying diseases in these patients and contributed to 50% of the deaths observed in this study. The general characteristics of the patients enrolled are presented in Table 1.

Overall detection rate of FilmArray RP v1.7

Among the 775 specimens, 428 (55.2%, 428/775) had a single organism, 198 (25.5%, 198/775) had multiple organisms, and 149 (19.2%, 149/775) had no organism. The overall positive rate of the specimens was 80.8% (626/775). Rhino/Entero was the most prevalent organism (25.5%, 198/775), followed by RSV (19.5%, 151/775) and Para 3 (14.8%, 115/775). The positivity rates of other organisms were as follows: ADV, 10.8% (84/775); *M. pneumoniae*, 10.6% (82/775); *B. pertussis*, 6.3% (49/775); FluA, 6.1% (47/775); FluB, 4.8% (37/775); hMPV, 4.8% (37/775); CoV, 4.3% (33/775); Para 1, 3.2% (25/775); Para 4, 1.3% (10/775); Para 2, 0.4% (3/775); and *C. pneumoniae*, 0.1% (1/775).

Table 1 General characteristics of the patients

Characteristic	Value for patients
Total	775
Age, No. (%)	
< 1 year	338 (43.6)
1–2 years	185 (23.9)
3–5 years	146 (18.9)
6–15 years	106 (13.7)
Sex, No. (%)	
Male	430 (55.5)
Female	345 (44.5)
Clinical diagnosis, No. (%)	
URI	50 (6.5)
LRI	725 (93.5)
Underlying diseases, No. (%)	
None	538 (69.4)
CHD	148 (19.1)
Congenital biliary atresia	25 (3.2)
Malignancy	19 (2.5)
Congenital immunodeficiency	6 (0.8)
Other diseases	39 (5.0)
Prognosis after treat, No. (%)	
Alive	731 (94.3)
Death[b]	12 (1.5)
Unknown[c]	32 (4.1)

[a]Abbreviations: *URI* Upper respiratory tract infection; *LRI* Lower respiratory tract infection; *CHD* Congenital heart disease

[b]Most of the children died from underlying diseases, including malignancy, congenital heart disease, Niemann-Pick Disease, etc.

[c]Including the patients who transfer to other hospitals for treatment or abandon treatment. Upon follow-up by phone, 7 patients showed clinical improvement after transfer to other hospitals, 11 patients died after giving up treatment and discharged from our hospital, and 14 patients cannot be contacted and their prognosis were finally unknown

Analysis of the positive rates and prevalence in different age groups

All the patients were grouped by age as follows: infants (age: < 1 year), toddlers (age: 1–2 years), preschoolers (age: 3–5 years) and school-aged children (age: 6–15 years) (Table 2). The highest specimen positivity rate, at 82.2% (278/338), was in the < 1-year age group, followed by 80.5% (149/185), 80.1% (117/146) and 77.4% (82/106) in the 1–2-year, 3–5-year and 6–15-year groups, respectively. There were no significant differences in the positivity rate of the different age groups. In contrast, the prevalence of organisms were different between the different age groups (Table 2). Rhino/Entero, Para 3, RSV and *B. pertussis* showed the highest prevalence in the < 1-year age group, while ADV, hMPV and FluA showed the highest prevalence in the 3–5-year age group. The most prevalent organism in the 6–15-year age group was *M. pneumoniae.* No organism showed a notably high prevalence in the 1–2-year age group. There was only one *C. pneumoniae*-positive patient during the study period, and this patient was in the 3–5-year age group.

Analysis of specimens detected with multiple organisms

Among the 775 specimens, 198 (25.5%, 198/775) were positive for more than one organism. The largest proportion (49.0%, 97/198) of multi-organism-positive specimens had combinations with Rhino/Entero. Rhino/Entero plus Para 3 was the most common combination, making up 10.6% (21/198) of all multi-organism-positive specimens, while the combination of Rhino/Entero plus ADV was the second most common type (6.1%, 12/198), followed by Rhino/Entero plus RSV (5.6%, 11/198). The multi-organism combinations are listed in Additional file 1: Table S1.

Seasonal prevalence of respiratory organisms from December 1, 2016 to November 30, 2017

The number of positive specimens was determined during different months of the year to demonstrate the epidemiology of the respiratory organisms. Regarding the atypical bacteria, *M. pneumoniae* was detected throughout the year, with the highest incidence occurring in September and three minor peaks in December, January and June (Fig. 1a). The highest incidences of *B. pertussis* were observed in March and May. Only one case of *C. pneumoniae* was detected in July.

The seasonal prevalence of viruses with high detection rates were as follows. Both FluA and hMPV had two peaks that occurred in January and March, and ADV showed a peak in January (Fig. 1b). The prevalence of Para 3 remained high from February–August. The peaks

Table 2 Prevalence of respiratory organisms tested in different age groups

Analyte	< 1 year		1-2 years		3-5 years		6-15 years		χ^2	*p*
	No. Pos	Prevalence (*n* = 338)	No. Pos	Prevalence (*n* = 185)	No. Pos	Prevalence (*n* = 146)	No. Pos	Prevalence (*n* = 106)		
ADV	17	5.0%	29	15.7%	27	18.5%	11	10.4%	25.157	0.000
CoV total	21	6.2%	7	3.8%	2	1.4%	3	2.8%	6.788	0.079
229E	4	1.2%	1	0.5%	0	0%	2	1.9%	2.750	0.339
HKU1	6	1.8%	1	0.5%	1	0.7%	1	0.9%	1.542	0.696
OC43	11	3.3%	5	2.7%	1	0.7%	0	0%	5.548	0.117
hMPV	9	2.7%	12	6.5%	14	9.6%	1	0.9%	15.751	0.001
Rhino/Entero	101	29.9%	48	25.9%	27	18.5%	22	20.8%	8.453	0.038
FluA total	12	3.6%	13	7.0%	15	10.3%	7	6.6%	8.647	0.034
H3	10	3.0%	11	5.9%	11	7.5%	7	6.6%	5.825	0.120
2009 H1	2	0.6%	2	1.1%	4	2.7%	0	0%	4.550	0.134
FluB	2	0.6%	8	4.3%	15	10.3%	12	11.3%	32.794	0.000
Para total	94	27.8%	36	19.5%	20	13.7%	4	3.8%	34.146	0.000
1	9	2.7%	8	4.3%	8	5.5%	1	0.9%	4.842	0.176
2	0	0%	1	0.5%	1	0.7%	1	0.9%	3.714	0.203
3	81	24.0%	24	13.0%	8	5.5%	2	1.9%	46.976	0.000
4	4	1.2%	3	1.6%	3	2.1%	0	0%	2.095	0.559
RSV	105	31.1%	32	17.3%	11	7.5%	3	2.8%	61.491	0.000
B. pertussis	45	13.3%	2	1.1%	1	0.7%	1	0.9%	49.486	0.000
C. pneumoniae	0	0%	0	0%	1	0.7%	0	0%	3.750	0.325
M. pneumoniae	16	4.7%	16	8.6%	17	11.6%	33	31.1%	60.438	0.000
Total	278	82.2%	149	80.5%	117	80.1%	82	77.4%	1.314	0.726

in RSV cases occurred in both the fall and the winter months. The number of Rhino/Entero cases was relatively high throughout the year regardless of season.

The detection rates for the NPS and sputum samples

Among the 775 patients in our study, NPS samples were collected from 662 (85.4%). Among the other 113 (14.6%) patients, 88 used ventilators, 13 were hypoxic, and 12 were cyanotic after spasmodic coughing or crying, preventing NPS samples from being obtained from these patients; instead, sputum samples were collected and sent for FilmArray RP detection. The positivity rates of the NPS and sputum samples were 83.5% (553/662) and 64.6% (73/113), respectively. Detailed organism information on the two sample types collected from the different age groups is provided in Additional file 2: Tables S2 and S3.

Respiratory organisms detected in patients with suspected pertussis

According to the government policy, all cases of positive pertussis have to be reported to CDC. Because no routine examination could distinguish the patients with pertussis from those with pertussis-like syndrome, we paid special attention to the 140 patients who were clinically diagnosed with suspected pertussis in the present study. Among these patients, 95.0% (133/140) were positive for at least one organism by FilmArray RP, with 50.0% (70/140) and 45.0% (63/140) having single and multiple organisms detected, respectively. Detailed information on the organisms detected is presented in Fig. 2. 49 in the 140 patients (35%) were detected pertussis positive, among whom 42 (85.7%) were under 6 months, and 25 (71.4%) were co-detected with at least one virus.

Discussion

In our study, 775 specimens were collected from pediatric patients with RTIs over a period of one year and analyzed with FilmArray RP v1.7. The overall results yielded a positivity rate of 80.8%, with multiple organisms detected in 25.5% of specimens, which is in accordance with Litwin and Piralla's reports [13, 14]. As in other studies, a notable variation in the pathogen prevalence with season and age was observed. Most viruses had their highest positivity rates in winter, except that Para 3 positivity rate was well distributed through the spring and summer, and the epidemiologic peaks for hMPV occurred 1 to 2 months later than those for RSV

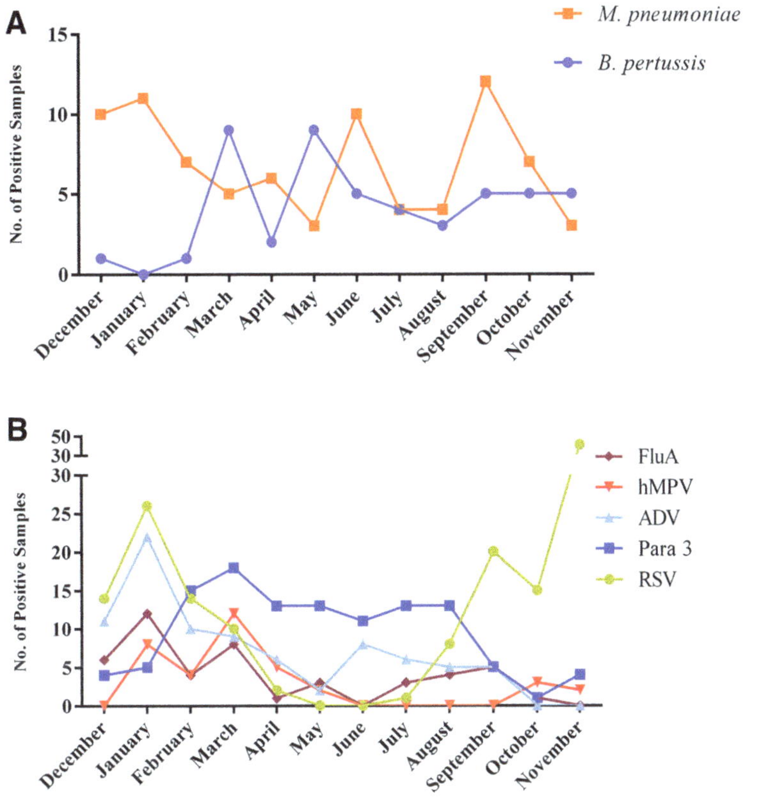

Fig. 1 Seasonal distribution of respiratory organisms detected by FilmArray RP. **a** Monthly prevalence of *B. pertussis* and *M. pneumoniae*. **b** Monthly prevalence of FluA, hMPV, ADV, Para 3 and RSV

[15, 16]. The majority of respiratory viruses were observed in children younger than 5 years old. Notably, RSV was the most prevalent virus in the < 1-year age group, and the prevalence decreased with age; while the incidence of *M. pneumoniae* increased with age [17].

Multiple respiratory organisms were detected in 25.5% of the specimens in our study, the largest proportion of which included Rhino/Entero. Other studies in adults reported lower multi-pathogen detection rates of approximately 8.7–15.9% [14, 18–20], suggesting that pediatric patients with RTIs are more likely to be infected by multiple pathogens than adults. However, the clinical significance, including disease severity and hospitalization time, of multi-pathogen infection, especially Rhino/Entero combination infections, is not clear. A previous report indicated that dual-positive results with RSV and Rhino/Entero specimens might be due to viral shedding from a previous Rhino/Entero infection [21]. Nokso-Koivisto et al. also found that rhinovirus was the most prevalent virus in asymptomatic carriers [22].

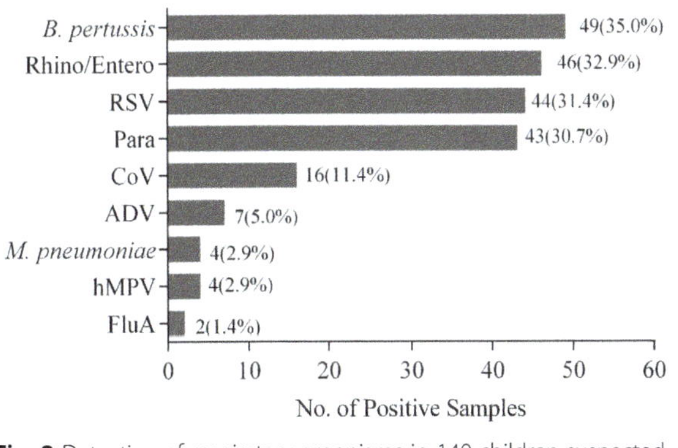

Fig. 2 Detection of respiratory organisms in 140 children suspected with pertussis. 35% (49/140) of the children were tested positive for *B. pertussis* with FilmArray RP

The most unexpected result in our study is the high detection rate of *B. pertussis*, with an overall detection rate of 6.32% in the group of 775 patients, further demonstrating the value of FilmArray RP in clinical application. At present, the diagnosis of pertussis in China is based on culture and serology results. However, both the CDC and World Health Organization (WHO) use positive PCR results as the criteria for diagnosis, suggesting that FilmArray RP testing, in addition to culture, can be considered for patients with suspected pertussis in order to better monitor disease outbreaks. Additionally, the early diagnosis of patients with *B. pertussis*, which is typically difficult to distinguish from pertussis-like syndrome, can also help to reduce unnecessary macrolide treatment. The limitation of the panel is the lack of *B.*

parapertussis, which contributes to more than 5% of pertussis cases [23]. However, it has been added to the second-generation panel, FilmArray RP2 v1.1 [24], and the prevalence of *B. parapertussis* in our patients is currently under investigation.

As stated in the manufacturer's instructions, "FilmArray Respiratory Panel (RP) is a multiplexed nucleic acid test intended for use with FilmArray systems for the simultaneous qualitative detection and identification of multiple respiratory viral and bacterial nucleic acids in nasopharyngeal swabs (NPS) obtained from individuals suspected of respiratory tract infections". Therefore, NPS samples are recommended for FilmArray RP, but there are also studies demonstrating a comparable or even higher detection rate in sputum [25, 26]. However, the detection rate in sputum in our study was lower than that in NPS samples. This might partially be attributed to the fact that most of the sputum samples (86.7%, 98/113) were from ICU patients, and the sputum-providing patients showed a higher positivity rate in their sputum culture than the NPS-providing patients (33.6% vs 20.5%). In addition to sputum, bronchoalveolar lavage fluid (BALF) is a common type of respiratory sample, and Azadah et al. showed that detection in BALF by FilmArray RP can provide new and useful microbiological information within 7 days after a negative NPS result is obtained [27]. Therefore, the choice of the most appropriate sample type and time-point for each patient, particularly in specific clinical contexts, such as undergoing fiberoptic bronchoscopy or ventilator use, may require further investigation.

As with other molecular methods, distinguishing whether the microbes detected in the FilmArray analysis, especially those that are also detected in asymptomatic children, such as human rhinovirus, are causative pathogens or colonizers is not feasible [28–30]. Therefore, the clinicians should take caution when judging pathogens because the results are sometimes "false positive". On the other hand, despite the high detection rate of FilmArray RP, a negative result does not mean the patient is not infected; moreover, a positive result does not mean there is no other co-infecting agent, especially in critically ill patients, in whom a bacterial co-infection often occurs. For this "false-negative" limitation, BioFire has a new pneumonia panel that also targets BALF/sputum and covers 9 common viruses, as well as 15 bacteria, including *Klebsiella pneumonia*, *Haemophilus influenza*, *Streptococcus pneumonia* and *Staphylococcus aureus*. Nevertheless, the FilmArray panel only aims to rapidly provide results for potential pathogens as a reference. A more appropriate method is to comprehensively consider the results from other examinations, such as routine blood testing, C-reactive protein (CRP), procalcitonin (PCT), the erythrocyte sedimentation rate (ESR), culture and radiography, as well as the patients, symptoms, including body temperature, breathing, blood oxygen, heart rate, and mental condition.

Our study also has several limitations. First, our study was performed in a single center and may not be representative of the entire Chinese pediatric population. Second, we did not have data from a more appropriate assay to evaluate the specificity of FilmArray RP. Additionally, we do not provide detailed information on the effects of FilmArray RP on the use of antibiotics, clinical outcomes and health economics, which require further investigation.

Conclusion

In conclusion, the FilmArray RP assay significantly expands our ability to diagnose multiple respiratory infections caused by viruses and atypical bacteria. The array can detect 19 respiratory organisms simultaneously, with a high detection rate, in 65 min. Our study provided the age groups and seasonal distributions of different organisms for pediatric RTI patients. This study also provides new insights into the current status of pertussis infection in China. Whether FilmArray RP can enhance clinical decision-making and limit the unnecessary use of antibiotics in China as in other countries still requires further investigation.

Abbreviations

ADV: Adenovirus; *B. pertussis*: *Bordetella pertussis*; *C. pneumoniae*: *Chlamydophila pneumoniae*; CAP: Community-acquired pneumonia; CoV: Coronaviruses; FilmArray RP: FilmArray Respiratory Panel; FluA: Influenza A viruses; FluB: Influenza B viruses; hMPV: Human metapneumovirus; *M. pneumoniae*: *Mycoplasma pneumoniae*; NPS: Nasopharyngeal swab; Para: Parainfluenza virus; PCR: Polymerase chain reaction; Rhino/Entero: Human rhinovirus/enterovirus; RITs: Respiratory tract infections; RSV: Respiratory syncytial virus; SCMC: Shanghai Children's Medical Center

Acknowledgements

We would like to thank the patients and their parents for the support and cooperation in publishing this work.

Funding

This work was financially supported by the Key Developing Disciplines Project from Shanghai Municipal Commission of Health and Family Planning (2016ZB0104), the Collaborative Innovation Center for Translational Medicine at Shanghai Jiaotong University School of Medicine (TM201616), and the Love Charity Foundation Research Project in Shanghai Children's Medical Center (2017SCMC-AY004).

Authors' contributions

QC and XM initiated the study. JL, YT, MYT and BLD performed the detection of respiratory organisms. JL, YT, MYT, QC and XM wrote the manuscript and analyzed the data. YJX provided technical support and assisted in the data analysis. All authors read and approved the final manuscript.

Consent for publication
Not applicable.

Competing interests
Yijun Xia is an employee of bioMérieux. He was involved in the technical support and data analysis. All the other authors declare they have no conflict of interests to disclose. All the other authors declare that they have no competing interests.

Author details
[1]Department of Infectious Diseases, Shanghai Children's Medical Center, Shanghai Jiaotong University School of Medicine, Shanghai, China. [2]The Laboratory of Pediatric Infectious Diseases, Pediatric Translational Medicine Institute, Shanghai Children's Medical Center, Shanghai Jiaotong University School of Medicine, Shanghai, China. [3]Medical Affairs, Great China | bioMérieux (Shanghai) Company, Limited, Shanghai, China.

References
1. Monto AS. Epidemiology of viral respiratory infections. Am J Med. 2002; 112(Suppl 6A):4S–12S.
2. Jain S, Williams DJ, Arnold SR, Ampofo K, Bramley AM, Reed C, Stockmann C, Anderson EJ, Grijalva CG, Self WH, et al. Community-acquired pneumonia requiring hospitalization among U.S. children. N Engl J Med. 2015;372(9): 835–45.
3. Liu WK, Liu Q, Chen DH, Liang HX, Chen XK, Chen MX, Qiu SY, Yang ZY, Zhou R. Epidemiology of acute respiratory infections in children in Guangzhou: a three-year study. PLoS One. 2014;9(5):e96674.
4. Xu Y, Wang L, Xu J, Wang X, Wei C, Luo P, Ma X, Hou Q, Wang J. Seroprevalence of pertussis in China: need to improve vaccination strategies. Hum Vaccin Immunother. 2014;10(1):192–8.
5. Zhang Q, Zheng H, Liu M, Han K, Shu J, Wu C, Xu N, He Q, Luo H. The seroepidemiology of immunoglobulin G antibodies against pertussis toxin in China: a cross sectional study. BMC Infect Dis. 2012;12:138.
6. Brendish NJ, Malachira AK, Armstrong L, Houghton R, Aitken S, Nyimbili E, Ewings S, Lillie PJ, Clark TW. Routine molecular point-of-care testing for respiratory viruses in adults presenting to hospital with acute respiratory illness (ResPOC): a pragmatic, open-label, randomised controlled trial. Lancet Respir Med. 2017;5(5):401–11.
7. Caliendo AM. Multiplex PCR and emerging technologies for the detection of respiratory pathogens. Clin Infect Dis. 2011;52(Suppl 4):S326–30.
8. Poritz MA, Blaschke AJ, Byington CL, Meyers L, Nilsson K, Jones DE, Thatcher SA, Robbins T, Lingenfelter B, Amiott E, et al. FilmArray, an automated nested multiplex PCR system for multi-pathogen detection: development and application to respiratory tract infection. PLoS One. 2011;6(10):e26047.
9. Wahrenbrock MG, Matushek S, Boonlayangoor S, Tesic V, Beavis KG, Charnot-Katsikas A. Comparison of Cepheid Xpert flu/RSV XC and BioFire FilmArray for detection of influenza a, influenza B, and respiratory syncytial virus. J Clin Microbiol. 2016;54(7):1902–3.
10. Andersson ME, Olofsson S, Lindh M. Comparison of the FilmArray assay and in-house real-time PCR for detection of respiratory infection. Scand J Infect Dis. 2014;46(12):897–901.
11. Renaud C, Crowley J, Jerome KR, Kuypers J. Comparison of FilmArray respiratory panel and laboratory-developed real-time reverse transcription-polymerase chain reaction assays for respiratory virus detection. Diagn Microbiol Infect Dis. 2012;74(4):379–83.
12. Loeffelholz MJ, Pong DL, Pyles RB, Xiong Y, Miller AL, Bufton KK, Chonmaitree T. Comparison of the FilmArray respiratory panel and Prodesse real-time PCR assays for detection of respiratory pathogens. J Clin Microbiol. 2011;49(12):4083–8.
13. Piralla A, Lunghi G, Percivalle E, Vigano C, Nasta T, Pugni L, Mosca F, Stronati M, Torresani E, Baldanti F. FilmArray(R) respiratory panel performance in respiratory samples from neonatal care units. Diagn Microbiol Infect Dis. 2014;79(2):183–6.
14. Litwin CM, Bosley JG. Seasonality and prevalence of respiratory pathogens detected by multiplex PCR at a tertiary care medical center. Arch Virol. 2014; 159(1):65–72.
15. Aberle JH, Aberle SW, Redlberger-Fritz M, Sandhofer MJ, Popow-Kraupp T. Human metapneumovirus subgroup changes and seasonality during epidemics. Pediatr Infect Dis J. 2010;29(11):1016–8.
16. Madhi SA, Ludewick H, Kuwanda L, van Niekerk N, Cutland C, Klugman KP. Seasonality, incidence, and repeat human metapneumovirus lower respiratory tract infections in an area with a high prevalence of human immunodeficiency virus type-1 infection. Pediatr Infect Dis J. 2007;26(8):693–9.
17. Jiang W, Wu M, Zhou J, Wang Y, Hao C, Ji W, Zhang X, Gu W, Shao X. Etiologic spectrum and occurrence of coinfections in children hospitalized with community-acquired pneumonia. BMC Infect Dis. 2017;17(1):787.
18. Bierbaum S, Konigsfeld N, Besazza N, Blessing K, Rucker G, Kontny U, Berner R, Schumacher M, Forster J, Falcone V, et al. Performance of a novel microarray multiplex PCR for the detection of 23 respiratory pathogens (SYMP-ARI study). Eur J Clin Microbiol Infect Dis. 2012;31(10):2851–61.
19. Olofsson S, Brittain-Long R, Andersson LM, Westin J, Lindh M. PCR for detection of respiratory viruses: seasonal variations of virus infections. Expert Rev Anti-Infect Ther. 2011;9(8):615–26.
20. Mahony JB. Detection of respiratory viruses by molecular methods. Clin Microbiol Rev. 2008;21(4):716–47.
21. Brittain-Long R, Westin J, Olofsson S, Lindh M, Andersson LM. Prospective evaluation of a novel multiplex real-time PCR assay for detection of fifteen respiratory pathogens-duration of symptoms significantly affects detection rate. J Clin Virol. 2010;47(3):263–7.
22. Nokso-Koivisto J, Kinnari TJ, Lindahl P, Hovi T, Pitkaranta A. Human picornavirus and coronavirus RNA in nasopharynx of children without concurrent respiratory symptoms. J Med Virol. 2002;66(3):417–20.
23. Hong JY. Update on pertussis and pertussis immunization. Korean J Pediatr. 2010;53(5):629–33.
24. Leber AL, Everhart K, Daly JA, Hopper A, Harrington A, Schreckenberger P, McKinley K, Jones M, Holmberg K, Kensinger B. Multicenter evaluation of BioFire FilmArray respiratory panel 2 for detection of viruses and Bacteria in nasopharyngeal swab samples. J Clin Microbiol. 2018;56(6):e01945–17.
25. Branche AR, Walsh EE, Formica MA, Falsey AR. Detection of respiratory viruses in sputum from adults by use of automated multiplex PCR. J Clin Microbiol. 2014;52(10):3590–6.
26. Doern CD, Lacey D, Huang R, Haag C. Evaluation and implementation of FilmArray version 1.7 for improved detection of adenovirus respiratory tract infection. J Clin Microbiol. 2013;51(12):4036–9.
27. Azadeh N, Sakata KK, Brighton AM, Vikram HR, Grys TE. FilmArray respiratory panel assay: comparison of nasopharyngeal swabs and Bronchoalveolar lavage samples. J Clin Microbiol. 2015;53(12):3784–7.
28. Self WH, Williams DJ, Zhu Y, Ampofo K, Pavia AT, Chappell JD, Hymas WC, Stockmann C, Bramley AM, Schneider E, et al. Respiratory viral detection in children and adults: comparing asymptomatic controls and patients with community-acquired pneumonia. J Infect Dis. 2016;213(4):584–91.
29. Korten I, Mika M, Klenja S, Kieninger E, Mack I, Barbani MT, Gorgievski M, Frey U, Hilty M, Latzin P. Interactions of respiratory viruses and the nasal microbiota during the first year of life in healthy infants. mSphere. 2016;1(6): e00312-16.
30. Shann F. Etiology of severe pneumonia in children in developing countries. Pediatr Infect Dis. 1986;5(2):247–52.

16

Multiplex PCR point of care testing versus routine, laboratory-based testing in the treatment of adults with respiratory tract infections: a quasi-randomised study assessing impact on length of stay and antimicrobial use

Denise Andrews[1], Yumela Chetty[1], Ben S. Cooper[2,3], Manjinder Virk[4], Stephen K Glass[5], Andrew Letters[6], Philip A. Kelly[1], Malur Sudhanva[4] and Dakshika Jeyaratnam[5*]

Abstract

Background: Laboratory-based respiratory pathogen (RP) results are often available too late to influence clinical decisions such as hospitalisation or antibiotic treatment due to time delay in transport of specimens and testing schedules. Ward-based i.e. point of care (POC) testing providing rapid results may alter the clinical management pathway.

Methods: FilmArray® RP polymerase chain reaction (PCR) systems were placed in three in-patient and out-patient medical areas. Patients presenting with influenza-like illness /upper respiratory tract infection +/− lower RTI were recruited between January–July 2015. FilmArray® POC testing occurred on even days of the month (intervention) or routine, laboratory-based RP PCR testing +/− atypical serology on odd days (control). The primary outcome was length of hospital stay. The secondary outcomes were impact on the use of antimicrobials, readmissions, all-cause mortality, length of ward stay and turn-around time (TAT) (time to result from admission).

Results: Of 606 eligible patients, 545 (89.9%) were included; 211 in the control arm and 334 in the intervention arm. 20% of control arm patients and 24% of intervention arm patients had an RP detected. POC testing was not associated with the primary outcome measure, length of stay, but reduced the TAT from 39.5 h to 19.0 h, $p < 0.001$. Only the prescribing decision differed between study arms, $p < 0.001$. When antivirals were given, the intervention was associated with a reduction in the median time to the first dose of 36 h and allowed appropriate treatment of mycoplasma infection.

(Continued on next page)

* Correspondence: d.jeyaratnam@nhs.net
[5]Department of Medical Microbiology, Cheyne Wing, King's College Hospital NHS Foundation Trust, Denmark Hill, London SE5 9RS, UK
Full list of author information is available at the end of the article

(Continued from previous page)

Conclusions: We found no association between respiratory PCR POC testing and length of stay or most of the secondary outcomes except the antimicrobial prescribing decision. This was probably due to a delay in initiating FilmArray® testing. Despite this, POC testing allowed time-critical antivirals to be given significantly faster, appropriate mycoplasma treatment and results were available considerably faster than routine, laboratory-based testing. Ward-staff of all grades performed POC testing without difficulty suggesting potential use across many divergent healthcare settings. Further studies evaluating the implementation of rapid respiratory PCR POC testing and the effect on length of stay and antimicrobial use are required.

Keywords: Point of care, FilmArray®, Respiratory pathogens, Respiratory viruses, Respiratory tract infection, Length of stay, Multiplex PCR, Antimicrobial stewardship, Adults

Background

Respiratory tract infections (RTI) place a significant burden on health systems globally, particularly during the annual respiratory season epidemics [1]. Diagnostic tests for respiratory pathogens (RP) are usually laboratory–based with an inherent delay in time to result relating to specimen in transit to the laboratory and laboratory testing schedules, for example once a day, and/or not performed on weekends and holidays. For this reason or due to the nature of the test (culture, serology or batch molecular testing) results are rarely available to the clinician when the patient is first assessed. Consequently, though respiratory viruses are frequently isolated in community acquired pneumonia (CAP) [2] and are reported to be responsible for 12.8% of CAP cases admitted to UK hospitals [3], the decision to manage as a viral RTI or treat for bacterial infection including *Mycoplasma pneumoniae* or *Chlamydia pneumoniae* ('atypical bacteria') is based upon the clinical scenario and severity criteria such as the CURB-65 score. Thus a proportion of infections will be inappropriately managed with antibiotics or the result may arrive too late for influenza treatment to be effective [4]. The World Health Organization (WHO) states that antimicrobial resistance threatens the effective prevention and treatment of an ever-increasing range of infections [5]. The Centre for Evidence Based Medicine highlights the considerable number of new diagnostic technologies in development to underpin the rational prescribing of antibiotics [6], which extends to antivirals.

Point of care (POC) tests eliminate the need for specimen transportation to the testing laboratory and can be performed on demand by ward staff. By providing faster results, POC tests may influence early treatment decisions such as hospital admission and allow earlier discharge, targeted antimicrobial prescriptions and better antimicrobial stewardship. POC testing should also reduce cross-transmission and subsequent nosocomial outbreaks related to viral RTI cases that are undiagnosed and patients not placed in appropriate isolation. However, current POC tests for respiratory viruses are generally antigen detection tests, usually only detect influenza and respiratory syncytial virus (RSV) and their sensitivity can be suboptimal [7, 8]. The BioFire FilmArray® respiratory panel (BioFire Diagnostics, Salt Lake City, UT, a bioMerieux Company) detects 14 respiratory viruses: influenza virus types A and B (with influenza A subtyping), adenovirus, coronaviruses HKU1, NL63, 229E and OC43, human metapneumovirus, human rhinovirus/enterovirus, parainfluenza virus types 1–4 and RSV and 3 bacteria: *Mycoplasma pneumoniae, Chlamydia pneumoniae* and *Bordetella pertussis*. FilmArray® lends itself to POC testing as it is a small, desktop, fully-automated nested multiplex PCR in an enclosed disposable pouch requiring only 2 min of hands-on time with results available in about 1 hour [9]. Though more expensive than single or low multiplex laboratory or POC tests, clinical outcomes such as a reduced length of stay and reduction in inappropriate antimicrobial usage resulting from the rapid and extended panel may offset test costs. Thus understanding FilmArray®'s clinical utility as a POC test early in a patient's admission is important.

We undertook a study to assess the FilmArray® RP panel as a POC test compared to routine, laboratory-based detection methods in order to assess the impact on length of stay and antibiotic utilization. It is the first study, to our knowledge, in which ward-staff were performing the FilmArray® RP panel as a POC test.

Methods

Study aims

The aim of the study was to determine whether in adults presenting with upper respiratory tract infection (URTI)/ influenza-like illness (ILI) +/– lower respiratory tract infection (LRTI), FilmArray® RP panel POC testing, when compared to the routine, laboratory-based RP testing was associated with length of hospital stay or antimicrobial use.

Study setting

The study took place in a 900 bedded teaching and tertiary referral site of a two-site 1450 bedded acute NHS hospital Trust in London.Four FilmArray® systems were placed in side-rooms across three adult (>16 years) wards: two Acute Medical Units (AMUs) and the Medical Assessment Centre (MAC). The AMUs are 28 and 30 bedded short-stay, acute medical wards to which patients are admitted from the Emergency Department (ED). The MAC is an area to which out-patients can be referred for review by clinicians. It is open daily from 8 am to 10 pm. MAC patients are assessed and then admitted to an AMU or discharged.

Study design

A quasi-randomised trial design was used such that patients were enrolled in to the control arm on odd days of the month and in to the intervention arm on even days of the month. This was the most pragmatic design that could be implemented on the study wards. The study was not blinded.

Study-ward staff were educated about the study and consent taking, given a staff information sheet and trained to use the FilmArray® respiratory panel as per manufacturer's instructions. Competency assessments were conducted. All staff were required to don personal protective equipment when performing each assay. FilmArray® tests were to be ordered and performed by study-ward staff, however if they were unable to do the testing e.g. due to clinical duties, the study investigators, who worked on weekdays until 7 pm and a half-day on weekends and bank holidays, performed the FilmArray® test. In order to interpret the FilmArray® results out of hours, study-ward staff consulted a standard operating procedure describing each pathogen, the type of diseases associated with it, the groups at risk of severe infection, any medical management and the infection control precautions required, if at all. They also had direct contact numbers for the study investigators who were available at all hours. Eligible patients were identified by ward staff or study staff. Written informed consent was obtained by ward staff before patient participation.

In the control arm, combined nose and throat flocculated swabs (Copan Diagnostics, Italy), were placed in viral transport medium (VTM, Copan) which was transported to the laboratory by hospital porters as is routine. The standard, routine diagnostic assays for viral pathogens used in the control arm are in-house developed real-time PCRs with 4 separate multiplex assays (influenza A (H1N1) pdm09 matrix gene RNA[1] and H1 RNA, influenza A virus RNA, influenza B virus RNA, rhinovirus RNA, RSV subgroup A and subgroup B RNA, parainfluenza viruses 1, 2 and 3 RNA and human metapneumovirus RNA) and an adenovirus monoplex [10–12]. Outside this study, there is no rapid/POC RP testing at this hospital. If requested by the clinical team, *Mycoplasma pneumoniae* and *Chlamydia pneumoniae* were tested for in the control arm using the laboratory's routine, complement fixation tests (CFT) (Launch Diagnostics, Kent, UK and TCS Biosciences, Buckingham, UK). A comparison of the pathogens detected by the FilmArray® and the routine diagnostic tests is shown in Table 1. The routine tests were performed on site by qualified Health Care Scientists. PCR results were available at

Table 1 FilmArray® panel compared to the routine laboratory-based PCR and non-PCR methods

	Control		Intervention
Pathogen	Routine PCR	Serology/culture	FilmArray®
Adenovirus	✓	–	✓
Coronavirus HKU1, NL63, 229E, OC43	Not tested	–	✓
Human metapneumovirus	✓	–	✓
Human rhinovirus/ enterovirus	✓	–	✓
Influenza A virus	✓	–	✓
Influenza A virus H1	✓	–	✓
Influenza A virus H3	✓	–	✓
Influenza A virus H1–2009	✓	–	✓
Influenza B virus	✓	–	✓
Parainfluenza virus 1,2,3	✓	–	✓
Parainfluenza virus 4	Not tested	–	✓
Respiratory syncytial virus	Subgroups A/B	–	✓
Bordetella pertussis	Not tested	Culture	✓
Chlamydia pneumoniae	Not tested	Complement Fixation test (CFT)	✓
Mycoplasma pneumoniae	Not tested	Complement Fixation test (CFT)	✓

around 4 PM every weekday and on weekends. Routine serology testing was batch-tested once per week.

In the intervention arm, combined nose and throat flocculated swabs (Copan Diagnostics, Italy), were placed in viral transport medium (VTM, Copan) and thereafter a rehydration buffer and 200 μl of the VTM was introduced into the FilmArray® pouch by ward-based staff (POC testing) on even days of the month (intervention arm). FilmArray® was validated against the routine method to ensure satisfactory performance characteristics but a head to head comparison was not included as part of this study. External (Quality Control for Molecular Diagnostics [QCMD], Glasgow, UK) and internal quality control specimens were tested by FilmArray® during the study. The use of the FilmArray® was approved by the Trust Point of Care Testing Committee.

All results were uploaded to the hospital results reporting system. Positive results for both study arms were telephoned by a microbiologist or virologist to the health care provider. Antimicrobial stewardship activities did not change during the study.

All other diagnostic specimens e.g. for bacterial culture were sent to the laboratory as usual for both study arms. These results were not included in the analysis.

Eligible patients

The inclusion criteria were that patients were ≥16 years of age, with mental capacity to give written informed consent and presenting with URTI/ILI defined as symptoms including fever or feeling feverish (chills), cough, sore throat, runny or stuffy nose, muscle-aches or body-aches, headaches, fatigue (tiredness) and possibly vomiting or diarrhoea [13] +/− LRTI. Patients who did not meet inclusion criteria or with evidence or suspicion of bacterial infection affecting sites other than the respiratory tract were excluded from the opportunity to participate in the study. Patients who requested withdrawal from the study were excluded from the analysis.

Primary and secondary outcomes

The primary outcome studied was the length of hospital stay defined as the time between hospital admission and hospital discharge. The FilmArray® RP panel is relatively expensive (£89–£133 for the consumables and £28, 000-£33,000 for the capital purchase of the system depending upon the country) compared to currently employed routine tests, (£50 per test for our standard laboratory method). However the average cost for managing pneumonia in the community is estimated at £100 per episode compared with £1700–5100 for hospitalised patients in the UK [14] and $8000 in the US [15]. Thus if a FilmArray® POC result allows earlier discharge, the consequent financial savings from the shorter hospital stay may offset the extra test costs and prove cost-beneficial, hence our choice of primary outcome. The secondary outcomes were antimicrobial prescription/s (antibiotics: any versus none, duration, time to prescription within the first 72 h of the patient's stay and prescribing decisions within 24 h after the the diagnostic results under investigation: start, stop, de-escalation, escalation and continued use, as assessed by the Chief Investigator), readmission rates and all-cause mortality (both within 30 days of the test) and length of study-ward stay (i.e. removing the length of stay on subsequent wards to which the patient was transferred, where relevant). Escalation was defined as the addition of an antibiotic/s to the existing antibiotic therapy or the substitution of the current agent with a broader agent. De-escalation was the cessation of ≥1 antibiotic when >1 antibiotic was prescribed or the substitution with a narrower agent. We collected these data prospectively and retrospectively from the electronic patient record (EPR) and the electronic patient medicines administration system (EPMA). In some cases, enrolment of the patient into the hospital administrative system occurred after examination and initiation of antibiotic therapy by the physician on the ward or in the ED. Therefore, a negative time to antibiotic administration on the ward was corrected to zero hours to antibiotics. We defined the turn-around time (TAT) of the tests as the time between hospital admission and the time of the result on the FilmArray® system (intervention) or the time of the result on the EPR (control).

For each patient, we collected demographic data, Charlson co-morbidity score, and at the time of admission, CURB-65 score for patients with a diagnosis of community-acquired pneumonia, an early warning score (EWS) [16], peripheral white cell count (WCC), C-reactive protein (CRP) and the day of the week of admission. The type of LRTI e.g. infective exacerbation of chronic obstructive pulmonary disease (COPD), bronchitis, pneumonia was not recorded.

Statistical methods

The power calculation was based upon length of stay, which had previously been observed to be 3.2 days on the study wards. Rapid pathogen identification has been associated with a reduction of mean hospital length of stay, in one study from 11.9 days to 9.3 days (approx. 20%) (p = 0.1) [17]. For a 20% reduction in length of stay (LOS) in the intervention arm, sample size calculations indicated that sample sizes of 1131 cases in each arm were required to achieve 90% power to detect a difference of 0.6 between the null hypothesis that both group means are 3.2 days (76.8 h, based upon data collected from the study wards) and the alternative hypothesis that the mean of group 2 is 2.6 days (62.4 h) with known group standard deviations of 5.2 and 5.2 and with a significance level (alpha) of 0.05.

The primary outcome was analysed with a linear regression model (after log-transformation of length of stay data) according to a pre-specified analysis plan with an individual patient taken as the unit of analysis. Secondary outcomes were analysed using linear regression models for continuous outcome data, logistic regression for binary outcomes, and negative binomial regression for count outcome data. For all these patient-related outcomes we adjusted for multiple pre-specified potential confounders (age, sex, Charlson score, EWS, WCC, CRP). Pearson's Chi-squared test was used to test for differences between the arms in categorical antibiotic prescribing decisions with p-values calculated by 10,000 Monte Carlo replicates (to avoid problems associated with small cell counts associated with the usual asymptotic p-values). A t-test was used to compare the time to test between the two arms. A planned subgroup analysis was performed as above for primary and secondary outcomes excluding patients who had infection proven elsewhere after enrolment as it is plausible that a respiratory pathogen POC result would not alter LOS or antibiotic use when the patient had another infective diagnosis made. Analysis was conducted in *R* [18]. Multiple imputation was used to account for missing data using the package *mice* [19].

Results

The study ran from 5th January 2015 until 1st July 2015 as planned. No changes were made to the study protocol. During this time 606 patients met eligibility criteria (Fig. 1). Sixty-one (10.1%) of these patients were not included (33 in the intervention arm, 28 in the control arm) because 20 were discharged before enrolment, an interpreter was unavailable for three, 34 declined participation, one patient died before being approached, one patient consented but the test was not performed and information is missing for two patients. No patients withdrew from the study. Thus 545 (89.9%) patients were enrolled and included in the analysis, 211 in the control arm and 334 in the intervention arm. All statistical analyses were pre-specified; there were no post-hoc analyses.

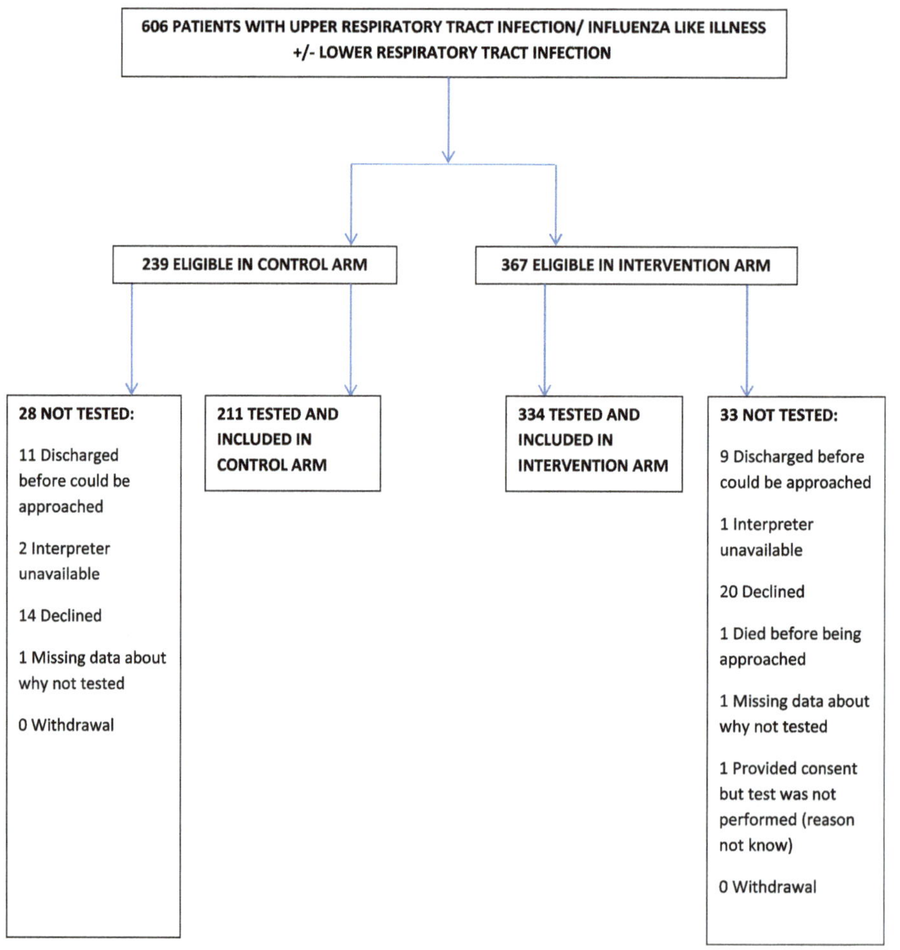

Fig. 1 Flow of study participants through the trial. N.B. The total number of patients screened for eligibility was not collected

Baseline characteristics were similar between the two study arms (Table 2). CURB-65 score was missing for 62.9% of patients for whom it was relevant and was omitted from the analysis. One hundred and sixty-five (30%) patients had a negative time to antibiotics changed to 0 h (median - 1.5 h [IQR -3.5 to -0.8]).

The median time to result from admission was substantially shorter in the intervention arm compared to the control arm (control arm 39.5 h (IQR 25.4–57.6), intervention arm 19.0 h (IQR 8.1–31.7)), two-sample t-test assuming unequal variances, $p < 0.001$. Ward staff of all grades performed 28% of POC tests, 68% of the samples were tested by study investigators and there is no record for 4%. No adverse events were reported.

Overall, 124 (22.8%) of the 545 patients had a positive result (Table 3), 43 (20.4%) in the control arm and 81 (24.3%) in the intervention arm. The viruses and bacteria detected are shown in Table 3. Every virus on the panels was identified except parainfluenza virus type 1, type 2 and type 4. Only single pathogens were detected by routine testing but FilmArray® detected dual infections in five samples. FilmArray® also detected coronaviruses, not detected using standard tests. There were three and four invalid tests in the control and intervention arms respectively, the remaining tests were negative (78.2% control, 74.6% intervention).

M. pneumoniae was the only bacterium on the panels which was identified. Four patients in the control arm had an elevated *Mycoplasma* CFT (1:64, 1:64, 1:32, >1:16). Convalescent serology was not sent, rendering results uninterpretable. All of these results were available after ward discharge, three after hospital discharge, and did not influence management. The TAT was 8–13 days. Five patients in the intervention arm had *M. pneumoniae* detected by FilmArray®. Antibiotics were started for 2 of these cases and extended in 2 after discussion with the Microbiologist.

There was no evidence that the length of hospital stay, the primary endpoint, was reduced by POC testing. The median length of hospital stay was 79.6 h (IQR 41.9–188.9) in the control arm and 98.6 h (IQR 48.1–218.4) in the intervention arm. In the linear model (for log-transformed length of stay data, adjusting for potential confounders) the rapid test was associated with an absolute difference in the natural logarithm of the length of stay of 0.108 (95% CI [-0.089, 0.305]; $p = 0.28$). This corresponds to an 11% (95% CI [-9%, 36%]) increase in length of stay associated with the rapid test arm. Six of 33 patients tested on the MAC in the control arm (18%) and 13 of 67 patients tested in the MAC in the intervention arm (19.4%) were discharged without admission to a hospital ward.

For all but one of the secondary outcomes, there was no evidence that the intervention had an effect (Table 4). Only the prescribing decision within 24 h following the diagnostic results under investigation showed evidence of a difference between study arms (Table 5, $p < 0.001$, Pearson's Chi-squared test, p-value calculated by 10,000 Monte Carlo replicates).

Table 2 Baseline characteristics

	Control	Intervention
Male gender	52% (110/211)	52% (172/334)
Age (years)[a]	61 (47–73)	67 (47–77)
Charlson score[a]	0 (0–2)	1 (0–3)
White cell count ($\times 10^9$/L)[a]	9.6 (6.8–13.7)	9.6 (6.9–13.1)
C-Reactive protein (mg/L)[a]	38.3 (9.4–123.1)	39.5 (15.4–124.5)
Early warning score[a]	2 (1–4)	2 (1–4)
Admitted on the weekend	22% (47/211)	22% (73/334)

[a]median (IQR), Early Warning Score: Six physiological parameters routinely recorded: i) respiratory rate, ii) oxygen saturations, iii) temperature, iv) systolic blood pressure, v) pulse rate and vi) level of consciousness. In addition, a weighting score of 2 should be added for any patient requiring supplemental oxygen (oxygen delivery by mask or nasal cannulae)

Table 3 Summary of respiratory pathogen testing results

Result	Routine PCR /serology/ culture (Control)	FilmArray® (Intervention)
Total	211	334
Invalid or Inhibitory	3 (1.4)	4 (1.2)
Negative (%)	165 (78.2)	249 (74.6)
Positive (%)	43 (20.4)	81 (24.3)
Positive for a virus (%)	43 (20.4)	76 (22.8)
Positive for a bacterium (%)	0 (0)	5 (1.5)
Influenza A	6	13 (2 dual)
Influenza B	15	18 (1 dual)
Adenovirus	2	3
Parainfluenza virus 1	0	0
Parainfluenza virus 2	0	0
Parainfluenza virus 3	5	8 (1 dual)
Parainfluenza virus 4	Not tested	0
Human metapneumovirus	2	2
Rhinovirus (/enterovirus)	12	16
Respiratory syncytial virus	1	6 (1 dual)
Coronavirus 229E	Not tested	3 (2 dual)
Coronavirus HKU1	Not tested	4 (2 dual)
Coronavirus NL63	Not tested	5
Coronavirus OC43	Not tested	3 (1 dual)
Mycoplasma pneumonia	0	5
Bordetella pertussis	0	0
Chlamydia pneumoniae	0	0

Dual infections: Coronavirus HKU1 & Influenza A, Coronavirus 229E & HKU1, Parainfluenza 3 & Coronavirus 229E, Coronavirus OC43 & RSV and Influenza A & Influenza B

Table 4 Summary of secondary outcome measures

Outcome		Control	Intervention	Estimated intervention effect	Adjusted p value
Antibiotic use at any time during the hospital stay post-enrolment[a]	Percentage	77% (152/198)	75% (243/324)	aOR (95% CI)1.0 (0.6, 1.5)	0.99
Duration of antibiotic usage (days)[b]	median (IQR)	6.0 (5.0, 7.3)	6.0 (4.0, 7.0)	Absolute difference in natural logarithm of duration (95% CI)-0.08 (−0.22, 0.054)	0.23
Time to antibiotic within the first 72 h of stay (hours)[c]	median (IQR)	0.0 (0.0–3.0)	0.0 (0.0–6.0)	Absolute difference in days (95% CI)2.2 (−1.4,5.8)	0.21
Readmission within 30 days of study participation[a]	Percentage	20% (42/211)	19% (64/333)	aOR (95% CI)0.9 (0.6, 1.4)	0.70
Mortality 30 days post-enrolment[a]	Percentage	4% (9/211)	4% (14/333)	aOR (95% CI)0.9 (0.3, 2.2)	0.79
Length of study ward inpatient stay (hours)[c]	median (IQR)	54 (23, 99)	61 (24, 115)	Absolute difference in natural logarithm of length of stay (95% CI) 0.05 (−0.16, 0.25)	0.66

[a]Based on a logistic regression analysis
[b]Analysed with a linear model (after log transformation)
[c]Analysed with a negative binomial regression
All models adjusted for age, sex, Charlson and Potts scores, day of week, and admission values of WCC and CRP and used multiple imputation to account for missing data. The CURB-65 score was not available for 59% of patients, and was therefore not adjusted for in statistical models. There was less than 5% missing data for all covariates. Missing outcome variables 1) Antibiotics within 72 h and 2) Antibiotics at any time: missing data for 13 patients in the control arm and 10 patients in the intervention arm, 3) Time to antibiotics in the first 72 h: missing data for 1 patient in the intervention arm, 4) duration of antibiotics: missing data for 4 patients in the control arm and 13 in the intervention arm, 5) readmission: missing data for 1 patient in intervention arm, 6) mortality: missing data for 1 patient in intervention arm

Fifty-one patients had influenza A virus and/or influenza B virus detected by either the routine assay (21) or by the FilmArray® (30). Of these patients, 13 of 21 (62%) in the control arm and 24 of 30 (80%) in the intervention arm were given antivirals. The time to the first dose from the time of admission was known for all but one patient in each arm and was considerably reduced in the intervention arm: median of 60.4 h in the control arm (IQR 22.7–85.2) and 24 h in the intervention arm (IQR 11.6–33.0). Only one patient in each arm was given empiric antivirals but had a no viruses detected.

The planned subgroup analysis excluding patients who had infection proven elsewhere after enrolment e.g. urinary tract infection (n = 33) did not substantially alter any of the above results.

Discussion

We found no evidence for an association between respiratory multiplex PCR (BioFire FilmArray®) POC testing and length of hospital stay when compared to our routine, laboratory-based respiratory PCR and serology testing. There was an association between POC testing and the antibiotic prescribing decision within 24 h after the result. POC testing also produced results considerably faster than laboratory-based assays. We did not investigate whether the POC results actually influenced decision making and the association with the prescribing decision may only reflect that the FilmArray® result was available before the antibiotics were prescribed and not that the prescriber considered the FilmArray® result in their decision making. Similar percentages of patients

Table 5 Effect of RP Result on Antibiotic Prescribing

Antibiotic Prescribing Decision Category	Control		Intervention		Total
	number	percent of control arm	number	percent intervention arm	
Continue	128	60.7	165	49.4	293
De-escalate	5	2.4	6	1.8	11
Escalate	4	1.9	26	7.8	30
Start	1	0.5	17	5.1	18
Stop	7	3.3	15	4.5	22
Remain off antibiotics	51	24.1	95	28.4	146
Missing data about decision	15	7.1	10	3.0	25
Total	211		334		545

Control arm de-escalate: 2 stop ≥1 antimicrobial, 3 substitution of Beta-lactam with narrower spectrum Beta-lactam. Intervention arm de-escalate: 2 stop ≥1 antimicrobial, 2 substitution of Beta-lactam with narrower spectrum Beta-lactam, 2 substitution of Beta-lactam with narrower spectrum Beta-lactam and atypical agent was stopped. Control arm escalate: 4 add antibiotic to existing antibiotics (all agents against atypical pneumonia). Intervention arm escalate: 19 add antibiotics to existing antibiotics (14 agents against atypical pneumonia, 5 addition of agents against 'typical pneumonia' to atypical agent e.g. Beta-lactam or teicoplanin with ciprofloxacin if penicillin allergic), 7 substitution of Beta-lactam with broader spectrum Beta-lactam received antibiotics in both study arms. There were no significant differences for the remaining secondary outcomes between the two study arms.

The hypothesis was that POC testing would reduce the length of stay. However, though the POC test was 1 day faster than laboratory-based testing, the results were available later than anticipated. This was not due to testing performance of FilmArray®, which took only 65 min but related to a delay in the processing of the specimen by the clinical staff on the ward. Sixty-eight percent of POC tests were performed by study investigators reflecting the fact that the study protocol was not initiated by clinical staff as soon as the patient was admitted to the study ward in many cases. Instead testing was delayed until the study investigators visiting the study wards initiated the study protocol. This resulted in a significant delay in time to results. This is in contrast to a trial of MRSA POC screening by our AMU ward staff that had a TAT from admission of 3.7 h [20]. MRSA testing is mandatory and most patients were eligible for inclusion. The delay in the present study may be related to screening for more complex eligibility criteria than the MRSA study and an additional reliance on study investigators present on the ward to perform the test. If this is the case, the TAT would be faster if FilmArray® was embedded as a routine, diagnostic POC test. When ward staff did perform the test, they were from all grades and they performed it without incident. Others report a TAT of 2.3 h for FilmArray® POC testing, though the TAT was from the time of decision to test to the time of result and testing was conducted by trial staff [21]. Thus FilmArray® POC testing can be successfully implemented but this study failed to achieve the optimum TAT.

POC testing was associated with a reduction in time to antivirals for those identified with influenza virus. Antivirals were given a day and a half quicker in the intervention arm and within a day of admission. Given that these drugs are of clinical benefit only if administered within 48 h of symptom onset [4], this is a key, clinical outcome. POC testing allowed changes to therapy for the appropriate treatment of mycoplasma infection; in the control arm, positive results were uninterpretable and were predominantly available after discharge. The ability of FilmArray® to detect coronaviruses allowed for a diagnosis to be made in 15 samples that would have been missed using routine methods. Routine testing only identified single pathogens as opposed to FilmArray® which identified dual infection in 5 patients, of importance for infection control and virus surveillance. Parainfluenza virus types 1, 2 and 4, *Chlamydia pneumoniae* and *Bordetella pertussis* were not detected during the course of this study which did not span the entire winter.

The positive impact on antivirals of the faster time to detection of influenza with FilmArray® was reported by an observational study of paediatric patients, 81% of who were given oseltamivir in a timely manner, which was not possible with the comparator test [22]. An observational study reported a faster time to a negative influenza result with FilmArray® compared to another RT-PCR (46.4 h versus 3.1 h) which shortened unnecessary oseltamivir use by 2 days with an estimated cost saving per patient of $34.16 US [23].

Seventy-five percent of the POC results were negative, providing no information about the aetiology of the infection or the predicted clinical course. Negative results would not be expected to expedite discharge or antibiotic cessation, the main outcomes under consideration here. A paediatric observational study found that patients with a positive respiratory virus PCR result had a 42% shorter duration of intravenous antibiotics [24]. A retrospective study noted a reduced length of stay in children with a positive FilmArray® result reported within 4 h, not seen with negative tests [25]. The reduced time to detection of influenza with laboratory-based FilmArray® was associated with significantly lower odds ratios for admission, length of stay, duration of antibiotics and chest X-rays when compared to positive routine tests in a retrospective study of adults [26]. A randomised trial noted that patients with positive FilmArray® POC results received shorter courses of antibiotics and had shorter hospital stays than those with negative POC results [21]. Our 20–24% positive yield may be because our study was seasonally limited and extended in to the summer months. Further, we did not record the types of RTI, which may have resulted in this lower than expected percentage. Another UK, adult study between September 2012 and February 2014 identified viruses in 30% of patients with lower RTI [27].

The POC result was too slow to influence initial antibiotic decision making as the median time to antibiotics from admission was 0 h. This rapid initiation of antibiotics was also found in a randomised trial of FilmArray® POC testing [21] and is consistent with guidelines that recommend antibiotic treatment for CAP within 4 h of presentation to hospital [3]. Therefore, we would expect almost all patients to be initially started on an antibiotic. However with the delay in POC testing we would not expect this parameter to be impacted, i.e. if testing had been done in an appropriate time frame (<4 h after patient evaluation) the subsequent initiation or discontinuation may have been significantly influenced. Some of this reflects a continuation on the study wards of antibiotics started in the ED. Even with a positive POC result, AMU doctors may be dissuaded on safety grounds from stopping or de-escalating antibiotics that were started on the basis of a clinical assessment that they did not witness in the ED. Our findings are consistent with a randomised trial of FilmArray® POC testing, which found that the mean duration of antibiotics did not differ between the FilmArray® and control arms. However that group identified that a greater proportion of patients in the intervention arm (with a POC result) than in the control arm received only a single dose of antibiotics or <48 h of antibiotics [21], something that we did not assess in the present study. Other trials of RP diagnostics in adults, including FilmArray®, have found that PCR detection of only a viral pathogen coupled with a low procalcitonin level led to antibiotic cessation in only 32% of cases [28] or a trend towards fewer days of antibiotic treatment off-set by only 4/18 patients having their antibiotics stopped [29]. The authors of the latter study advocate real-time stewardship with RP results, which was omitted from the intervention in the present study. Rapid pathogen identification with antimicrobial stewardship has been associated with a significant reduction of hospital costs for adult in-patients [17].

This study has other limitations, nearly all due to limited resources. We employed a pragmatic quasi-randomised design, allocating patients to the intervention arm on even days making the study vulnerable to bias due to differences in patients allocated to the study arms. Though we found no evidence for such differences, and the outcome analysis adjusted for several pre-specified potential confounders, a fully randomised design would have provided a stronger level of evidence. There were more patients in the intervention arm suggesting that the patient recruitment processes in the two arms were not equivalent and this may reflect enthusiasm for the FilmArray®. This may also reflect increased disease severity in the intervention arm and a need to identify the cause of the disease, thereby resulting in a biased use of the FilmArray® in this cohort. CURB-65 scores were not assessed and therefore an accurate comparison of the severity of the pneumonia in the two arms of the study could not be determined. Further, we did not collect data on the type of RTI; a randomised trial of FilmArray® POC testing recorded a shorter duration of antibiotics for patients with asthma and COPD who were in the intervention arm versus the control and a shorter length of stay for COPD patients in the FilmArray® arm [21]. The ED does not routinely use EPMA and so we do not know exactly how many patients received antibiotics there. A negative time to antibiotics, due to administrative errors, was changed to 0 h in 30% of patients however the median was small (−1.5 h) and this phenomenon occurred in both study arms. As in other similar studies on this subject [21] we did not include routine bacteriology results in the analysis however the hypothesis had greater dependence upon the predominantly viral panel results under investigation and bacteriology results would not be expected to differ between the study arms and thus influence results. Finally, the number of eligible patients admitted to the study wards was less than predicted by the data used to plan the study and hence the number of cases recruited fell short of the statistical calculation that required 1131 patients in each arm to detect a fall of 0.6 days. It is not clear why this was the case but may be related to patients bypassing the study wards during the busy winter months of January to March and due to the inclusion of some summer months in the study.

We have selected for patients who required admission and possibly antibiotics by placing the FilmArray® systems on hospital wards. A panel which includes common bacterial causes of lower RTI would probably have identified more pathogens in this setting. A recent study in the UK identified bacteria in lower respiratory tract specimens from 81% of patients with pneumonia [27]. Though we did not record the type of RTI in this study, as in-patients, most patients probably had a lower RTI. A study in the ED might have tested a greater number of patients with a viral illness. There, POC results could provide reassurance that discharge is reasonable. With a rapid result and the broader RP panel afforded by FilmArray®, it is plausible that safety-netting antibiotic prescriptions would have reduced. Due to the mandated maximum 4-h wait for patients in English EDs [30] and a perceived lack of understanding of these results vocalised by our ED staff (because with laboratory-based testing the patient has left ED when results are available), we moved the study one step in to the hospital. This highlights an important knowledge gap. An ED-based study of POC testing incorporating decision making support is therefore advisable.

Conclusion

We found no association between respiratory multiplex PCR (BioFire FilmArray®) POC testing and length of hospital stay when compared to our routine, laboratory-based respiratory PCR and serology testing. This result was most likely influenced by the delay in the rapid POC testing. POC testing produced results considerably faster than the routine tests but the results were not rapid as designed to be. This was not the fault of the POC test, but highlights the fact that new technology itself is not enough: the correct systems must be in place in order to reap their benefits. Patients who had the POC test received time-critical antivirals for influenza significantly faster and appropriate therapy for mycoplasma infection, not seen in the control arm. Ward staff of all grades performed the POC test without incident meaning that this test has potential across a range of healthcare. Further studies are required that focus on implementing respiratory multiplex PCR POC testing with rapid results, in order to fully assess the impact on length of stay and antibiotic use.

Abbreviations

AMUs: Acute Medical Units; CAP: Community acquired pneumonia; CFT: Complement fixation test; CRP: C-reactive protein; ED: Emergency Department; EPMA: Electronic patient medicines administration system; EPR: Electronic patient record; EWS: Early warning score; MAC: Medical Assessment Centre; PCR: Polymerase chain reaction; POC: Point of care; RP: Respiratory pathogen; RSV: Respiratory syncytial virus; RTI: Respiratory tract infection; TAT: Turn-around time; WCC: Peripheral white cell count

Acknowledgements

Ann-Louise Caress, James Beresford-Davies, BioFire and bioMérieux (Nadia Albrecht, Ryan Anderson, Sam Bozette, Christine Ginocchio, Marie-Francoise Gros, Karen Jordan, Alasdair Macmillan, Wade Stevenson), Nergish Desai, British Lung Foundation Central Manchester Breathe Easy patient/carer support group, Chandan Kainth, staff and patients of the study wards, Pei Jun Wu.

Previous presentation acknowledgement

The theory behind the study and the turn-around times were an oral presentation at the bioMérieux Integrated Symposium entitled 'From single to syndromic testing: the new paradigm in microbiology' at the 26th ECCMID, Amsterdam, Netherlands, April 9–12, 2016 and at a FilmArray® Users' Group at biomérieux, Annency, France in October 2015. The results and the analysis were not presented at either meeting. A poster concerning the turn-around times and staff undertaking the test (analysis of the first 3 month's data) entitled 'First ever use of BioFire FilmArray® respiratory panel at the point of care' was at the Interscience Conference on Antimicrobial Agents and Chemotherapy (ICAAC) ICAAC 2015: 55th ICAAC September 18 — 21, 2015. San Diego, CA. Again, the results and the analysis were not presented.

Funding

The research was funded bioMérieux and by the National Institute for Health Research (NIHR) Collaboration for Leadership in Applied Health Research and Care South London at King's College Hospital NHS Foundation Trust. The views expressed are those of the author(s) and not necessarily those of the NHS, the NIHR or the Department of Health.

Authors' contributions

All authors contributed to the execution of the study and/or study analysis, and/or writing of the manuscript and all approved the manuscript.

Consent for publication

Not applicable

Competing interests

DJ has received speaker's fees from bioMérieux.

Author details

[1]Division of Acute Medicine, King's College Hospital NHS Foundation Trust, London SE5 9RS, UK. [2]Mahidol-Oxford Tropical Medicine Research Unit, Faculty of Tropical Medicine, Mahidol University, Bangkok 10400, Thailand. [3]Centre for Tropical Medicine and Global Health, Nuffield Department of Clinical Medicine, University of Oxford, Oxford, UK. [4]South London Specialist Virology Centre, King's College Hospital NHS Foundation Trust, London SE5 9RS, UK. [5]Department of Medical Microbiology, Cheyne Wing, King's College Hospital NHS Foundation Trust, Denmark Hill, London SE5 9RS, UK. [6]Infection, Prevention and Control Team, King's College Hospital NHS Foundation Trust, London SE5 9RS, UK.

References

1. Surveillance of influenza and other respiratory viruses, including novel respiratory viruses, in the United Kingdom: winter 2012/13, Public Health England. http://webarchive.nationalarchives.gov.uk/20140714084352/http://www.hpa.org.uk/webc/HPAwebFile/HPAweb_C/1317139321787 Accessed on 15 Mar 2017.
2. Musher DM, Thorner AR. Community-acquired pneumonia. N Engl J Med. 2015;372(3):294.
3. Lim WS, Baudouin SV, George RC, Hill AT, Jamieson C, Le Jeune I, Macfarlane JT, Read RC, Roberts HJ, Levy ML, Wani M, Woodhead MA. Guidelines for the Management of Community Acquired Pneumonia in adults: update 2009. Thorax 2009. Volume 64. Supplement III.
4. Muthuri SG, Venkatesan S, Myles PR, Leonardi-Bee J, Al Khuwaitir TS, Al Mamun A, et al. PRIDE Consortium Investigators. Effectiveness of neuraminidase inhibitors in reducing mortality in patients admitted to hospital with influenza a H1N1pdm09 virus infection: a meta-analysis of individual participant data. Lancet Respir Med. 2014;2(5):395–404.
5. WHO Antimicrobial resistance fact sheet http://www.who.int/mediacentre/factsheets/fs194/en/ Accessed on 14 Dec 2016.
6. Pluddemann A, Onakpoya I, Harrison S, Shinkins B, Tompson A, Davis R, et al. Position paper on anti-microbial resistance diagnostics – Centre for Evidence-Based Medicine. Oxford: University of Oxford June 2015. http://www.cebm.net/wp-content/uploads/2015/07/AMR-Diagnostic-technologies_10-June-2015.pdf Accessed on 15 Mar 2017.
7. Centers for Disease Control and Prevention. Rapid diagnostic testing for influenza: information for health care professionals. Page last updated: August 4, 2016. http://www.cdc.gov/flu/professionals/diagnosis/rapidclin.htm. Accessed on 8 Sept 2016.
8. Clark NM, Lynch JP 3rd. Influenza: epidemiology, clinical features, therapy, and prevention. Semin Respir Crit Care Med. 2011;32(4):373–92.
9. Poritz MA, Blaschke AJ, Byington CL, Meyers L, Nilsson K, Jones DE, et al. FilmArray, an automated nested multiplex PCR system for multi-pathogen detection: development and application to respiratory tract infection. PLoS One. 2011;6(10):e26047. https://doi.org/10.1371/annotation/468cfdcd-184c-42f7-a1d0-3b72a2f6a558.
10. Auburn H, Zuckerman M, Broughton S, Greenough A, Smith M. Detection of nine respiratory RNA viruses using three multiplex RT-PCR assays incorporating a novel RNA internal control transcript. J Virol Methods. 2011 Sep;176(1–2):9–13.
11. Heim A, Ebnet C, Harste G, Pring-Akerblom P. Rapid and quantitative detection of human adenovirus DNA by real-time PCR. J Med Virol. 2003; 70(2):228–39.
12. CDC protocol of real-time RTPCR for influenza a(H1N1) 28 April 2009 revision 1 (30 April 2009) revision 2 (6 October 2009) http://www.who.int/csr/resources/publications/swineflu/CDCRealtimeRTPCR_SwineH1Assay-2009_20090430.pdf?ua=1 Accessed on 06 Feb 2017.
13. https://www.cdc.gov/flu/keyfacts.htm last accessed 9 Aug 2017.
14. Guest JF, Morris A. Community-acquired pneumonia: the annual cost to the National Health Service in the UK. Eur Respir J. 1997;10:1530–4.
15. Merchant S, Mullins CD, Shih YC. Factors associated with hospitalization costs for patients with community-acquired pneumonia. Clin Ther. 2003; 25(2):593–610.
16. Royal College of Physicians. National Early Warning Score (NEWS): Standardising the assessment of acute illness severity in the NHS. Report of a working party. London: RCP, 2012. file:///C:/Users/dakshika%20jeyaratnam/Downloads/National%20Early%20Warning%20Score%20(NEWS)%20-%20Standardising%20the%20assessment%20of%20acute-illness%20severity%20in%20the%20NHS_0%20(1).pdf Accessed on 15 March 2017.
17. Perez K, Olsen RJ, Musick WL, Cernoch PL, Davis JR, Land GA, et al. Integrating rapid pathogen identification and antimicrobial stewardship significantly decreases hospital costs. Arch Pathol Lab Med. 2013 Sep;137(9):1247–54.
18. R Core Team (2015). R: a language and environment for statistical computing. R foundation for statistical computing, Vienna, Austria. https://www.R-project.org/.
19. Van Buuren S, Groothuis-Oudshoorn K. Mice: multivariate imputation by chained equations in R. J Stat Softw. 2011;45(3):1–67. http://www.jstatsoft.org/v45/i03/

20. Wu PJ, Jeyaratnam D, Tosas O, Cooper BS, French GL. Point-of-care universal screening for meticillin-resistant Staphylococcus Aureus: a cluster-randomized cross-over trial. J Hosp Infect. 2017;95(3):245–52.
21. Brendish NJ, Malachira AK, Armstrong L, Houghton R, Aitken S, Nyimbili E, et al. Routine molecular point-of-care testing for respiratory viruses in adults presenting to hospital with acute respiratory illness (ResPOC): a pragmatic, open-label, randomised controlled trial. Lancet Respir Med. 2017;5:401–11.
22. Xu M, Qin X, Astion ML, Rutledge JC, Simpson J, Jerome KR, et al. Implementation of Filmarray respiratory viral panel in a core laboratory improves testing turnaround time and patient care. Am J Clin Pathol. 2013; 139(1):118–23.
23. Pettit N, Matushek S, Charnot-Katsikas A, Tesic V, Boonlayangoor S, Brielmaier B, et al. Comparison of turnaround time and time to oseltamivir discontinuation between two respiratory viral panel testing methodologies. J Med Microbiol. 2015;64(Pt 3):312–3.
24. Schulert GS, Lu Z, Wingo T, Tang YW, Saville BR, Hain PD. Role of a respiratory viral panel in the clinical management of pediatric inpatients. Pediatr Infect Dis J. 2013;32(5):467–72.
25. Rogers BB, Shankar P, Jerris RC, Kotzbauer D, Anderson EJ, Watson JR, et al. Impact of a rapid respiratory panel test on patient outcomes. Arch Pathol Lab Med. 2015;139:636.
26. Rappo U, Schuetz AN, Jenkins SG, Calfee DP, Walsh TJ, Wells MT, et al. Impact of early detection of respiratory viruses by multiplex PCR assay on clinical outcomes in adult patients. J Clin Microbiol. 2016;54(8):2096–103.
27. Gadsby NJ, Russell CD, McHugh MP, Mark H, Morris AC, Laurenson IF, et al. Comprehensive molecular testing for respiratory pathogens in community-acquired pneumonia. Clin Infect Dis. 2016;62(7):817–23.
28. Gilbert D, Gelfer G, Wang L, Myers J, Bajema K, Johnston M, et al. The potential of molecular diagnostics and serum procalcitonin levels to change the antibiotic management of community-acquired pneumonia. Diagn Microbiol Infect Dis. 2016;86(1):102–7.
29. Gelfer G, Leggett J, Myers J, Wang L, Gilbert DN. The clinical impact of the detection of potential etiologic pathogens of community-acquired pneumonia. Diagn Microbiol Infect Dis. 2015;83(4):400–6.
30. House of Commons Committee of Public Accounts. Department of Health: improving emergency care in England. Sixteenth report of session 2004–05. Report, together with formal minutes, oral and written evidence. Ordered by The House of Commons to be printed 9 March 2005. http://www.publications.parliament.uk/pa/cm200405/cmselect/cmpubacc/445/445.pdf Accessed on 8 Sept 2016.

17

Genetic diversity of drug resistant *Mycobacterium Tuberculosis* in local area of Southwest China

Tao Shi[1*†], Tongxin Li[2†], Jungang Li[2], Jing Wang[2] and Zehua Zhang[3*]

Abstract

Background: By 2014 although tuberculosis (TB) incidence had fallen by an average of 1.5% per year since 2000 and was 18% lower than the level of in 2000, 1.5 million people died for TB in that year. One of reason was that drug resistant *Mycobacterium tuberculosis* (DRTB) spread. This study aims to determine drug resistant characteristics and genotype of DRTB that isolated from patients in a tuberculosis referral hospital of southwest China.

Methods: Five hundred thirty-eight drug resistant tuberculosis samples were collected from July 2013 to March 2015. All the isolates were identified by genomic deletions in region of difference 105 (RD105) and genotyped by mycobacterial interspersed repetitive unit-variable number tandem repeat typing (MIRU-VNTR). Polymorphism and cluster analysis of each locus was carried out using Bionumerics Version 3.0 and phyloviz software.

Results: Five hundred thirty-eight TB strains included 503 *Mycobacterium tuberculosis* (MTB) isolates and 35 non *Mycobacterium tuberculosis* (NMTB) isolates. Of 503 isolates Beijing family type was 447 (88.9%, 447/503) and non-Beijing family type was 56 (11.1%, 56/503). Five hundred three DRTB isolates were divided into 345 genotypes, of which 265 isolates were single genotype and the remaining 238 strains were classified into 80 clusters with cluster rate of 47.3% and cluster ratio of 31.4%. Sixty-nine clusters belonged to Beijing family with cluster rate was 48.3% and clustering ratio was 32.9%. The non - Beijing family had 11 clusters with a cluster rate of 39.3% and the clustering ratio of 19.6%. Beijing genotype had a significant correlation with the age ($P < 0.05$), the retreatment patients ($P < 0.05$) and the city of Chongqing ($P < 0.05$), not with gender ($P > 0.05$). In the 9 Beijing genotype clusters each cluster contained some patients who lived in the same region.

Conclusions: Beijing genotype was the predominant in the patients with DRTB in our hospital. In Chongqing retreatment patients with Beijing genotype MTB may be patient with DRTB. Drug resistance test (DST), regular medication and strict follow-up are very important for patients with Beijing genotype MTB. In Chongqing control and treatment of DRTB should be paid attention. Transmission and relations of patients with DRTB need to be further research.

Keywords: *Mycobacterium tuberculosis*, Drug resistance, Genetic diversity, Transmission

* Correspondence: shitaostone@163.com; shitaostone@163.com; zhangzehuatmmu@163.com

†Tao Shi and Tongxin Li contributed equally to this work.

[1]Department of Orthopedics, The Third Affiliated Hospital of Chongqing Medical University (Gener Hospital), No. 1, Shuanghu Branch Road, Yubei District, Chongqing 401120, China

[3]Department of Orthopedics, Southwest Hospital, Third Military Medical University, No. 30, Gaotanyan Main Street, Shapingba District, Chongqing 400038, China

Full list of author information is available at the end of the article

Background

With the development of tuberculosis diagnosis and treatment methods, the prevention and control of tuberculosis has made great progress. In 2014 tuberculosis (TB) incidence had fallen by an average of 1.5% per year since 2000 and was 18% lower than the level of 2000 according to the "Global Tuberculosis Report 2015" from the World Health Organization (WHO) [1]. Unfortunately about 3.3% of new cases and 20% of previously treated cases were drug resistant *Mycobacterium tuberculosis* (DRTB) [1]. In 2014 about approximately 1.5 million people died of DRTB [1].

China is one of the world's 22 high tuberculosis burden countries and faces the challenge of DRTB, which accounted for 22 to 30% of all cases of tuberculosis [1]. It is unknown whether the spread of DRTB originates from acquire resistance or primary resistance, especially multidrug-resistant tuberculosis (MDR-TB) and extensive drug resistance tuberculosis (XDR-TB). MDR-TB is defined as resistance to at least isoniazid and rifampin, while XDR-TB is defined as having resistance to rifampin and isoniazid as well as any member of the quinolone family and at least one of the remaining second-line anti-TB injectable drugs. The traditional epidemiology investigation lack optimal way to gain answer about this problem.

Early molecular epidemiological tools had provided a reliable way to investigate molecular evolution over shorter and longer periods of time [2–5]. Although IS*6110*-restriction fragment length polymorphism DNA fingerprinting had been the genotyping technique used most widely for MTB and was considered a "gold standard", it is no longer widely used due to time-consuming, technically demanding and requirement of large quantities of high-quality DNA [6]. According to comparison results of different ways, spoligotyping or RD105 was a reliable standard for identifying strains as belonging to the Beijing family because it is simple, highly reproducible and applicable to a digital format and mycobacterial interspersed repetitive unit–variable number tandem repeat typing (MIRU-VNTR) was the most reliable method for the genetic differentiation of MTB isolates because the discriminatory power of this method can be comparable to that of IS*6110* typing [7–9].

Chongqing is the largest municipality located in southwestern China and a city of high incidence of tuberculosis. An epidemiological study demonstrated that the rates of primary and acquired MDR-TB were 3.8 and 26.9%, respectively [10]. Sichuan Province is an adjacent area at the northwest Chongqing and also a high incidence of tuberculosis [8]. Nevertheless; we still have no knowledge of the potential transmission profile of DRTB in these areas. In this study in order to determine drug resistant characteristics, genotype and spread of DRTB, we genotyped the DRTB isolates using RD105 and MIRU-VNTR. The relationship between the molecular characteristics and transmission of DRTB was also analyzed.

Methods

Bacterial strains and culture conditions

From July 2013 to March 2015 a total of 753 samples from The Public Health Medical Center and the 12th People's Hospital of Chongqing were collected. Various *M. tuberculosis* culture and identification systems were used during the study period. The bacterial strains and culture conditions were the same as what Weng described [11]. The first was the BACTEC MGIT 960 system (Becton Dickinson, Sparks, Maryland, USA). Clinical specimens were processed, and the centrifuged sediment was inoculated onto Löwensteine-Jensen (LJ) medium (BBL; Becton Dickinson, Sparks, MD, USA) and Middlebrook 7H9 broth (BBL; Becton Dickinson). The cultures were incubated at 35 °C in 5% carbon dioxide for up to 8 weeks. Identification of *M. tuberculosis* was based on colony morphology and biochemical reactions (nitrate reduction and niacin test). Bacterial cells were isolated from LJ medium.

Drug susceptibility testing

The isolates were determined by conventional proportional drug susceptibility test. The concentrations of drugs in media were as follows: isoniazid (INH) 0.2 μg/ml, rifampicin (RFP) 40 μg/ml, ethambutol (EMB) 2 μg/ml, streptomycin (SM) 4 μg/ml, amikacin (AMK) 30 μg/ml, capreomycin (Cm) 40 μg/ml, levofloxacin (Lofx) 2 μg/ml, protionamide (Pto) 40 μg/ml and dipasic (PAIN) 0.1 μg/ml [10]. A strain was declared resistant to a drug when the growth rate was > 1% compared with the control. MDR-TB strains were defined as those resistant to both isoniazid and rifampicin. In addition, isolates resistant to rifampicin and isoniazid as well as any member of the quinolone family and at least one of the remaining second-line anti-TB injectable drugs were defined as XDR-TB.

Genomic DNA extraction

Genomic DNA was extracted from freshly cultured bacteria. Following centrifugation at 13000 rpm for 2 min, the bacterial cells were transferred to a microcentrifuge tube containing 500 ml Trisethylenediaminetetraacetic acid (TE) buffer. The supernatant was discarded and the pellet was resuspended in 500 ml TE buffer and heated in a 95 °C water bath for 1 h. The cellular debris was isolated by centrifugation at 13000 rpm for 5 min and the DNA in the supernatant was used for PCR amplification reactions.

Genotyping

The identification of genomic deletions in region of difference 105 (RD105) was performed by PCR to distinguish Beijing type from non-Beijing type. Briefly, each PCR mixture was prepared in a volume of 20 μl containing 19 μl RD105 PCR Mix and 1 μl DNA template. The amplification cycle was 10 min at 95 °C followed by 25 cycles of 30 s at 94 °C, 30 s at 68 °C, and 3 min at 72 °C, with a final step for 7 min at 72 °C.

To identify a suitable MIRU-VNTR loci set for genotyping *M. tuberculosis* in this area, the number of tandem repeats was determined in 12 MIRU-VNTR genetic loci: four original MIRU-VNTR loci: MIRU-10, MIRU-26, MIRU-31, MIRU-40; one loci of exact tandem repeats (ETRs): ETR- F; two Mtub loci: Mtub-04, Mtub-21; five Queen's University of Belfast (QUBs) loci: QUB-11b, -18,-26, -4156 and 1895. QUB-11b, QUB-18, QUB-26, QUB-4156, MIRU26, MIRU31, MIRU10, Mtub21 and Mtub04 locus of MTB isolates was amplified separately by PCR using specific primers. Briefly, 1 μl of DNA was added to 19 μl of reagent mix. The amplification parameters consisted of 10 min at 95 °C, followed by 30 cycles of 30 s at 94 °C, 30 s at 58 °C, and 90 s at 72 °C, with a final extension at 72 °C for 7 min. QUB-1895, MIRU40 and ETR-F locus of MTB isolates was amplified separately by PCR using specific primers. Briefly, 1 μl of DNA was added to 19 μl of reagent mix. The amplification parameters consisted of 10 min at 95 °C, followed by 30 cycles of 30 s at 94 °C, 30 s at 64 °C, and 90 s at 72 °C, with a final extension at 72 °C for 7 min. The PCR products were electrophoresed on a 1% agarose gel. The H37Rv strain was assayed in the same manner as a control. The Hunter–Gaston discriminatory index (HGDI) was used to evaluate the discriminatory power of the MIRU-VNTR loci. BioNumerics (version 5.0, Applied Maths, Sint-Martens-Latem, Belgium) was used to construct the Minimal Spanning Trees (MSTs) based on VNTR data. A dendrogram was constructed based on the chi square test and the software package MEGA (version 6.0).

Statistical analysis

All data were presented as mean ± standard deviation (SD) or frequency. Statistical analysis for possible significant association between the different symptoms and different genotype *M. tuberculosis* was performed using Chi-square test. All tests were set as two sides and a P value of < 0.05 was considered statistical significant.

Results

In the 753 samples there were 215 (28.6%) negative culture samples and 538 (71.4%) positive culture samples that included 503 *Mycobacterium tuberculosis (*MTB) isolates and 35 non *Mycobacterium tuberculosis* (NMTB) isolates.

Demography

The mean age of 503 patients including 189 female and 314 male was 38.9 ± 14.9 years old (16–78 years old). There were 201 new patients and 302 previously treated patients. Table 1 displayed distribution of patients in different regions. There are 19 districts and 19 counties in Chongqing and 21 cities in Sichuan Province. Most patients lived in Chongqing regions or near the Chongqing and few patients lived out of Chongqing, but all the patients lived in Chongqing when they suffered from DRTB. Patients from Chongqing accounted for 82.1, 16.1% from Sichuan Province and 1.8% from other regions.

Table 1 Distribution of 503 patients in different regions ($n = 503$)

Chongqing ($n = 413$)						Sichuan Province ($n = 81$)		Other regions ($n = 9$)	
Pengshui	62	Tongliang	10	Dazu	2	Dazhou	44	Tibet	1
Shapingba	33	Yuzhong	10	Fengjie	2	Guangan	23	Jilin Province	1
Banan	29	Wulong	9	Youyang	2	Ziyang	4	Hubei Province	1
Yubei	25	Dadukou	9	Yunyang	2	Yibin	3	Heilongjiang Province	1
Fengdu	21	Yongchuan	6	Wushan	2	Guangyuan	2	Guizhou Dejiang	1
Nanan	20	Jiangjin	6	Tongnan	2	Luzhou	2	Guizhou Fenggang	1
Beibei	20	Nanchuan	6	Rongchang	1	Neijiang	2	Guizhou Qianxi	1
Changshou	19	Bishan	5	Shizhu	1	Chengdu	1	Guizhou Tongren	1
Zhong	16	Kai	5	Wanzhou	1			Guizhou Yinjiang	1
Fuling	15	Qijiang	5	Xiushan	1				
Hechuan	15	Liangping	5	Qiangjiang	1				
Jiulongpo	14	Wansheng	4						
Dianjiang	13	Wuxi	4						

Characteristics of DRTB

All the 503 isolates were MDR-TB. There were 75 (14.9%) XDR-TB in the 503 isolates. Of 503 patients there were some special varieties of resistant drugs. There were 34(6.8%) patients with only resistance to INH and RFP including 27(5.4%) new and 7(1.4%) retreatment patients; 61(12.1%) only resistance to first-line drug including 43(8.5%) new and 18(3.6%) retreatment patients; 54(10.7%) resistance to INH, RFP and any second-line drug including 15(3.0%) new and 39(7.7%) retreatment patients; 17(3.4%) resistance to all test drugs including 5(1.0%) new and 12(2.4%) retreatment patients. The numbers of new and retreatment of patients resistant to Lofx, Pto and PAIN were a significant statistical difference, retreatment patients were more obviously resistant to the above three drugs than new cases (Fig. 1a). Male patients of resistant to AMK and PAIN had a significant statistical difference with female patients; the male was more obviously resistant than the female resistant to AMK and PAIN (Fig. 1b). Resistance to PAIN was more common than the other anti-TB drugs in the retreatment patients and male patients.

The identification of genomic RD105

The collection of 503 DRTB isolates was analyzed by RD105 in this study. 447 (88.9%) isolates belonged to the Beijing genotype, while 56 (11.1%) were from non-Beijing families, demonstrating that Beijing is the predominant genotype.

MIRU-VNTR profiles and genotypes

Five hundred three strains were divided into 345 genotypes that included 265 strains were a single genotype and the remaining 230 strains were classified into 80 clusters (2–24 isolates per cluster). The cluster rate was 47.3% and the cluster ratio was 31.4%. Four hundred forty-seven Beijing genotype isolates were clustered into 69 genotypes and 56 non-Beijing genotype isolates were clustered into 11 genotypes. The cumulative clustering rates of Beijing genotype and non-Beijing genotype strains were 48.3 and 39.3%, respectively. The both clustering ratio were 32.9 and 19.6%, respectively. The non-Beijing genotype isolates came from the newly diagnosed patients.

The details of 80 clusters were displayed in the Table 2 and Fig. 2. Figure 3 displayed the minimum spanning tree of 503 DRTB isolates according to MIRU-VNTR results.

HGDI showed that the 12-site combination had a total resolution index of 0.99. The allelic diversity of each MIRU-VNTR locus was evaluated using the HGDI (Table 3). Overall, the HGDI of four loci (QUB18, Mtub21, QUB26 and QUB11b) exceeded 0.6, classified as highly discriminating loci. The six loci (QUB1895, QUB4156, MIRU26, MIRU31, MIRU40 and Mtub04) showed moderate discrimination (0.3 < HGDI< 0.6). The MIRU10 and ERT-F showed low discrimination loci. A dendrogram was generated based on the genotypes of the 503 isolates using 12 loci.

Comparison between demographic characteristics and DRTB

Clinical factors, including age, gender and treatment history were analyzed between the Beijing and non-Beijing family (Table 4). Beijing genotype had a significant correlation with the age ($P < 0.05$), the retreatment patients ($P < 0.05$) and Chongqing ($P < 0.05$), not with gender ($P > 0.05$). In particular, isolates from patients with retreatment were all Beijing genotype, and there was no statistical result.

Distribution of DRTB

All patients lived in the above regions. The living regions of patients carrying clustering isolates were analyzed. Although all the patients carrying non-Beijing genotype clustering isolates came from different regions of Chongqing, some patients carrying Beijing genotype clustering isolates came from the same regions of Chongqing. Table 5 displayed regional distribution of some patients with Beijing genotype. The patients of the remaining Beijing genotype clusters came from different regions of Chongqing. In each non-Beijing genotype cluster there were no patients who come from the same region. In our study Pengshui, Shapingba and Banan were three regions of high incidence in Chongqing and locate in the southeast Chongqing, while Dazhou and Guangan were two regions of high incidence in Sichuan Province and locate in northeast Sichuan Province (Table 1).

Discussion

The Beijing genotype of *Mycobacterium tuberculosis* was first discovered by Soolingen in 1995 [12]. Since then, several studies have reported that Beijing genotype MTB is the main pathogen type of TB and DRTB patients [13–18]. In our study, a large number of patients with multiple MDR patients in Chongqing were collected. The basic types of DRTB were analyzed systematically. The results showed that DRTB in this region was mainly Beijing family type, accounting for 93.4%, which is similar to most of the current DRTB molecular type of research reports but not exactly the same. The results of the national tuberculosis drug resistance baseline analysis showed that the DR ratio of Beijing genotype strains was 63.97% in China and 59.97% in the southwest China [19], while our study showed the DR ratio of Beijing genotype strains was 88.9% that was significantly higher than the levels of nationwide and southwest

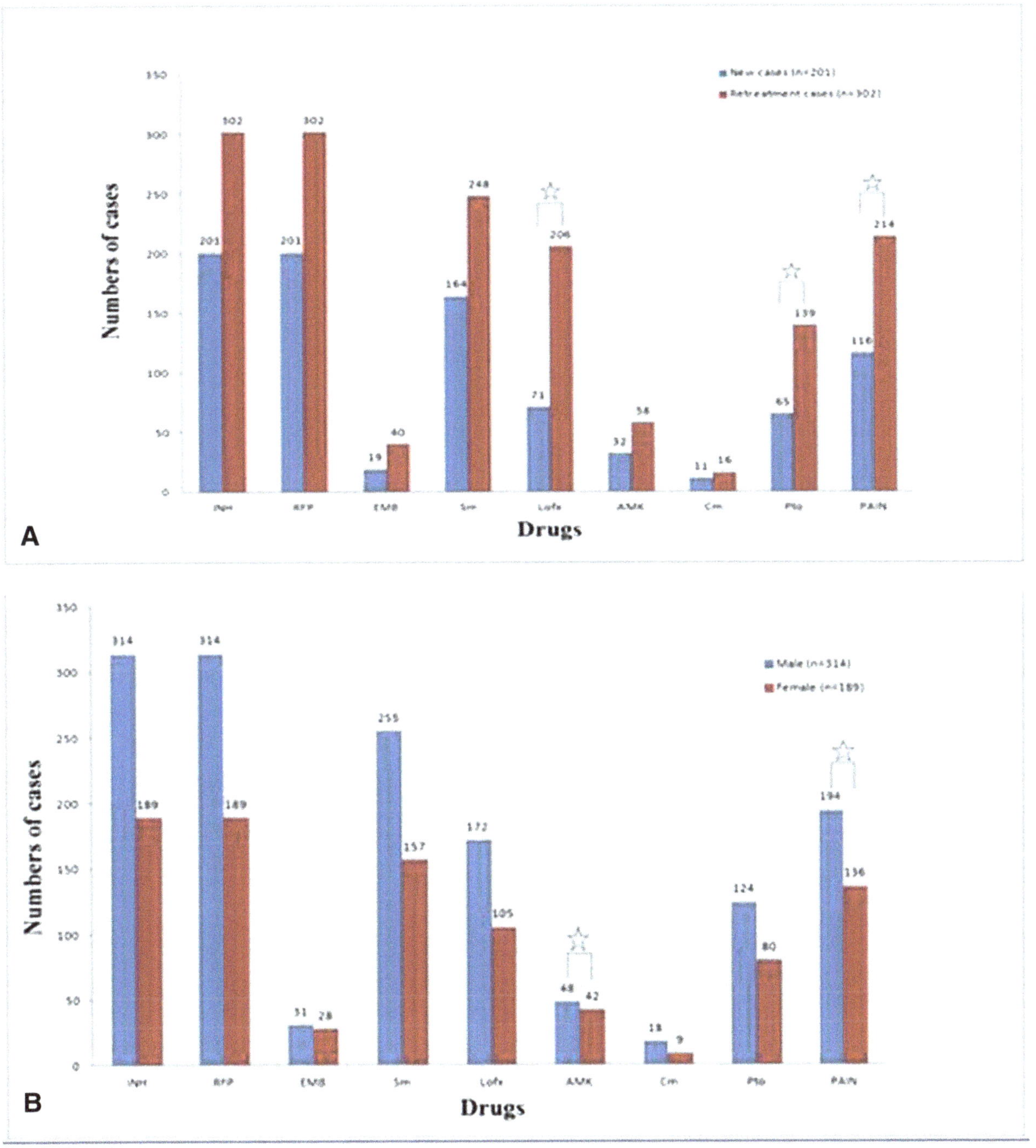

Fig. 1 a Distribution of the new cases and retreatment cases in the different anti-TB drugs. **b** Distribution of femal and male patients in the different anti-TB drugs. ☆ Means $P < 0.05$

China. This suggests that the prevalence of the Beijing genotype family in Chongqing may result in the spread of DRTB.

Anti-TB chemotherapy is the cornerstone of treatment of patients with MTB [20]. Unfortunately, evolution of TB leads to be resistant to anti-TB drugs. DRTB is a big challenge to anti-TB treatment. Many researchers studied the DR characteristics of DRTB. Fox example, according to Kapil's research the DR ratio of INH, RFP and SM were 92.7, 81.9 and 69.3%, respectively [21]. Another article showed SM and EMB were most common resistant drugs [10]. In this study INH, RFP and SM were three most common first-line anti-TB resistant drugs and Lofx and PAIN were common second-line

Table 2 Details of 80 clusters

Genotype	No. of cluster	No. of strains in each cluster
Beijing-type		
	1	26
	1	11
	1	10
	1	9
	1	8
	1	7
	4	4
	9	3
	50	2
Non-Beijing-type		
	11	2

anti-TB resistant drugs. In addition DR ratio of Lofx, Pto and PAIN in the retreatment patients was higher than in the new case and resistance to AMK and PAIN was more common in male patients than female. These results may be helpful for treatment of patients with DRTB in southwest China. Different studies have shown the DR ration of different anti-TB drugs varied by regions.

In this study, 503 cases of DRTB strains were divided into 80 clusters and 345 genotypes with a clustering rate of 47.3%. Two hundred sixty-five patients were isolated as a single genotype, accounting for 52.7% of all patients (265/503), which may be considered to be independent isolates and no mutual transmission between patients, but rather independent infection or endogenous recurrent disease. The remaining 238 strains were classified in to 80 clusters, that the largest cluster of which contained 26 Beijing genotype isolates, including 22 isolates from the Chongqing Municipal Public Health Medical Treatment Center and 4 isolates from the Twelfth People's Hospital of Chongqing. By analyzing the redidential regions of patients in the clusters that contained ≥3 isolates, we found some isolates transmitted within one region and had tendency transmitting to an adjacent area. There was a study about MDR transmitting across countries [22]. All these researches suggested the DRTB were transmitting more and more widely. Additional, each cluster of DRTB highly suggested that these isolates belonged to their respective groups and in each group isolates had a certain relationship according to results of MIRU-VNTR. Cross analysis results of MIRU-VNTR and living locations of patients suggested that patients with DRTB were cross-infection, that is, these patients with DRTB are primary resistant, rather than due to withdrawal and relapse. Continue to track these patients to determine the cause of resistance, such as whether patients with the same genotype are relative, contact

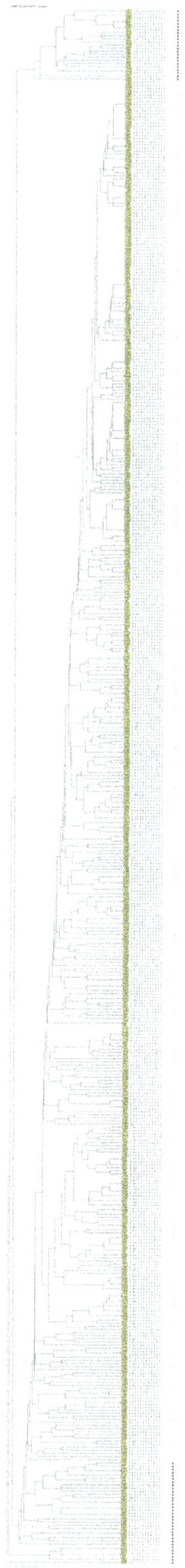

Fig. 2 Dendrogram of 503 DRTB isolates. The phylogenetic tree was generated from the MIRU-VNTR profile

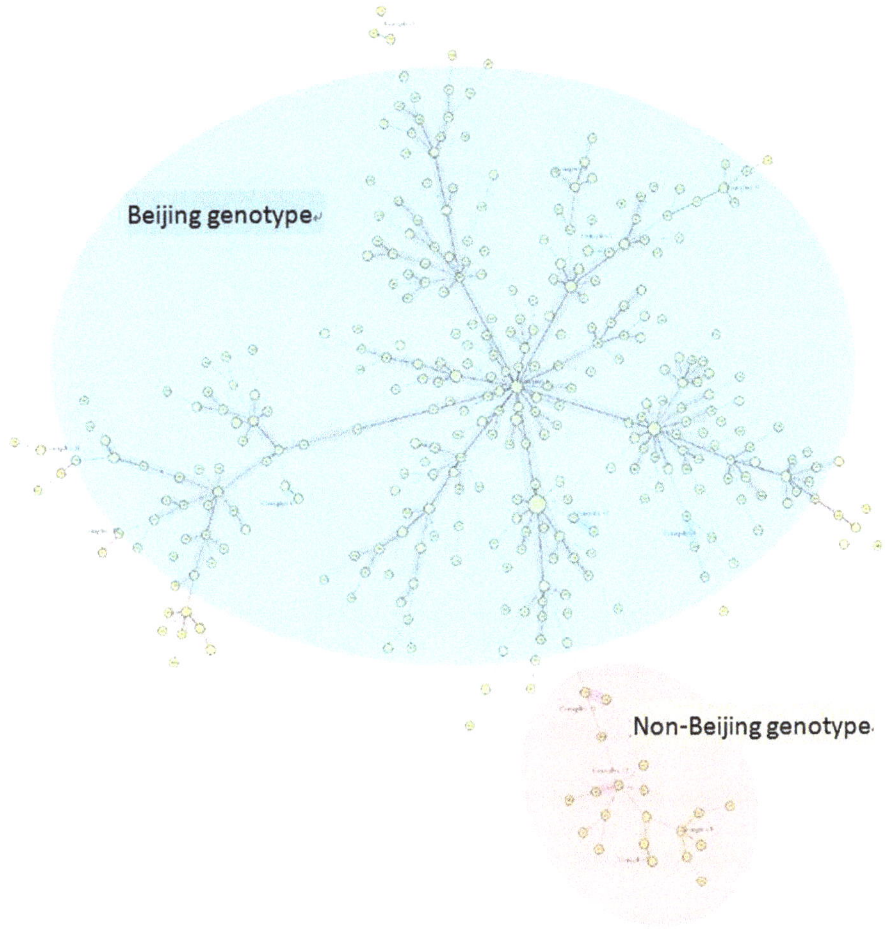

Fig. 3 Minimum spanning tree (MST) of 503 DRTB isolates. The MST was generated from the MIRU-VNTR profile

Table 3 Allelic diversity of 12 different MIRU-VNTR loci among Mycobacterium tuberculosis strains

	Locus	HGDI
1	QUB-11b	0.62
2	QUB-18	0.65
3	QUB-26	0.66
4	QUB-4156	0.37
5	QUB-1895	0.37
6	MIRU26	0.57
7	MIRU31	0.47
8	MIRU10	0.26
9	MIRU40	0.44
10	Mtub21	0.62
11	Mtub04	0.55
12	ETR-F	0.26

history and living in the same community, which is the focus of our follow-up study.

MTB genotyping can explain the epidemiology, infection, pathogenesis and DR of MTB from the molecular level and it is important in TB epidemiological investigation, surveillance and transmission source discovery and transmission pathways. MIRU-VNTR was classified according to the difference of the number of copies between different strains. The method was simple, the result was digitized and the resolution was high, which was convenient for comparison between different laboratories. Compared to IS*6110*-RFLP which used to be the "gold standard" for DNA fingerprints of MTB, MIRU-VNTR has obviously advantages. Using the MIRU-VNTR 191 Beijing family-type MTB were divided into 110 unique genotype and 27 clusters in China [8] and in Sichuan 191 Beijing Mycobacterium tuberculosis has 65 unique genotypes and 8 clusters [23]. In addition, Chinese Center for Disease Control and Prevention analyzed 4017 MTB isolates from 31 different provinces that were divided into 161 clusters and 407 isolates using spoligotyping and

Table 4 Clinical characteristics of the Beijing and non-Beijing family strains

Characteristics	Total	Beijing family	Non-Beijing family	χ^2	*P*-value
Age, years					
≤30	153	150	3	784.00	< 0.05
30–60	306	279	27		
≥60	44	41	3		
Gender					
Male	314	289	25	2.68	> 0.05
Female	189	181	8		
Treatment history					
New cases	201	168	33	214.40	< 0.05
Retreatment	302	302	0		
Regions					
Chongqing	413	402	11	25.40	< 0.05
Sichuan Province	81	78	3		
Other regions	9	6	3		

MIRU-VNTR [24]. According to the results of a study comparing different methods RD105 or spoligotyping is a reliable method for identifying whether the strain belongs to the Beijing cluster, although the identification ability may be not comparable to that of IS*6110*-RFLP. MIRU-VNTR was the most reliable method for the genetic differentiation of MTB isolates because the discriminatory power of this method is also comparable to that of IS*6110* typing [7–9]. The different research purposes of MTB molecular epidemiology study should select the appropriate technological choice ways based on different research purposes, or combined variety of ways in order to improve work efficiency and accuracy of the results.

The discrimination of the MIRU-VNTR depends on the resolution of the site used and the VNTR loci should be selected according to the genetic polymorphism of MTB in different regions. The reports had displayed that QUB18, Mtub21, QUB26, QUB11b, QUB11a, and MIRU26 were highly discriminating loci in Chongqing [25] and Mtub04, Mtub21, Mtub39, QUB26, QUB11b, MIRU10, MIRU26, MIRU39, MIRU40, ETRA and ETRE were highly discriminating loci in Sichuan province [26]. In this study, VNTR genotyping was carried out at 12 sites, which were representative of both international and domestic locations. By analyzing the allelic polymorphism of the isolates, the HGDI of polymorphism of 12 loci was between 0.29 and 0.67. The results showed that the seven loci including QUB-11b, QUB-18, QUB-26, MIRU26, MIRU31, Mtub21 and Mtub04 had high discrimination in MTB in Chongqing area. But the discrimination of MIRU10 in Chongqing is lower than that of Sichuan province. Compared with the typing of Yongchuan in Chongqing the Mtub04 loci selected in this study have a relatively high resolution [10], while

Table 5 Regional Distribution of some patients with Beijing genotype

No. of strains in one cluster	Region	No. of patients	No. of strains in one cluster	Region	No. of patients
26	Pengshui	7	8	Fengjie	2
	Beibei	2		Yubei	2
	Zhong	2		others	4
	others	15	7	Guangan	3
11	Nanan	2		others	4
	Banan	2	4	Zhong	3
	others	7		others	1
10	Pengshui	2	3	Shapingba	2
	others	8		others	1
9	Beibei	3	3	Jiangbei	2
	others	6		others	1

"others" mean "the rest patients came from different regions and only one patient in one region"

MIRU10 and ETR-F are relatively low, which may be related to the size of the selected study sample range. Therefore, in the future the classification work will select high polymorphic combination of sites including QUB-11b, QUB-18, QUB-26, MIRU26, MIRU31, Mtub21 and Mtub04 that is a great help for increasing classification efficiency.

Conclusions

Beijing genotype was the predominant in the patients with DRTB in our hospital. In Chongqing retreatment patients with Beijing genotype MTB may be patient with DRTB. DST, regular medication and strict follow-up are very important for patients with Beijing genotype MTB. In Chongqing control and treatment of DRTB should be paid attention. Transmission and relations of patients with DRTB need to be further research.

Abbreviations

AMK: Amikacin; Cm: Capreomycin; DNA: Deoxyribonucleic acid; DRTB: Drug resistant Mycobacterium tuberculosis; DST: Drug susceptibility testing; EMB: Ethambutol; ETRs: Exact tandem repeats; HGDI: Hunter–Gaston discriminatory index; INH: Isoniazid; Lofx: Levofloxacin; MDR-TB: Multi-drug resistance Tuberculosis; MGIT: Mycobacterium Growth Indicator Tube; MIRU-VNTR: Mycobacterial interspersed repetitive unit-variable number tandem repeat typing; MSTs: Minimal Spanning Trees; NMTB: Non Mycobacterium tuberculosis; PAIN: Dipasic; PCR: Polymerase chain reaction; Pto: Protionamide; QUB: Queen's University of Belfast; RD105: Region of difference 105; RFP: rifampicin; SM: Streptomycin; TB: Tuberculosis; WHO: World Health Organization; XDR-TB: Extensive drug resistance tuberculosis

Acknowledgements

We thank the patients' agreement to participate in this research.

Funding

ZHZ is supported by the Natural Science Foundation of China (grant number: 81772365). The funding sources had no role in the study design, data collection, data analysis, or writing of the report.

Authors' contributions

Conceived and designed the study: TS, TXL. Collected the data: TXL, JGL, JW and ZHZ. Analyzed the data: TXL, JGL, JW. Wrote the paper: TS. Interpreted the results: TXL, JGL, JW. Acquisition of funding: ZHZ. All authors have read and approved the final manuscript.

Consent for publication

Not applicable.

Competing interests

The authors declare that they have no competing interests.

Author details

[1]Department of Orthopedics, The Third Affiliated Hospital of Chongqing Medical University (Gener Hospital), No. 1, Shuanghu Branch Road, Yubei District, Chongqing 401120, China. [2]Department of Clinical Laboratory, Public Health Medical Center, No. 109, Baoyu Road, Shapingba District, Chongqing 400036, China. [3]Department of Orthopedics, Southwest Hospital, Third Military Medical University, No. 30, Gaotanyan Main Street, Shapingba District, Chongqing 400038, China.

References

1. World Health Organization (WHO). Global tuberculosis report 2015. Geneva: World Health. Organization; 2015.
2. McAdam RA, Hermans PW, van Soolingen D, Zainuddin ZF, Catty D, van Embden JD, et al. Characterization of a Mycobacterium tuberculosis insertion sequence belonging to the IS3 family. Mol Microbiol. 1990;4:1607–13.
3. Supply P, Allix C, Lesjean S, Cardoso-Oelemann M, Rüsch-Gerdes S, Willery E, et al. Proposal for standardization of optimized mycobacterial interspersed repetitive unit–variable-number tandem repeat typing of Mycobacterium tuberculosis. J Clin Microbiol. 2006;44:4498–510.
4. Van Embden JD, Cave MD, Crawford JT, Dale JW, Eisenach KD, Gicquel B, et al. Strain identification of Mycobacterium tuberculosis by DNA fingerprinting: recommendations for a standardized methodology. J Clin Microbiol. 1993;31:406–9.
5. Arnold C. Molecular evolution of Mycobacterium tuberculosis. Clin Microbiol Infect. 2007;13:120–8.
6. Thierry D, Cave MD, Eisenach KD, Crawford JT, Bates JH, Gicquel B, et al. IS6110, an IS-like element of Mycobacterium tuberculosis complex. Nucleic Acids Res. 1990;18:188.
7. Liu Q, Yang D, Xu W, Wang J, LV B, Shao Y, et al. Molecular typing of mycobacterium tuberculosis isolates circulating in Jiangsu Province, China. BMC Infect Dis. 2011;11:288.
8. Guo J-h, Xiang W-l, Zhang G, Luo T, Xie N, Yang ZR, et al. Mycobacterial Interspersed Repetitive Unit typing in Mycobacterium tuberculosis isolates from Sichuan Province in China. Indian J Med Res. 2011;134:362–8.
9. Kam KM, Yip CW, Tse LW, Wong KL, Lam TK, Kremer K, et al. Utility of mycobacterial interspersed repetitive unit typing for differentiating multidrug-resistant Mycobacterium tuberculosis isolates of the Beijing family. J Clin Microbiol. 2005;43(1):306–13.
10. Zhang D, An J, Wang J, Hu C, Wang Z, Zhang R, et al. Molecular typing and drug susceptibility of Mycobacterium tuberculosis isolates from Chongqing municipality, China. Infect Genet Evol. 2013;13:310–6.
11. Weng CY, Ho CM, Dou HY, Ho MW, Lin HS, Chang HL, et al. Molecular typing of Mycobacterium tuberculosis isolated from adult patients with tubercular spondylitis. J Microbiol Immunol Infect. 2013;46(1):19–23.
12. Van Soolingen D, Qian L, de Haas PE, Douglas JT, Traore H, Portaels F, et al. Predominance of a single genotype of Mycobacterium tuberculosis in countries of East Asia. J Clin Microbiol. 1995;33(12):3234–338.
13. Park YK, Shin S, Ryu S, Cho SN, Koh WJ, Kwon OJ, et al. Comparison of drug resistance genotypes between Beijing and non-Beijing family strains of Mycobacterium tuberculosis in Korea. J Microbiol Methods. 2005;63(2):165–72.
14. Ghebremichael S, Groenheit R, Pennhag A, Koivula T, Andersson E, Bruchfeld J, et al. Drug resistant Mycobacterium tuberculosis of the Beijing genotype does not spread in Sweden. PLoS One. 2010;5(5):e10893.
15. Mokrousov I, Jiao WW, Sun GZ, Liu JW, Valcheva V, Li M, et al. Evolution of drug resistance in different sublineages of Mycobacterium tuberculosis Beijing genotype. Antimicrob Agents Chemother. 2006;50(8):2820–3.
16. Liu Y, Tian M, Wang X, Goldbogen J, Southall B. Genotypic diversity analysis of Mycobacterium tuberculosis strains collected from Beijing in 2009, using Spoligotyping and VNTR typing. PLoS One. 2014;9(9):e106787.
17. Chen YY, Chang JR, Kuo SC, Tseng FC, Huang WC, Huang TS, et al. Molecular epidemiology of tuberculosis in Kaohsiung City located at southern Taiwan, 2000–2008. PLoS ONE. 2015;10(1):e0117061.
18. Wang Q, Lau SK, Liu F, Zhao Y, Li HM, Li BX, et al. Molecular epidemiology and clinical characteristics of drug-resistant Mycobacterium tuberculosis in a tuberculosis referral hospital in China. PLoS One. 2014;9(10):e110209.
19. Wang SF, Zhou Y, Pang Y, Zhao YL. Epidemic characteristics of Mycobacterium tuberculosis of Beijing genotype strains and its association

with drug resistance—analysis of the data from national drug resistant tuberculosis baseline survey in 2007. Chin J Antitubercul. 2015;37(8):836–42.
20. Tuli SM. Tuberculosis of the spine: a historical review. Clin Orthop Relat Res. 2007;460:29–38.
21. Mohan K, Rawall S, Pawar UM, Sadani M, Nagad P, Nene A, et al. Drug resistance patterns in 111 cases of drug-resistant tuberculosis spine. Eur Spine J. 2013;22(Suppl 4):S647–52.
22. Moonan PK, Teeter LD, Salcedo K, Ghosh S, Ahuja SD, Flood J, et al. Transmission of multidrug-resistant tuberculosis in the USA: a cross-sectional study. Lancet Infect Dis. 2013;13(9):777–84.
23. Guo JH, Xiang WL, Zhang G, Luo T, Xie N, Yang ZR, et al. Mycobacterial interspersed repetitive unit typing in Mycobacterium tuberculosis isolates from Sichuan Province in China. Indian J Med Res. 2011;134:362–8.
24. Pang Y, Zhou Y, Zhao B, Liu G, Jiang G, Xia H, et al. 2012. Spoligotyping and drug resistance analysis of Mycobacterium tuberculosis strains from national survey in China. PLoS One. 2012;7(3):e32976.
25. Zhang D, An J, Wang Y, Pang Y. Genetic diversity of multidrug-resistant tuberculosis in a resource-limited region of China. Int. J Infect Dis. 2014;29: 7–11.
26. Liu HC, Deng JP, Dong HY, Xiao TQ, Zhao XQ, Zhang ZD, et al. Molecular typing characteristic and drug susceptibility analysis of Mycobacterium tuberculosis isolates from Zigong, China. Biomed Res Int. 2016;2016: 6790985.

18

Tuberculosis-Human Immunodeficiency Virus (HIV) co-infection in Ethiopia

Mebrahtu Teweldemedhin[1*], Negasi Asres[2], Hailay Gebreyesus[2] and Solomon Weldegebreal Asgedom[3]

Abstract

Background: Human Immunodeficiency Virus (HIV) and Tuberculosis (TB) are the double burden diseases of the world. The African continent takes a great share of TB-HIV cases worldwide. This study was aimed to determine the prevalence of TB-HIV co-infection in Ethiopia, using a meta-analysis based on a systematic review of published articles.

Methods: An electronic search was conducted in databases including PubMed, HINARI, EMBASE, Cochrane library and Google Scholar to extract the articles. Articles published between 1995 and November 2017 had been searched for using different keywords. The analysis was performed using MetaXL software and R statistical software (version 3.2.3).

Result: Our searches returned a total of ($n = 26,746$) records from 30 articles of which 21 were cross-sectional, 7 were retrospectives and 2 were prospective studies. The range of prevalence of TB-HIV co-infection was found to be from 6 to 52.1% with random effects pooled prevalence of 22% (95% CI 19–24%) and with substantial heterogeneity chi-square ($X^2) = 746.0$, $p < 0.001$, ($I^2 = 95.84\%$).

Conclusion: Our analysis indicated that the prevalence of TB-HIV co-infection is high in Ethiopia with substantial regional variation. An integrated, facility-based and community-based effort towards the prevention, early detection and management of cases should be further strengthened throughout the country to mitigate the double burden disease.

Keywords: Tuberculosis, Human immunodeficiency virus, Co-infection, Prevalence, Meta-analysis

Background

Human Immunodeficiency Virus (HIV) remained as the leading cause of mortality and morbidity; in 2016 for instance, 1.8 million people were newly infected and 1 million AIDS-related deaths were registered [1]. HIV/AIDS and TB (Tuberculosis) are considered as the double burden diseases of the world. According to the World health organization (WHO) report, there were 1.5 million deaths attributed to TB out of which 26% were due to HIV-associated TB [2]. In developing countries, particularly in sub-Saharan Africa, TB is increasing due to the burden of HIV [3]. Hence, the African continent takes the greater share (74%) of the 1.2 million TB-HIV cases worldwide [2]. In Ethiopia, 4 in 100 people die due to TB-HIV co-infection and the incidence of Multidrug-resistant Tuberculosis (MDR-TB) was estimated to be 5.8 per 1000 people [4].

The burden of TB is still alarming due to the emergences of drug-resistant strains. Recent studies indicated that the prevalence of MDR-TB in Ethiopia is particularly noticeable (15%) in previously treated TB cases [5]. Among laboratory-confirmed TB cases in the Oromo region, for instance, 33% of the cases were found to be MDR-TB, majorly among the adult population [6]. This increase in MDR-TB, especially among people living with HIV is a great burden to the healthcare system; challenging the management efforts of the disease through drug interaction and immune reaction [7–9].

* Correspondence: mebrie1216@gmail.com
[1]Department of Medical Laboratory Sciences, College of Health Sciences, Aksum University, PO.BOX 298, Aksum, Tigray, Ethiopia
Full list of author information is available at the end of the article

The associated morbidity and mortality related to noticeable economic loss of the productive society and the socioeconomic status of the country at large. In developing countries, it is estimated that around 30% of the annual household income is taken by TB and HIV associated disease [10].

In general, people living with HIV are 20 times riskier to be infected with TB as compared to HIV negative people [11], with case fatality rate of 16–35%, which is almost 4 times higher than HIV free individuals [12]. The incidence of co-infection is determined by many factors including smoking, family size, the clinical stage of HIV, use of antiretroviral therapy (ART), injectable drug use and anemia [13–15]. In addition, it is evident that HIV positivity, alcohol intake, farming occupation and previous TB contact are contributing factors for MDR-TB [6].TB and HIV co-infection has various health outcomes limiting the life expectancy of the infected host; accelerated by malnutrition, rapid progression of the disease, atypical TB presentations, delayed diagnosis and a low treatment response [16]. Active tuberculosis facilitates the transcription of HIV genes resulting in increased diversity and replication of HIV [17]. On the other hand, as the clinical stage of HIV progresses, there is an increased dissemination and extra-pulmonary TB manifestations [18]. Finally, patients suffer due to frequent pyrexia, diarrhea, severe weight loss and wasting [19, 20].

In high burden and resource-limited countries like Ethiopia, integrating health services on TB and HIV has paramount importance in order to increase the effectiveness of the diagnosis and to improve the management approaches [21]. Considering this, the WHO introduced collaborative strategies to control HIV associated TB and Ethiopia is one of the countries exercising this program as part of the health care system [22]. The Centers for Disease Control (CDC) program in Ethiopia (opened in 2001) is providing guidance and technical support towards TB-HIV co-infection and MDR-TB services. As a result, large improvements have been achieved in HIV testing, ART provision and diagnostic potential. Studying the prevalence of TB-HIV co-infection is important for programmatic changes or further improvements on the existing programs. Therefore, this study was aimed to determine the prevalence of TB-HIV co-infection in Ethiopia, using a meta-analysis based on a systematic review of published articles.

Methods

Search strategy and inclusion criteria

An electronic search was conducted to retrieve and recruit studies. Published articles of cross-sectional, prospective and retrospective cohort studies were included, which focused on the "Prevalence of TB-HIV co-infection in Ethiopia". Databases PubMed, HINARI, EMBASE, Cochrane library, and Google Scholar search engine were used to extract journals. Articles published between 1995 and November 2017 had been searched

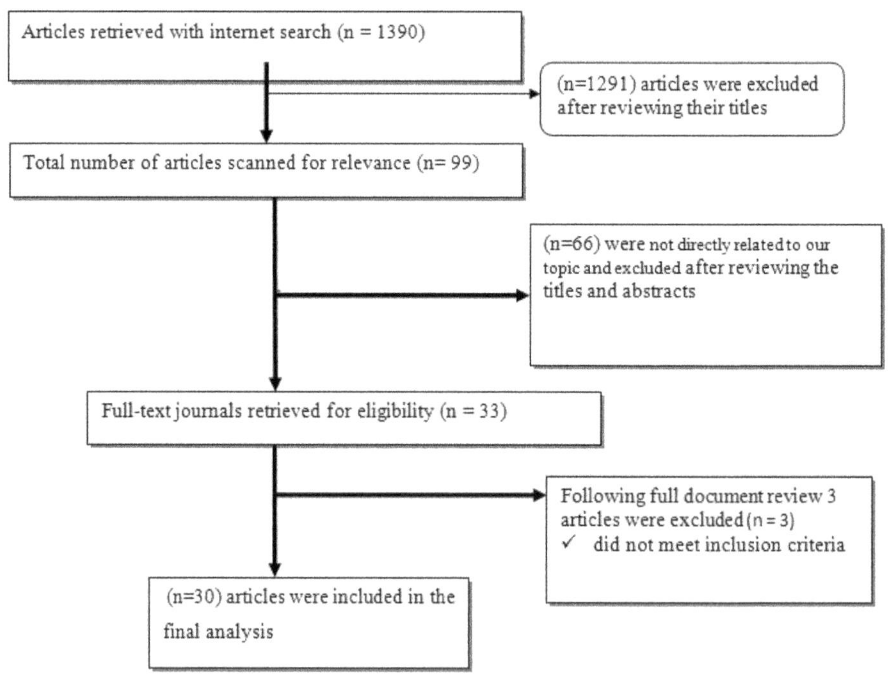

Fig. 1 Flow diagram of articles selection process

Table 1 Summary of the studies in the review

Author, Year, (Ref.)	Study setting/region	Study design	Study population/participants	Prev. of TB-HIV co-infection
Alemayehu et al., 2014 [29]	Amhara Region, Gondar University; Hospital based	Cross-sectional	HIV patients, aged 18 years and above, $n = 250$	6%
Alemie & Gebreselassie, 2014 [30]	Amhara Region; selected private health institutions	Cross-sectional	TB patients, $n = 1153$	20%
Alemu, etal,2016 [31]	Amhara Region, West Gojjam and South Gondar, Population based	Retrospective	HIV patients, children aged less than 15, $n = 645$	12%
Ali et al.,2016 [32]	Across Ethiopia, Population based	Cross- sectional	HIV patients, aged 15–90, $n = 575$	29.4%
Balcha et al.,2014 [33]	Oromia Region, Adama; Population based	Prospective	HIV-patients, aged 18 years and above, $n = 812$	17.9%
Belay et al.,2015 [34]	Afar and Dessie Town; in 5 health facilities.	Cross-sectional	TB patients, aged above 18 $n = 110$	40%
Datiko et al.,2008 [35]	Southern Ethiopia, heath facilities	Cross-sectional	TB patients, $n = 1261$,	18%
Dengetu & dolamo, 2014 [36]	Addis Ababa; governmental health facilities	Facility-based Cross-sectional	TB patients, children aged 15–17 years, $n = 579$	35%
Deribew, et al.,2011 [37]	Addis Ababa; primary health care units	Facility based cross-sectional	TB patients, $n = 298$	27.2%
Fanosie et al.,2016 [38]	Amhara Region, University of Gondar Hospital	Institution based cross-sectional	TB patients, $n = 141$	14.1%
Fekadu et al., 2015 [39]	South Ethiopia	Retrospective	HIV/AIDS patients, $n = 499$	18.2%)
Belay et al., 2014 [40]	Afar region	Cross sectional	TB patients, $n = 287$	28.6%
Taddesse et al., 2013 [41]	Amhara region	Cross sectional	TB patients, $n = 301$	18.3%
Gebrecherkos et al., 2016 [42]	Amhara Region, North Gondar zone	Cross-sectional	TB patients, $n = 282$	27%
Gebreegziabiher et al., 2017 [28]	Tigray Region, Mekelle, Public health institutions	Cross-sectional	TB pregnant mother, $n = 201$	21.8%
Gebremariam, et al., 2016 [43]	Southern Rgion, Arsi Negele Health Center	Retrospective	TB patients, $n = 1562$	10%
Kassu et al.,2007 [44]	Amhara, Gondar University	Cross-sectional	TB patients, $n = 257$,	52.1%
Kebede et al., 2014 [45]	Oromiya, Este welega	Cross- sectional	TB patients, $n = 406$	33.7%
Kifle et al., 2014 [46]	Amhara, Northwest Shewa	Cross- sectional	TB patients, $n = 335$	28.7%
Ligidi et al.,2011 [47]	Oremiya, Adama Hospital based	Cross- sectional	TB patients, $n = 258$	26.4%
Mekonnen et al.,2015 [48]	Tigray Rgion,Southern zone	Retrospective	TB patients, $n = 973$	24.3%
Mihret et al., 2014 [49]	Addis Ababa Ethiopia	Cross-sectional	TB patients, $n = 418$	23.2%
Mitku et al. 2016 [50]	Amhara Region, Hospital based	Retrospective	HIV positive, $n = 571$	27.7%
Skogmar et al.,2014 [51]	Across Ethiopia	Cross-sectional	TB patients, $n = 1116$	27.5%
Tarekegne et al.,2016 [52]	Amhara Rgion, Metema Hospital	Retrospective	TB patients, $n = 2005$	20.1%
Teklu et al., 2012 [53]	Sothern Ethiopia, Sedo, institution based	Retrospective	HIV patients, $n = 459$	7.8%
Wondimeneh et al., 2012 [54]	Amhara Region, Gondar university, Hospital based	Cross sectional	HIV patients, $n = 400$,	7.5%
Yassin et al., 2004 [55]	Southern region of Ethiopia., health facilities	Prospective epidemiological	HIV patients, $n = 261$	19%
Degu J. et al. [56]	Southern Ethiopia, Arba Minch Hospital	Cross- sectional	TB patients, $n = 190$	20.1%

Table 1 Summary of the studies in the review *(Continued)*

Author, Year, (Ref.)	Study setting/region	Study design	Study population/participants	Prev. of TB-HIV co-infection
Alemie G.A. et al., 2014 [30]	Amhara Region, private health institutions	Cross-sectional	TB patient, $n = 808$	20%
EHNRI, 2014 [57]	Across Ethiopia	Survey in public health facilities	TB patients, $n = 13{,}684$	20%
EPHI, 2015 [58]	Across Ethiopia	Survey in public health facilities	TB patients, $n = 7987$	17.5%

EHNRI Ethiopian Health and Nutrition Research Institite, *EPHI* Ethiopian Public Health Institute.

for and their full-text was retrieved by two independent reviewers.

Inclusion criteria

The predetermined inclusion criteria for this analysis were: 1) studies conducted in Ethiopia, 2) either longitudinal/cohort or cross-sectional studies which assessed the prevalence of TB/HIV co-infection in Ethiopia and has a sample size of greater than 100 ($n > 100$). 3) Studies written in English. 4) Articles which were published and available online.

Based on these inclusion criteria, 30 articles were selected and analyzed (Fig. 1).

Data extraction and synthesis

We developed a data collection tool to collect the findings from the published articles. The data collection tool was pretested on 5 articles and an amendment was done accordingly. After the preliminary data extraction, a careful analysis was made to record the type of the study, study setting/region, author and year of publication, number of patients/participants and the main outcomes of the study on the data collection tool.

Description of studies

As summarized in Fig. 1, the literature search with the chosen search terms firstly identified 1390 citations. We repossess 99 articles after reviewing the proximity of the title to the predetermined objectives, and after further reading the abstracts of each article, only 33 of the articles were subjected to document review. Lastly, 30 articles met the inclusion criteria for this systematic review and the meta-analysis (Fig. 1).

Statistical analysis

We performed all analyses in Meta-XL software and R statistical software (version 3.2.3). When working on binary data with low prevalence, the inverse variance weight in fixed-effects meta-analyses is sub-optimum. Hence, the estimated prevalence was determined using the variance stabilizing double arcsine transformation [23]. Wilson method was used to calculate the 95% confidence intervals; the Cochran's Q and I^2 statistic were used to determine heterogeneity [24–26]. The I^2 does not essentially depend on the number of studies included. Therefore, a high, moderate and low degree of heterogeneity indicates an I^2 value of 75, 50, and 25% respectively. In this study, the I^2 was greater than 75% and hence the summary statistics were made using the random-effects models in which the individual study weight is the sum of the weight used in the fixed effects model and the between-study variability [27]. To analyze the basis of heterogeneity, we performed a sensitivity analysis by excluding one largest study [28] and by analyzing the groups according to the geographic area.

Results

Study characteristics

Our searches returned a total of ($n = 26{,}746$) records from 30 articles of which 21 were cross-sectional, 7 were retrospectives and 2 were prospective studies. Furthermore, 17 studies had more than 500 participants; 12 studies were conducted in the Amhara region, 6 in southern Ethiopia, 2 in Tigray, 3 in Oromia, 3 in Addis Ababa, 2 in Afar and 2 across Ethiopia.

Nineteen [19] studies determined HIV infection among TB patients ($n = 21{,}376$) and 11 studies determined TB among HIV/AIDS patients (5370) (see Table 1).

Estimates of TB-HIV co-infection prevalence ranged from 6 to 52.1% (Fig. 2). The random effects pooled prevalence of TB-HIV co-infection was 22% (95% CI 179–24%) with substantial heterogeneity chi-square (X^2) = 746.0, $p = 0.0001$, (*I^2 = 95.85% 95% CI: 94.9–96.6*) (Fig. 2). Prevalence of TB/HIV co-infection was 20% (95% CI 16–24) in the Amhara region, 26% (95% CI 16–36) in the Oromia region, 24% (95% CI 24.21–26.0–) in the Tigray Region, 15% (95% CI 9–21) in Southern Ethiopia, 28% (95% CI 21–36) in Addis Ababa and 34% (95% CI 23–45) in the Afar region (Fig. 3).

As part of our sensitivity analyses, we excluded one large study [28]; estimates of TB-HIV co-infection prevalence did not change.

Discussion

This systematic review and meta-analysis of TB-HIV co-infection identified 30 studies of 26,746 individuals in

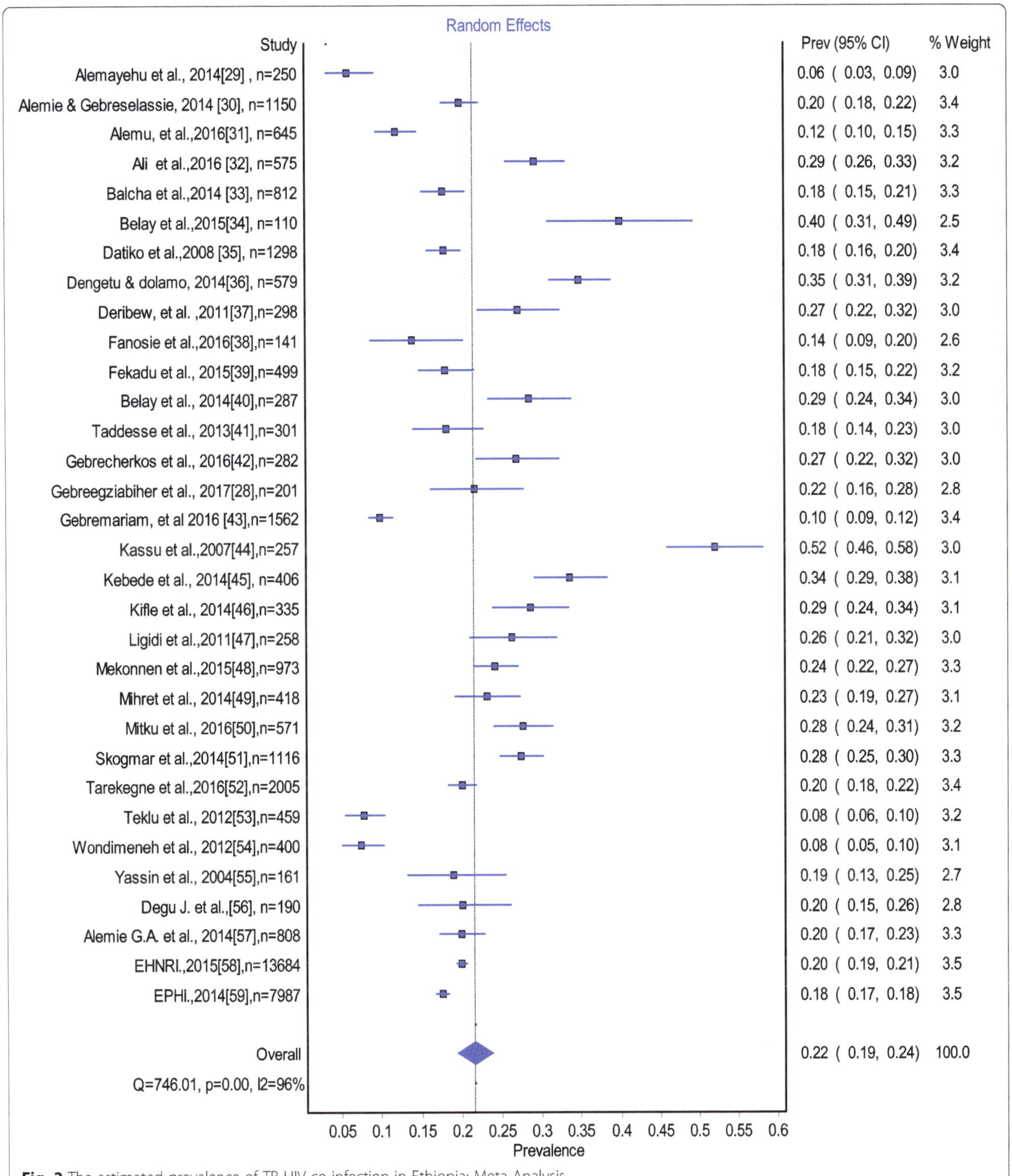

Fig. 2 The estimated prevalence of TB-HIV co-infection in Ethiopia: Meta-Analysis

Ethiopia. Our pooled results confirmed that the prevalence of TB-HIV co- infection is 22% in Ethiopia. Furthermore, the high prevalence of HIV/AIDS in the general population is related to a higher prevalence of TB-HIV co-infection. This result is almost consistent with one global study [59] but higher than the finding in China (11%) [60], Nigeria (17.5%) [61] and Ghana (18.2%) [62].

According to the subgroup analysis, the highest prevalence was found in the Addis Ababa region (31%), followed by the Afar regional state (29%), whereas the lowest prevalence was found in southern Ethiopia (18%).

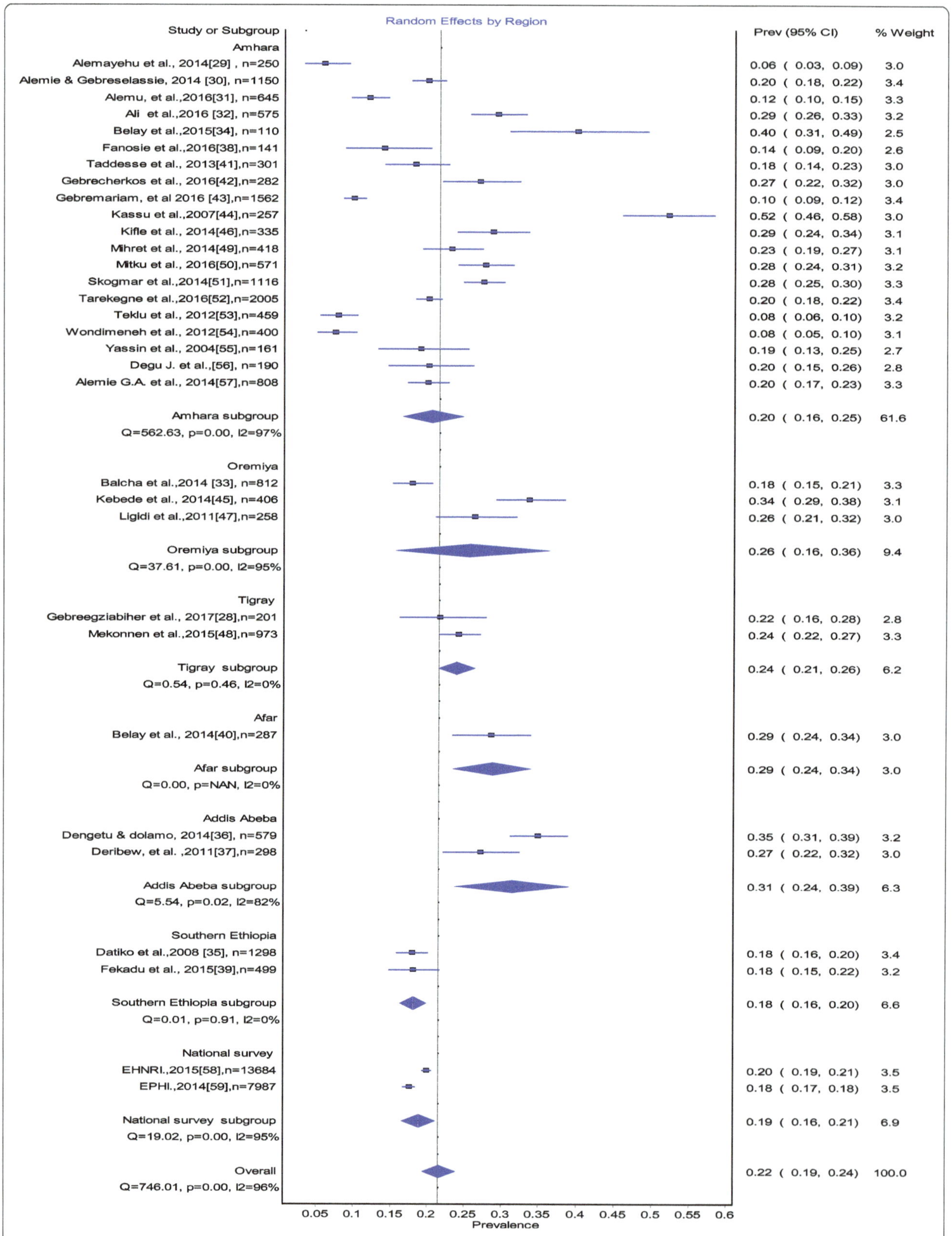

Fig. 3 The estimated prevalence of TB-HIV co-infection in Ethiopia by Region Meta-analysis

The substantial difference between the regions might be due to the difference in the socio-cultural and demographic characteristics of the population and associated HIV prevalence [63, 64]. Supporting this, the rank of the regions based on the prevalence of HIV evidenced in the Ethiopian Demographic Health Survey (EDHS) 2016 report [64], is majorly consistent with the rank of the regions in this pooled analysis. This is logically sounding because HIV is the driving factor for TB infection as a result of the immunosuppression.

As Ethiopia is among the high burden countries for TB and HIV, it may be expected to find a high prevalence of TB-HIV co-infection. However, the pooled prevalence of TB-HIV co-infection (22%) is still higher than the WHO estimated figure (8%) in 2017 [65]. The pooled prevalence of TB-HIV co-infection in the current study is bothersome considering the feared complications and emergence of drug resistance; in Ethiopia, the estimated prevalence of MDR-TB is particularly high in previously treated cases (14%) [65]. In addition to this, HIV had been significantly associated with MDR-TB; studies indicate that there was a high rate of MDR-TB among HIV positive individuals; 14% in Addis Ababa [66], 19.4% in the Amhara region [67] and 19.5% in the Oromia region [68]. However, only 70% of those with MDR-TB are thought to be started on second-line treatment and the coverage of ART initiation was 88% in those confirmed to have TB [65]. Moreover, as part of the millennium development goals and now the health sector transformation plan, Ethiopia has been working to reduce HIV and TB associated morbidity and mortalities. Therefore, the pooled prevalence in the current study is still alarming despite the previous efforts. It implicates that efforts are still needed in reducing HIV associated TB which may include prevention, early detection and comprehensive management of cases. As part of the early detection of cases, TB contact household based screening may have a significant input to augment the facility-based screening of TB among HIV positive individuals [69]. In addition to the prevention, early diagnosis helps the early initiation of ART which in turn significantly increases the success rate of TB treatment among HIV patients [70].

TB-HIV co-infection has a great impact on the health outcome of the victims due to accelerated progression. Co-infected individuals have significantly lower years of survival as compared to those HIV positive only [60]. Witnessing this, though the case fatality ratio of TB in Ethiopia is 0.17, the case fatality ratio of TB-HIV together is estimated to be 0.28 [65]. The simultaneous occurrence of the two infections results in different immunological changes, such as the polyclonal activation of HIV harboring lymphocytes and an increased survival of the bacilli inside macrophages [71]. In addition, there is a clear impact on treatment success rate; as compared to TB alone or HIV alone, co-infected patients are more vulnerable to treatment failure and there is a low rate of treatment success [61]. Poor treatment outcome is 2 times higher among TB-HIV patients [48]. Therefore, this TB treatment failure, poor adherence to ART, the progression of the two diseases and the presence of other co-morbidities may significantly facilitate the death of TB-HIV patients [72]. As a limitation, this study did not explain the heterogeneity in terms of differences in the study setting, population or year. In addition, due to differences in the design and population of the studies, this study did not present the analysis of the trends of prevalence over the years.

Conclusion

Our analysis indicated that the prevalence of TB-HIV co-infection is high in Ethiopia with substantial regional variation. Therefore, an integrated and consistent facility-based as well as community-based effort addressing the prevention, early detection and management of TB and HIV infection should be further strengthened throughout the country to mitigate the double burden disease.

Abbreviations

AIDS: Acquired Immunodeficiency Syndrome; ART: Antiretroviral Therapy; CDC: Centers for Disease Control; HIV: Human Immunodeficiency Virus; MDR-TB: Multidrug-Resistant Tuberculosis; TB: Tuberculosis; WHO: World Health Organization

Acknowledgements

We would like to acknowledge Aksum University College of Health Sciences for providing the internet access.

Funding

This work was not funded by any external funding agent.

Authors' contributions

MT&NA: Conceived and designed the review, made the literature search, did the statistical analysis and wrote the manuscript; SW &HG: participated in statistical analysis. All authors read and approved the final manuscript.

Consent for publication

Not applicable.

Competing interests

The authors declare that they have no competing interests.

Author details

[1]Department of Medical Laboratory Sciences, College of Health Sciences, Aksum University, PO.BOX 298, Aksum, Tigray, Ethiopia. [2]Department of Public Health, College of Health Sciences, Aksum University, Aksum, Tigray, Ethiopia. [3]School of Pharmacy, College of Health Sciences, Mekelle University, Mekelle, Tigray, Ethiopia.

References

1. The Joint United nation Program on HIV/AIDS (UNAIDS). Global summary of the AIDS epidemic. Geneva: UNAIDS; 2017.
2. World Health Organization. Global TB report, 2016. Geneva, Switzerland: WHO; 2016.
3. Nachega JB, RE C. drug resistance: a global threat. Clin Infect Dis. 2003;36(1):524–30.
4. World Health Organization. Global TB report, 2017. Geneva: WHO; 2017.
5. Eshetie S, Gizachew M, Dagnew M, Kumera G, Woldie H, Ambaw F, et al. Multidrug resistant tuberculosis in Ethiopian settings and its association with previous history of anti-tuberculosis treatment: a systematic review and meta-analysis. BMC Infectious Diseases. 2017;17:219.
6. Mulisa G, Workneh T, Hordof N, Suaudi M, Abebe G, Jarso G. Multidrug-resistant Mycobacterium tuberculosis and associated risk factors in Oromia Region of Ethiopia. Int J Infect Dis. 2015;39:57–6.
7. World Health Organization. Towards universal access to diagnosis and treatment of multidrug-resistant and extensively drug-resistant tuberculosis by 2015. In: WHO Progress Report 2011. Geneva: WHO. p. 2011.
8. Breen R, Smith C, Bettinson H. Paradoxical Reactions during Tuberculosis Treatment in Patients with and without HIV Co-Infection. Thorax. 2004;59: 704–7.
9. Havlir D, Kendall M, Ive P, Kumwenda J, Swindells S, Qasba S. Timing of Antiretroviral Therapy for HIV-1 Infection and Tuberculosis. N Engl J Meds. 2011;365:482–91.
10. Russell S. The economic burden of illness for households in developing countries: a review of studies focusing on malaria, tuberculosis, and human immunodeficiency virus/acquired immunodeficiency syndrome. Am J Trop Med Hyg. 2004;71(Suppl 2):147–55.
11. Melkamu H, Seyoum B, Dessie Y. Determinants of Tuberculosis Infection among Adult HIV Positives Attending Clinical Care in Western Ethiopia: A Case-Control Study. AIDS Res Treat. 2013;2013:1–7.
12. Mukadi YD, Maher D, Harries A. Tuberculosis case fatality rates in high HIV prevalence populations in sub-Saharan Africa. AIDS. 2001;15:143–52.
13. Mulugeta Dalbo TA. Incidence and Predictors of Tuberculosis among HIV/AIDS Infected Patients: A Five-Year Retrospective Follow-Up Study. Adv Infect Dis. 2016;6:70–81.
14. Sterling TR, et al. Risk Factors for Tuberculosis after Highly Active Antiretroviral Therapy Initiation in the United States and Canada: Implications for Tuberculosis Screening. J Infect Dis. 2011;204:893–901.
15. Seyler C, et al. Risk Factors for Active Tuberculosis after Antiretroviral Treatment Initiation in Abidjan. Amer-ican. J Respir Crit Care Med. 2005;17:123–7.
16. Sharma SK, Mohan A, Kadhiravan T. HIV-TB co-infection: Epidemiology, diagnosis & management. Indian J Med Res. 2005;121:550–67.
17. Toossi Z. Virological and immunological impact of tuberculosis on human immunodeficiency virus type 1 disease. J Infect Dis. 2003;188:1146–55.
18. Sharma SK, Kadhiravan T, Banga A, Goyal T, Bhatia I, Saha PK. Spectrum of clinical disease in a cohort of 135 hospitalised HIV-infected patients from north India. BMC Infect Dis. 2004;4:52.
19. Zumla A, Malon P, Henderson J, Grange JM. Impact of HIV infection on tuberculosis. Postgrad Med J. 2000;76:259–68.
20. Rupali P, Abraham OC, Zachariah A, Subramanian S, Mathai D. Aetiology of prolonged fever in antiretroviralnaive human immunodeficiency virus-infected adults. Natl Med J India. 2003;16:193–9.
21. Howard AA, El-Sadr WM. Integration of Tuberculosis and HIV Services in Sub-Saharan Africa: Lessons Learned. CID. 2010;50(S3):S238–44.
22. World Health Organization. Strategic framework to decrease the burden of TB/HIV. Geneva: World Health Organization; 2002.
23. Freeman MF, Tukey JW. Transformations Related to the Angular and the Square Root. Ann Math Stats. 1950;21:607–11.
24. Wilson EB. Probable Inference, the Law of Succession, and Statistical Inference. J Am Stat Assoc. 1927;22:209–12.
25. Newcombe RG. Two-Sided Confidence Intervals for The Single Proportion: Comparison of Seven Methods. Stat Med. 1998;17:857–72.
26. Higgins JP, Thompson SG. Quantifying heterogeneity in a meta-analysis. Stat Med. 2002;21(1539–1558).
27. Higgins JP, Thompson SG, Deeks JJ, Altman DG. Measuring inconsistency in meta-analyses. BMJ. 2003;327:557–60.
28. Gebreegziabiher D, Adane K. Abebe M. A survey on undiagnosed active pulmonary tuberculosis among pregnant mothers in mekelle and surrounding Districts in Tigray, Ethiopia. Int J Mycobacteriol. 2017;6(1):43–6.
29. Alemayehu M, Gelaw B, Abate E, Wassie L, Belyhun Y, Bekele S, et al. Active tuberculosis case finding and detection of drug resistance among HIV-infected patients: A cross-sectional study in a TB endemic area, Gondar, Northwest Ethiopia. Int J Mycobacteriol. 2014;3(2):132–8.
30. Alemie GA, Gebreselassie F. Common types of tuberculosis and co-infection with HIV at private health institutions in Ethiopia: a cross sectional study. BMC public health. 2014;14:319.
31. Alemu YM, Andargie G, Gebeye E. High Incidence of Tuberculosis in the Absence of Isoniazid and Cotrimoxazole Preventive Therapy in Children Living with HIV in Northern Ethiopia: A Retrospective Follow-Up Study. PloS One. 2016;11(4):e0152941.
32. Ali SA, Mavundla TR, Fantu R, Awoke T. Outcomes of TB treatment in HIV co-infected TB patients in Ethiopia: a cross-sectional analytic study. BMC Infect Dis. 2016;16(1):640.
33. Balcha TT, Sturegard E, Winqvist N, Skogmar S, Reepalu A, Jemal ZH, et al. Intensified tuberculosis case-finding in HIV-positive adults managed at Ethiopian health centers: diagnostic yield of Xpert MTB/RIF compared with smear microscopy and liquid culture. PloS one. 2014;9(1):e85478.
34. Belay M, Bjune G, Abebe F. Prevalence of tuberculosis, HIV, and TB-HIV co-infection among pulmonary tuberculosis suspects in a predominantly pastoralist area, northeast Ethiopia. Global Health Action. 2015;8(1): 27949.
35. Datiko DG, Yassin MA, Chekol LT, Kabeto LE, Lindtjorn B. The rate of TB-HIV co-infection depends on the prevalence of HIV infection in a community. BMC public health. 2008;8:266.
36. Denegetu AW. Dolamo BL. HIV screening among TB patients and co-trimoxazole preventive therapy for TB/HIV patients in Addis Ababa: facility based descriptive study. PloS One. 2014;9(2):e86614.
37. Deribew A, Negussu N, Melaku Z, Deribe K. Investigation outcomes of tuberculosis suspects in the health centers of Addis Ababa, Ethiopia. PloS One. 2011;6(4):e18614.
38. Fanosie A, Gelaw B, Tessema B, Tesfay W, Admasu A, Yitayew G. Mycobacterium tuberculosis Complex and HIV Co-Infection among Extrapulmonary Tuberculosis Suspected Cases at the University of Gondar Hospital, Northwestern Ethiopia. PloS One. 2016;11(3):e0150646.
39. Fekadu S, Teshome W, Alemu G. Prevalence and determinants of Tuberculosis among HIV infected patients in south Ethiopia. J Infect Dev Ctries. 2015;9(8):898–904.
40. Belay M, Ameni G, Bjune G, Couvin D. Strain diversity of Mycobacterium tuberculosis isolates from pulmonary tuberculosis patients in Afar pastoral region of Ethiopia. Biomed Res Int. 2014;2014:238532.
41. Tadesse S, Tadesse T. HIV co-infection among tuberculosis patients in Dabat, northwest Ethiopia. J Infect Dis Immun. 2013;5(3):29–32.
42. Gebrecherkos T, Gelaw B, Tessema B. Smear positive pulmonary tuberculosis and HIV co-infection in prison settings of North Gondar Zone, Northwest Ethiopia. BMC Infect Dis. 2016;16(1):1091.
43. Gebremariam G, Asmamaw G, Hussen M, Hailemariam MZ, Asegu D, Astatkie A, et al. Impact of HIV Status on Treatment Outcome of Tuberculosis Patients Registered at Arsi Negele Health Center, Southern Ethiopia: A Six Year Retrospective Study. PloS One. 2016;11(4):e0153239.
44. Kassu A, Mengistu G, Ayele B, Diro E, Mekonnen F, Ketema D, et al. Coinfection and clinical manifestations of tuberculosis in human immunodeficiency virus-infected and -uninfected adults at a teaching hospital, northwest Ethiopia. J Microbiol Immunol Infect. 2007;40(2):116–22.
45. Kebede W, Keno F, Ewunetu T, Mamo G. Acceptance of Provider Initiated HIV Testing and Counseling among Tuberculosis Patients in East Wollega Administrative Zone, Oromia Regional State, Western Ethiopia. Tuberc Res Treat. 2014;2014:935713.
46. Keflie TS, Ameni G. Microscopic examination and smear negative pulmonary tuberculosis in Ethiopia. Pan Afr Med J. 2014;19:162.
47. Ligidi T, Gebre-Selassie S, Tsegaye A. The immunological status of newly diagnosed tuberculosis patients co-infected with human immunodeficiency virus-1 in Adama Hospital, Ethiopia. Ethiop Med J. 2011;49(2):75–83.
48. Mekonnen D, Derbie A, Desalegn E. TB/HIV co-infections and associated factors among patients on directly observed treatment short course in Northeastern Ethiopia: a 4 years retrospective study. BMC Res Notes. 2015;8(1):666.
49. Mihret A, Bekele Y, Aytenew M, Assefa Y, Wassie L, Abebe M, et al. Human immunodeficiency virus infection among new smear positive pulmonary tuberculosis patients in Addis Ababa, Ethiopia. Ethiopian Med J. 2014; 2014(Suppl 1):1–6.

50. Mitku AA, Dessie ZG, Muluneh EK, Workie DL. Prevalence and associated factors of TB/HIV co-infection among HIV Infected patients in Amhara region, Ethiopia. African health sciences. 2016;16(2):588–95.
51. Skogmar S, Balcha TT, Jemal ZH, Bjork J, Deressa W, Schon T, et al. Development of a clinical scoring system for assessment of immunosuppression in patients with tuberculosis and HIV infection without access to CD4 cell testing--results from a cross-sectional study in Ethiopia. Global Health Action. 2014;7:23105.
52. Tarekegne D, Jemal M, Atanaw T, Ebabu A, Endris M, Moges F, et al. Prevalence of human immunodeficiency virus infection in a cohort of tuberculosis patients at Metema Hospital, Northwest Ethiopia: a 3 years retrospective study. BMC Res Notes. 2016;9:192.
53. Teklu T, Belyhun Y, Tesfaye S, Medhin G. Trends of tuberculosis and HIV infections between 2004 and 2008 in Wolaita Sodo, southern Ethiopia. Ethiopian Med J. 2012;50(1):1–11.
54. Wondimeneh Y, Muluye D, Belyhun Y. Prevalence of pulmonary tuberculosis and immunological profile of HIV co-infected patients in Northwest Ethiopia. BMC Res Notes. 2012;5:331.
55. Yassin MA, Takele L, Gebresenbet S, Girma E, Lera M, Lendebo E, et al. HIV and tuberculosis coinfection in the southern region of Ethiopia: a prospective epidemiological study. Scand J Infect Dis. 2004;36(9):670–3.
56. Degu J, Aschalew E, Bernt L. Acceptability of HIV counselling and testing among tuberculosis patients in south Ethiopia. BMC Int Health Hum Rights. 2007;7(4).
57. Ethiopian Health and Nutrition Research Institute (EHNRI)/ Ministry of Health (MOH). National TB/HIV Sentinel surveillance one year report (July 2011–June 2012). Addis Ababa, Ethiopia, 2013. .
58. Ethiopian Public Health Institute (EPHI) Ministry of Health (MOH). National TB/HIV Sentinel Surveillance annual report (July–June 2015).
59. Gao J, Zheng P. Fu H. Prevalence of TB/HIV co-infection in countries except China: a systematic review and meta-analysis. PloS One. 2013;8(5):e64915.
60. Maimaiti R, Zhang Y, Pan K, Mijiti P, Wubili M, Musa M, Andersson R. High prevalence and low cure rate of tuberculosis among patients with HIV in Xinjiang,China. BMC Infect Dis. 2017;17(1):15.
61. Babatunde OI, Christiandolus EO, Bismarck EC, Emmanuel OI, Chike AC, Gabriel EI. Five years retrospective cohort analysis of treatment outcomes of TB-HIV patients at a PEPFAR/DOTS Centre in South Eastern Nigeria. African Health Sci. 2016;16(3):655–62.
62. Osei E, Der J, Owusu R, Kofie P, Axame WK. The burden of HIV on Tuberculosis patients in the Volta region of Ghana from 2012 to 2015: implication for Tuberculosis control. BMC Infect Dis. 2017;17(1):504.
63. Lakew Y, Benedict S, Haile D. Social determinants of HIV infection, hotspot areas and subpopulation groups in Ethiopia: evidence from the National Demographic and Health Survey in 2011. BMJ open. 2015;5(11):e008669.
64. Central Statistical Agency (CSA) [Ethiopia] and ICF. Ethiopia Demographic and Health Survey 2016: HIV Report. Addis Ababa, Ethiopia, and Rockville, Maryland: CSA and ICF. p. 2018.
65. World Health Organization. Global TB report, 2017.
66. Bruchfeld J, Aderaye G, Palme IB, Bjorvatn B, Ghebremichael S, Hoffner S, Lindquist L. Molecular epidemiology and drug resistance of Mycobacterium tuberculosis isolates from Ethiopian pulmonary tuberculosis patients with and without human immunodeficiency virus infection. J Clin Microbiol. 2002;40(5):1636–43.
67. Nigus DM, Lingerew W, Beyene B, Tamiru A, Lemma M, Melaku MY. Prevalence of multi drug resistant tuberculosis among presumptive multi drug resistant tuberculosis cases in Amhara National Regional State, Ethiopia. J Mycobac Dis. 2014;4(152):2161–1068.
68. Mulisa G, Workneh T, Hordofa N, Suaudi M, Abebe G, Jarso G. Multidrug-resistant Mycobacterium tuberculosis and associated risk factors in Oromia Region of Ethiopia. Int J Infect Dis. 2015;39:57–61.
69. Shapiro AE, Variava E, Rakgokong MH, Moodley N, Luke B, Salimi S, Chaisson RE, Golub JE, Martinson NA. Community-based targeted case finding for tuberculosis and HIV in household contacts of patients with tuberculosis in South Africa. Am J Respir Crit Care Med. 2012;185(10):1110 6.
70. Shastri S, Naik B, Shet A, Rewari B, De Costa A. TB treatment outcomes among TB-HIV co-infections in Karnataka, India: how do these compare with non-HIV tuberculosis outcomes in the province? BMC Public Health. 2013;13(1):838.
71. Rossouw T, Tucker JD, Zyl GU, Sikwesi K, Godfrey C. Barriers to HIV remission research in low-and middle-income countries. J Int AIDS Soc. 2017;20(1): 21521.
72. Agbor AA, Bigna JJ, Billong SC, Tejiokem MC, Ekali GL, Plottel CS, Noubiap JJ, Abessolo H, Toby R, Koulla-Shiro S. Factors associated with death during tuberculosis treatment of patients co-infected with HIV at the Yaoundé Central Hospital, Cameroon: an 8-year hospital-based retrospective cohort study (2006–2013). PloS One. 2014;15(9):12–e115211.

Case-control study of the epidemiological and clinical features of human adenovirus 55 and human adenovirus 7 infection in children with acute lower respiratory tract infections in Beijing, China, 2008–2013

Lili Xu[1†], Jun Liu[2†], Chunyan Liu[1], Yali Duan[1], Yun Zhu[1], Baoping Xu[2*] and Zhengde Xie[1*]

Abstract

Background: In adults, the emerging human adenovirus (HAdV) type 55 (HAdV-55) has been reported to cause more severe cases of adenovirus induced acute lower respiratory tract infections (ALRTIs) compared to other HAdV serotypes (HAdV-3, HAdV-7, HAdV-14). However, there is a dearth of comparative studies in children that address differences in the clinical epidemiological features between HAdV-55 and other HAdV serotypes that can also induce severe infection (such as HAdV-7).

Methods: We conducted a retrospective review of pediatric patients hospitalized at Beijing Children's Hospital with ALRTI from April 2008 to December 2013 who had adenovirus detected from nasopharyngeal or throat samples by PCR. We further compared pediatric patients infected with HAdV-55 to those infected with HAdV-7 using a case-control methodology by matching each subject with HAdV-55 infection to 4 patients with HAdV-7 infection within 2 months of each HAdV-55 infection. Demographic, clinical, and etiological data were collected and analyzed.

Results: Over the five-year period, HAdV was detected in 194 children. Of these, 8 were HAdV-55 positive. Epidemiological results showed that HAdV-55 infection was observed only in 4% of adenovirus infected children whereas HAdV-7 infection proportioned 53%. Most cases of HAdV-55 infection were identified during March and April, whereas HAdV-7 infection occurred throughout the year. Wheezing was significantly less frequent in the HAdV-55 group. No patients infected with HAdV-55 presented with vomiting or had any underlying disease. Coinfections with other respiratory tract pathogens were frequent among children infected with either HAdV-55 or HAdV-7.

Conclusions: HAdV-55 circulated in Beijing during spring and appeared to cause pediatric respiratory infections that were as severe as HAdV-7 infections. Broader surveillance studies are needed.

Keywords: HAdV-55, HAdV-7, Case-control study, Epidemiological feature, Clinical feature

* Correspondence: xubaoping@yahoo.com; xiezhengde@bch.com.cn
[†]Lili Xu and Jun Liu contributed equally to this work.
[2]National Clinical Research Center for Respiratory Diseases, Resiratory Department, Beijing Children's Hospital, Capital Medical University, National Center for Children's Health, Beijing, China
[1]Beijing Key Laboratory of Pediatric Respiratory Infection Diseases, Key Laboratory of Major Diseases in Children, Ministry of Education, National Clinical Research Center for Respiratory Diseases, National Key Discipline of Pediatrics (Capital Medical University), Beijing Pediatric Research Institute, Beijing Children's Hospital, Capital Medical University, National Center for Children's Health, Beijing, China

Background

Human adenovirus (HAdV) type 55 (HAdV-55)is an intertypic recombinant virus described originally as genome type 11a and identified from an outbreak of acute respiratory tract infection (ALRTI) in Shanxi Province, China, in 2006 [1]. In 2011, this pathogen apparently re-emerged and caused several cases of severe community-acquired pneumonia in adults in Beijing, China [2]. Research demonstrated that HAdV-55 showed the pathogenic properties of HAdV-14 but exhibited a neutralizing antigen epitope of HAdV-11 [3]. Further whole-genome sequencing verified that HAdV-55 had a HAdV-14 backbone and partial HAdV-11 hexon gene [4]; therefore, this pathogen was renamed HAdV-55 [5]. Comparative studies have shown that the ability of HAdV to cause severe disease may relate to HAdV serotypes. In adults, the emerging HAdV-55 has been reported to cause more severe cases of adenoviral pneumonia compared to other HAdV serotypes (HAdV-3, HAdV-7, HAdV-14) [6, 7]. However, there is a dearth of comparative studies, particularly in children, that address differences in clinical epidemiological features between HAdV-55 and other HAdV serotypes that can also induce severe infection (such as HAdV-7). In this study, we investigated whether HAdV-55 and HAdV-7(the most common adenovirus circulating in China that can cause severe or acute infection) have different epidemiological and clinical profiles in children, to assess if HAdV-55 virus can cause more severe infection than HAdV-7 as observed in adults.

Methods

Patient enrollment

We retrospectively enrolled pediatric patients with ALRTIs who were admitted to Beijing Children's Hospital from April 2008 to December 2013. Patients with signs and symptoms of respiratory tract infection (such as fever, coughing, expectoration), and lower respiratory signs (tachypnea, dyspnea, retractions, or wheezing/rales upon auscultation etc.) were defined as ALRTIs. Chest X-rays were taken for all patients. Nasopharyngeal aspirate or throat swab specimens were collected from each patient in virus transport media and stored at − 80 °C prior to use. No repeated samples were collected from any patient.

For each patient with HAdV-55 infection, we matched four neighbours with HAdV-7 infection as controls. Control subjects were collected within two months before and two months after the HAdV-55 cases. The nearest neighbours were recruited first.

Clinical information collection

Clinical information was collected using a standardized data form. A clinical scoring system for ALRTIs, which related with hospitalization time, pediatric intensive care unit (PICU) admitted time, oxygen supplemented time, maximal FIO_2, was used to assess severity of illness [8]. The score values ranged from 0 to 14. The median score value of 7 or greater was used to define severe ALRTIs infection and scores less than 7 were considered as mild or moderate disease.

Preparation of nucleic acids and detection of pathogens

NucliSens easyMAG system (bioMérieux, Marcy-l'Etoile, France) was used to extract viral nucleic acids in accordance with the manufacturer's instructions. cDNA was reverse transcribed from RNA using random primers and a SuperScript II reverse transcriptase (Invitrogen). Nineteen common respiratory viral pathogens and subtypes (influenza A (IFA); IFA subtype H1; IFA subtype H3; 2009 H1N1; influenza B (IFB); HAdV; human parainfluenza virus (HPIV) 1–4; respiratory syncytial virus (RSV) A and B; human metapneumovirus (HMPV); enteroviruses and rhinoviruses (EV/RhV); human coronavirus (HCoV) HKU1, 229E, NL63 and OC43; and human bocavirus (HBoV)) were detected by using the Luminex xTAG respiratory viral panel assay and a Luminex 200 instrument (Luminex, Austin, TX). HAdV-positive samples were further amplified using a nested PCR procedure that targeted hypervariable regions 1–6 of the hexon gene, as described previously [9]. PCR products were purified and sequenced for further confirmation. Meanwhile, bronchial alveolar lavage fluids (if available), blood, and cerebrospinal fluid (if available) from HAdV-55 and HAdV-7 infected patients during the entire hospital admission were plated onto selective agar plates to identify any bacteria or fungi.

Statistical analysis

Data analyses were performed using SPSS 19.0. A two-tailed independent-samples *t*-test method was used to compare continuous variables between two groups. Univariate analysis was conducted using χ^2 tests or Fisher's exact test for categorical data. Probability < 0.05 was considered to be statistically significant.

Results

From April 2008 to December 2013, 3428 pediatric patients with ALRTIs were identified. A total of 194 HAdV-positive cases were detected using the Luminex xTAG respiratory viral panel assay; the most prevalent HAdV serotype was HAdV-7 (102/194, 53%), followed by HAdV-3 (51/194, 26%). Eight cases (8/194, 4%) of HAdV-55 infection were detected. Other newly emerging and re-emergent serotypes or variants, such as HAdV-57 (3/194, 2%) and HAdV-14 (3/194, 2%), were also identified (Fig. 1).

Among the 8 HAdV-55 positive cases, 5 (63%) cases were detected in April, 2 (25%) cases were detected in March, and 1 (13%) case was detected in October. In contrast, HAdV-7 infections occurred throughout the year,

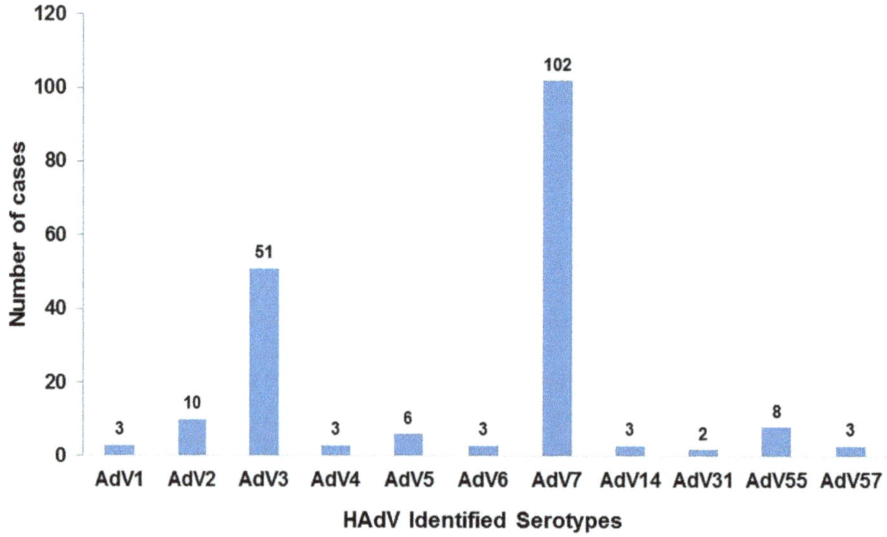

Fig. 1 The distribution of HAdV serotypes detected in pediatric ALRTIs cases in Beijing, China, 2008–2013

although such infections were also most frequent in April (19%) (Fig. 2).

Among the 8 HAdV-55 infected patients, one child was an outpatient, and we only knew her age and sex. Another patient left hospital in advance and without recovery, and her clinical features (except for the first blood test after admission to hospital) could not be documented. All 32 matched control subjects were inpatients.

Table 1 shows clinical characteristics of the patients with HAdV-55 infection and the control subjects with HAdV-7 infection. There were no cases of mortality in either group. Most clinical symptoms and signs, and blood parameters did not significantly differ between the two groups, with the exception of wheezing, which was observed in 17% of HAdV-55-infected patients and 63% of HAdV-7-infected patients ($P = 0.038$).

Furthermore, no patient infected with HAdV-55 exhibited vomiting or had any underlying disease; however, 3 (9%) patients vomited during the course of HAdV-7 infection, and 2 HAdV-7-infected patients had underlying disease (congenital heart disease and wheezing). Meanwhile, only 29% (2/7) of HAdV-55 infected patients developed respiratory failure, cardiac damage, or liver function damage, whereas in HAdV-7 infected group, the above mentioned complications arosed in more than half of the patients (56%, 18/32); however, this was not statistically significant ($P = 0.184$).

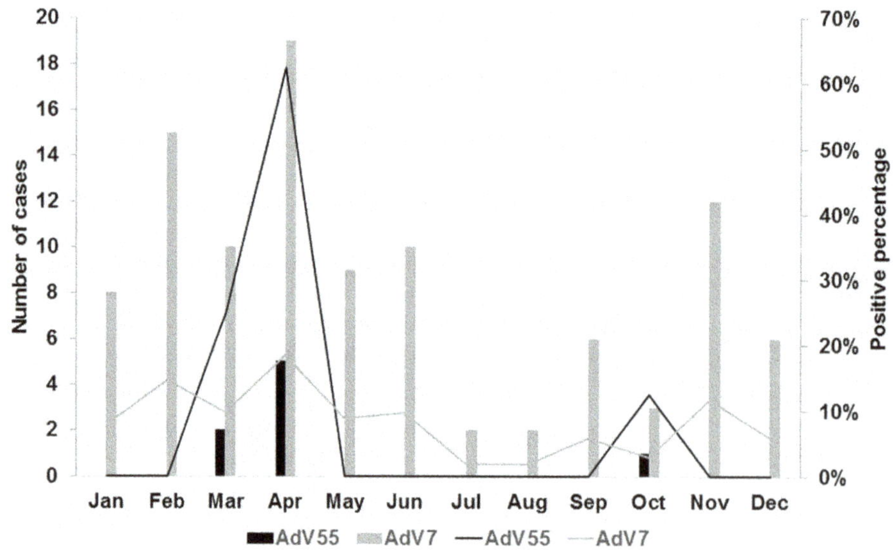

Fig. 2 The temporal distribution of HAdV-55 and HAdV-7 detection in pediatric ALRTIs cases in Beijing, China, 2008–2013

Table 1 Clinical features of patients infected with HAdV-55 or HAdV-7 in this study

	HAdV55 ($n = 8$)	HAdV7 ($n = 32$)	P
Age (yrs)	0.73 ± 0.78	2.48 ± 3.06	0.120
Male (%)	5/8 (63%)	26/32 (81%)	0.256
Any underlying diseases	0	2/32	0.529
Symptoms and signs			
Fever≥38 °C	7/7 [a] (100%)	32/32 (100%)	/
Maximum temperature (°C)	39.41 ± 0.94[b]	39.79 ± 0.64	0.161
Duration of fever (days)	14.5 ± 10.75[b]	15.14 ± 5.48	0.960
Cough	6/6[b] (100%)	32/32 (100%)	/
Rhinorrhea	2/6[b] (33%)	4/32 (13%)	0.199
Wheezing	1/6[b] (17%)	20/32 (63%)	0.038[c]
Swelling of tonsils	4/6[b] (67%)	13/32 (41%)	0.239
Rash	2/6[b] (33%)	5/32 (16%)	0.305
Vomiting	0[b]	3/32 (9%)	0.435
Diarrhea	1/6[b] (17%)	11/32 (34%)	0.392
Dyspnea	2/6[b] (33%)	10/32 (31%)	0.920
Lung infiltrates	4/6[b] (67%)	16/32 (50%)	0.453
Complication[d]	2/7[a] (29%)	18/32 (56%)	0.184
Laboratory detection			
WBC (10^9/L)	11.48 ± 3.08[a]	10.64 ± 5.71	0.709
Neutrophil %	63.20% ± 15.03%[a]	57.98% ± 17.46%	0.469
Lymphocyte %	29.26% ± 12.53%[a]	35.25% ± 17.59%	0.402
Platelet (10^9/L)	274.71 ± 184.61[a]	291.29 ± 146.87	0.801
CRP (mg/L)	26.53 ± 24.84[a]	33.42 ± 45.86	0.706
Treatment			
ICU admission	1/7[a] (14%)	5/32 (16%)	0.929
Mechanical ventilation	1/6[b] (17%)	9/32 (28%)	0.559
Immunoglobulin	2/7[a] (29%)	17/32 (53%)	0.239
Length of hospital stay (days)	11.33 ± 6.86[b]	19.10 ± 10.41	0.109
Clinical score[e]	6.43 ± 2.44[a]	8.21 ± 2.98	0.148

Note:
[a]One subject was an outpatient, and information about this subject was not documented
[b]There was a patient (other than the aforementioned outpatient) who left hospital in advance and without recovery, and her clinical features (except for the first blood test after admission to hospital) could not be documented
[c]Statistically significant ($P < 0.05$)
[d]Complications include respiratory failure, cardiac damage, or liver function damage
[e]A clinical scoring system for ALRTIs was used to assess severity of illness on the day of enrollment

Co-infections were observed in 75 and 94% of cases of HAdV-55 and HAdV-7 infections, respectively. HAdV-55 patients were most frequently coinfected with HPIV (25%); *Streptococcus pneumoniae* (17%), RhV (8%), IFA (8%), HCoV (8%), HBoV (8%), HMPV (8%), *Escherichia coli* (8%), and *Haemophilus influenzae* (8%) were also detected in cases involving multiple infection in the HAdV-55 group, in which the percentages of double, triple, and quadruple infection were each 33%. HAdV-7-infected patients were also most commonly coinfected with HPIV (40%); in the HAdV-7 group, multiple infections involving *Mycoplasma pneumoniae* (27%), RhV (23%), RSV (20%), viridans group *Streptococci* (17%), HBoV (10%), *Streptococcus pneumoniae* (10%), *Klebsiella pneumoniae* (10%), HCoV (7%), fungus (7%), IFA (3%), EBV (3%), *Acinetobacter baumannii* (3%), and *Haemophilus influenzae* (3%) were also detected. In that group, the percentages of double, triple, quadruple, quintuple, and sextuple infections were 56, 13, 13, 9, and 3%, respectively (Fig. 3).

Discussion

Epidemiological results in this study showed that in children, HAdV-55 infection was observed much less frequently than HAdV-7 infection. Most cases of HAdV-55

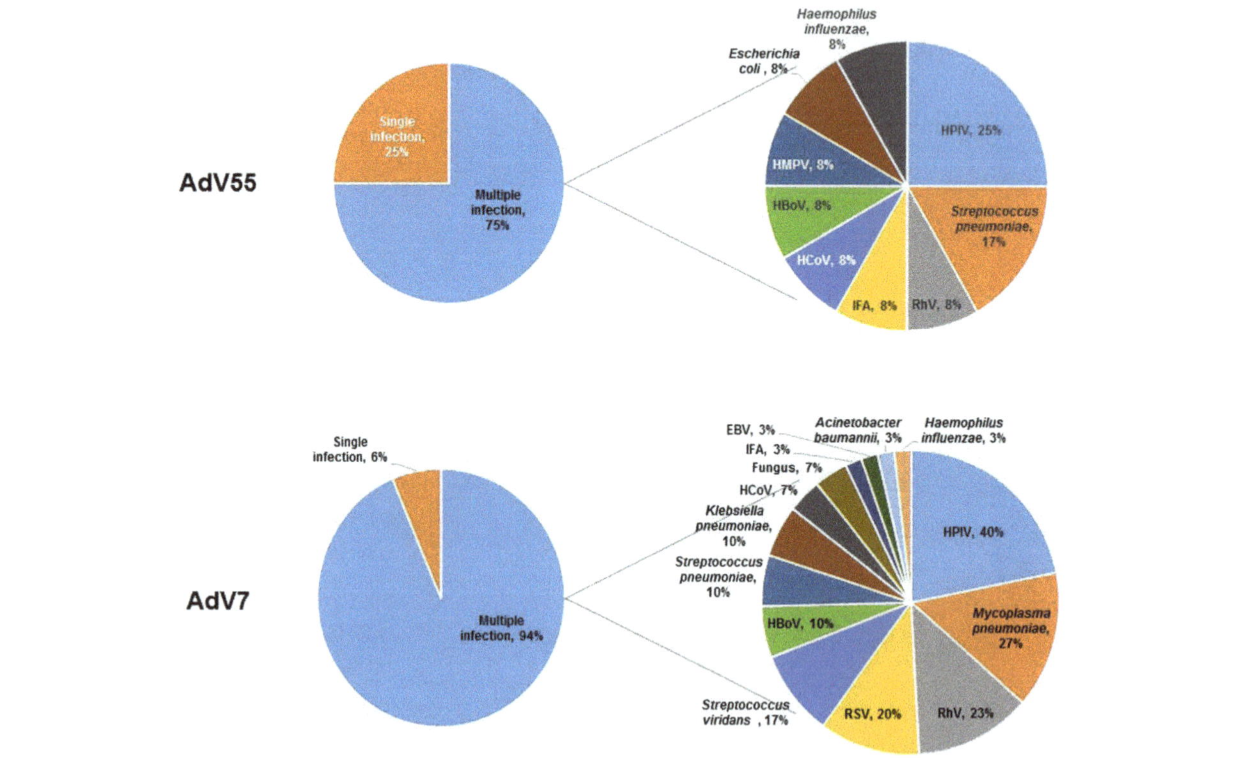

Fig. 3 Single and multiple infections involving HAdV-55 or HAdV-7 in pediatric ALRTIs cases in Beijing, China, 2008–2013

infection were identified during March and April, whereas HAdV-7 infection occurred throughout the year. These results were in accordance with previous reports about the typical adenoviruses season months [6, 10, 11].

A comparative study involving adult patients was conducted by Cao et al to discern epidemiological and clinical differences between HAdV-55 and other HAdV serotypes (HAdV-7, HAdV-3, HAdV-14, HAdV-50, and HAdV-C) [6]. Their results showed that most HAdV-55 cases were identified during February and March. They also found that patients with HAdV-55 infection had higher pneumonia severity index scores ($P = 0.030$) than patients infected with another HAdV serotype (HAdV-7, HAdV-3, HAdV-14, HAdV-50, or HAdV-C). Sun et al also found that HAdV-55 may cause severe acute respiratory distress syndrome (ARDS) in immunocompetent young men. They conducted a prospective, single-center observational study of pneumonia with ARDS with confirmed HAdV-55 infection in immunocompetent adults, and four (80%) of the five patients died despite receiving appropriate respiratory support [7]. However, our data showed that the HAdV-55 group had lower ALRTI clinical scores than the HAdV-7 group, although this difference was not significant.

Cao and Lu separately reported the presence of underlying diseases in 19.1 and 50% of HAdV-55 patients, respectively [6, 12]. We could not exclude the possibility that vomiting and underlying disease may be observed if our study is enlarged to include additional cases of HAdV-55 infection. One potential weakness of our data is that there were only 8 patients with HAdV-55 infection. However, these patients represented all positive cases of HAdV-55 infection in our hospital from April 2008 to December 2013. This result also indicated that HAdV-55 infection was less common than HAdV-7 infection in children.

Our results were consistent with those reported by Lu, who found that coinfections were frequent and observed coinfection in 83.3% of hospitalized children infected with HAdV-55 [12]. However, our data differed from Cao's data in certain respects. Their results showed that only 4 (19.1%) HAdV-55-infected patients were coinfected with other pathogens, with *Mycoplasma pneumoniae* detected in three patients and HPIV and IFB detected in one patient, and that only 1 HAdV-7-infected patient exhibited coinfection (with *Mycoplasma pneumoniae*) [6]. These inconsistent findings may be attributable to different pathogen detection methods. The Luminex xTAG respiratory viral panel assay is more sensitive and comprehensive than the approach used by Cao et al. Meanwhile, in our study, a nasopharyngeal aspirate or throat swab specimen was considered to be co-infected with one pathogen when either the Luminex xTAG respiratory viral panel assay or the selective agar plate culture showed positive result. Furthermore, respiratory tract specimens, blood, and cerebrospinal fluid collected during the entire hospital admission from patients were cultured to identify any bacteria or fungi. For these reasons, our study may have identified more co-infections than previous studies.

Conclusion

To our knowledge, our investigation is the only case-control study to date involving pediatric patients with HAdV-55 or HAdV-7 infection and comparisons of epidemiological and clinical features of HAdV-55-infected subjects and HAdV-7-infected subjects. We concluded that HAdV-55 circulated in Beijing during spring and appeared to cause pediatric respiratory infections that were as severe as HAdV-7 infections. Our data provide new insight into the epidemiology of HAdV-55 infection in pediatric ALRTIs patients. A wider or longer surveillance studies are needed to evaluate the spectrum of disease caused by this emerging pathogen in China.

Abbreviations

ALRTIs: Acute lower respiratory tract infections; ARDS: Acute respiratory distress syndrome; EV: Enteroviruses; HAdV: Human adenovirus; HBoV: Human bocavirus; HCoV: Human coronavirus; HMPV: Human metapneumovirus; HPIV: Human parainfluenza virus; IFA/IFB: Influenza A/B virus; PICU: Pediatric intensive care unit; RhV: Rhinoviruses; RSV: Respiratory syncytial virus

Acknowledgements

Not applicable.

Funding

This work was supported by grants from the National Major S & T Research Projects for the Control and Prevention of Major Infectious Diseases in China (2017ZX10103004-004, 2018ZX10305409-001-004), the Capital Health Research and Development of Special Projects (2016-2-1142), and Beijing Municipal Administration of Hospitals' Youth Programme (QML20171201). The funders had no role in study design, data collection and analysis, decision to publish, or preparation of the manuscript.

Authors' contributions

LLX made substantial contributions to conception and design, analysis and interpretation of data, and drafted the manuscript. JL acquired clinical data. CYL, YLD, and YZ participated in analysis and interpretation of data. ZDX and BPX conceived and designed the study. All authors read and approved the final version of the manuscript and agree to be accountable for all aspects of the work.

Competing interests

The authors have no potential conflicts of interest.

References

1. Zhu Z, Zhang Y, Xu S, Yu P, Tian X, Wang L, Liu Z, Tang L, Mao N, Ji Y, et al. Outbreak of acute respiratory disease in China caused by B2 species of adenovirus type 11. J Clin Microbiol. 2009;47(3):697–703.
2. Gu L, Liu Z, Li X, Qu J, Guan W, Liu Y, Song S, Yu X, Cao B. Severe community-acquired pneumonia caused by adenovirus type 11 in immunocompetent adults in Beijing. J Clin Virol. 2012;54(4):295–301.
3. Zhang Q, Seto D, Cao B, Zhao S, Wan C. Genome sequence of human adenovirus type 55, a re-emergent acute respiratory disease pathogen in China. J Virol. 2012;86(22):12441–2.
4. Yang Z, Zhu Z, Tang L, Wang L, Tan X, Yu P, Zhang Y, Tian X, Wang J, Zhang Y, et al. Genomic analyses of recombinant adenovirus type 11a in China. J Clin Microbiol. 2009;47(10):3082–90.
5. Walsh MP, Seto J, Jones MS, Chodosh J, Xu W, Seto D. Computational analysis identifies human adenovirus type 55 as a re-emergent acute respiratory disease pathogen. J Clin Microbiol. 2010;48(3):991–3.
6. Cao B, Huang GH, Pu ZH, Qu JX, Yu XM, Zhu Z, Dong JP, Gao Y, Zhang YX, Li XH, et al. Emergence of community-acquired adenovirus type 55 as a cause of community-onset pneumonia. Chest. 2014;145(1):79.
7. Sun B, He H, Wang Z, Qu J, Li X, Ban C, Wan J, Cao B, Tong Z, Wang C. Emergent severe acute respiratory distress syndrome caused by adenovirus type 55 in immunocompetent adults in 2013: a prospective observational study. Crit Care. 2014;18(4):456.
8. Larranaga CL, Ampuero SL, Luchsinger VF, Carrion FA, Aguilar NV, Morales PR, Palomino MA, Tapia LF, Avendano LF. Impaired immune response in severe human lower tract respiratory infection by respiratory syncytial virus. Pediatr Infect Dis J. 2009;28(10):867–73.
9. Lu X, Erdman DD. Molecular typing of human adenoviruses by PCR and sequencing of a partial region of the hexon gene. Arch Virol. 2006;151(8): 1587–602.
10. Liu C, Xiao Y, Zhang J, Ren L, Li J, Xie Z, Xu B, Yang Y, Qian S, Wang J, et al. Adenovirus infection in children with acute lower respiratory tract infections in Beijing, China, 2007 to 2012. BMC Infect Dis. 2015;15:408.
11. Moro MR, Bonville CA, Suryadevara M, Cummings E, Faddoul D, Kobayaa H, Branigan PJ, Domachowske JB. Clinical features, adenovirus types, and local production of inflammatory mediators in adenovirus infections. Pediatr Infect Dis J. 2009;28(5):376–80.
12. Lu QB, Tong YG, Wo Y, Wang HY, Liu EM, Gray GC, Liu W, Cao WC. Epidemiology of human adenovirus and molecular characterization of human adenovirus 55 in China, 2009-2012. Influenza Other Respir Viruses. 2014;8(3):302–8.

20

Probiotics *Streptococcus salivarius* 24SMB and *Streptococcus oralis* 89a interfere with biofilm formation of pathogens of the upper respiratory tract

Alessandro Bidossi[1], Roberta De Grandi[1], Marco Toscano[2], Marta Bottagisio[1], Elena De Vecchi[1], Matteo Gelardi[3] and Lorenzo Drago[1,2*]

Abstract

Background: Infections of the ears, paranasal sinuses, nose and throat are very common and represent a serious issue for the healthcare system. Bacterial biofilms have been linked to upper respiratory tract infections and antibiotic resistance, raising serious concerns regarding the therapeutic management of such infections. In this context, novel strategies able to fight biofilms may be therapeutically beneficial and offer a valid alternative to conventional antimicrobials. Biofilms consist of mixed microbial communities, which interact with other species in the surroundings and communicate through signaling molecules. These interactions may result in antagonistic effects, which can be exploited in the fight against infections in a sort of "bacteria therapy". *Streptococcus salivarius* and *Streptococcus oralis* are α-hemolytic streptococci isolated from the human pharynx of healthy individuals. Several studies on otitis-prone children demonstrated that their intranasal administration is safe and well tolerated and is able to reduce the risk of acute otitis media. The aim of this research is to assess *S. salivarius* 24SMB and *S. oralis* 89a for the ability to interfere with biofilm of typical upper respiratory tract pathogens.

Methods: To investigate if soluble substances secreted by the two streptococci could inhibit biofilm development of the selected pathogenic strains, co-cultures were performed with the use of transwell inserts. Mixed-species biofilms were also produced, in order to evaluate if the inhibition of biofilm formation might require direct contact. Biofilm production was investigated by means of a spectrophotometric assay and by confocal laser scanning microscopy.

Results: We observed that *S. salivarius* 24SMB and *S. oralis* 89a are able to inhibit the biofilm formation capacity of selected pathogens and even to disperse their pre-formed biofilms. Diffusible molecules secreted by the two streptococci and lowered pH of the medium revealed to be implied in the mechanisms of anti-biofilm activity.

Conclusions: *S. salivarius* 24SMB and *S. oralis* 89a possess desirable characteristics as probiotic for the treatment and prevention of infections of the upper airways. However, the nature of the inhibition appear to be multifactorial and additional studies are required to get further insights.

Keywords: Biofilm, *Streptococcus oralis*, *Streptococcus salivarius*, Probiotics, Respiratory tract infections

* Correspondence: Lorenzo.drago@unimi.it
[1]Laboratory of Clinical Chemistry and Microbiology, IRCCS Orthopedic Institute Galeazzi, Milan, Italy
[2]Department of Biomedical Sciences for Health, Laboratory of Clinical Microbiology, University of Milan, Milan, Italy
Full list of author information is available at the end of the article

Background

Despite the presence of mechanical barriers and host immune defenses, the upper respiratory tract offers an easy access to pathogens involved in acute and chronic infections of ears, paranasal sinuses, nose and throat. The majority of upper respiratory tract infections (URTIs) are commonly mild and caused by viruses; however, URTIs can also be mediated by bacteria, representing a clinical challenge related to a higher morbidity and a chronic progress of the disease [1]. Moreover, URTIs have been associated with the presence of microbial biofilm, which results in chronic infections characterized by remitting course and resistance to medical management [2, 3]. Biofilm is defined as a "structured community of microorganisms enveloped in a self-produced polymeric matrix, adherent to an inert or living surface" [4]. Once the biofilm is established, the infection becomes more and more difficult to eradicate, because the microbes residing into the matrix are protected from host immune system and antibiotics [5]. Consequently, the microbial biofilm makes infections persistent and more refractory to treatments.

Biofilms usually consist of mixed microbial communities able to interact with other species in the surroundings and to communicate through signaling molecules [6]. These interspecies interactions may result in either mutualistic or antagonistic effects [7, 8]. The importance of the normal microbiota in the protection against URTIs has been widely demonstrated. However, an imbalance in the physiological flora composition may lead to the colonization and infection of the mucosae by opportunistic pathogens.

For instance, it has been noted that otitis-prone children were characterized by a significantly lower number of α-hemolytic streptococci in their nasopharyngeal flora than non-otitis-prone ones [9, 10], opening the possibility to administer living microorganisms as probiotics to confer health benefits to the host [11]. Indeed, the use of bacterial species deriving from healthy human oral microbiota as a probiotic for the treatment of URTIs has been proposed as a valid alternative to antibiotics, contributing to the re-establishment of a balanced flora while reducing or preventing the adhesion and colonization of potential pathogens.

Alpha-hemolytic streptococci (i.e. *Streptococcus salivarius* and *Streptococcus oralis*) isolated from human pharynx are known to be early colonizers of upper respiratory mucosae and their numeric predominance is suggestive of a healthy flora [12, 13]. Furthermore, these species possess desirable characteristics, such as production of bacteriocin like Colicin V and bacteriocin-like peptides [14, 15] and both act as pioneer colonizer. Nonetheless, *S. salivarius* and *S. oralis* own a high affinity to human mucosae, protecting epithelial cells from pathogen adherence, internalization, and potential cytotoxic effects. For this reason, these α-hemolytic streptococci represent the predominant species in the upper respiratory healthy flora and they can selectively influence the composition of the microbiota [16–19]. In the past decades, several studies have demonstrated the intranasal administration of *S. salivarius* and *S. oralis* as safe and well-tolerated strategy to reduce the risk of new episodes of acute otitis media in otitis-prone children and to decrease middle ear fluids amount in children with secretory otitis media [19–23].

In this study, we tested the hypothesis that *S. salivarius* 24SMB and *S. oralis* 89a, both isolated from a commercial product (Rinogermina®, DMG Italia Srl, Pomezia, Italy), are able to interfere with biofilm formation in vitro and to eradicate pre-formed biofilm of typical upper respiratory tract pathogens, such as *Streptococcus pyogenes*, *Streptococcus pneumoniae*, *Moraxella catarrhalis*, *Staphylococcus aureus*, *Staphylococcus epidermidis* and *Propionibacterium acnes*. In addition, the mechanisms underlying the anti-biofilm activity of the probiotic streptococci were speculated.

Methods

Bacterial strains and culture media

Clinically relevant upper respiratory tract pathogens were isolated from patients with URTIs at the Laboratory of Clinical Chemistry and Microbiology of IRCCS Galeazzi Institute, where they were routinely collected and stored. In particular, biofilm-producing strains of *S. aureus*, *S. epidermidis*, *S. pyogenes*, *S. pneumoniae*, *M. catarrhalis* and *P. acnes* were selected. The identification of the isolates was carried out by means of the Vitek2 Compact (BioMerieux, Marcy L'Etoile, France) and further confirmed by pyrosequencing (PSQ96RA, Diatech, Jesi, Italy), as described elsewhere [24]. Biofilm production was assessed by means of the spectrophotometric assay described by Christensen et al. [25]. *S. salivarius* 24SMB and *S. oralis* 89a were isolated from the manufactured product and identified by biochemical assays and pyrosequencing, as described above. All strains were stored at − 80 °C in proper broths enriched with 10% glycerol (VWR Chemicals, Leuven, Belgium) until testing. Brain Heart Infusion broth (BHI, bioMérieux, Marci L'Etoile, France) was used for the culture of staphylococci, BHI plus 5% of defibrinated blood (Liofilchem, Roseto degli Abruzzi, Italy) for streptococci and *M. catarrhalis*, and thioglycollate broth (TH, Oxoid, Rodano, Italy) for *P. acnes*. When performing transwell and mixed species experiments (see below), *S. oralis* and *S. salivarius* were grown in the same medium needed for the tested pathogenic strain. Before the beginning of the study, the biofilm formation ability of *S. salivarius* 24SMB and *S. oralis* 89a was assessed in each of the above-mentioned culture media, finding no significant differences among them (data not shown).

Interaction between *S. salivarius* 24SMB and *S. oralis* 89a

To evaluate whether the reciprocal interactions between *S. salivarius* 24SMB and *S. oralis* 89a could inhibit their biofilm production, co-cultures were performed with the aid of transwell inserts (microporous PET membranes with pore diameter of 0.4 µm, 1.6×10^6 pores/cm^2) designed for 24-well plates (Falcon®, Corning, New York, NY, USA), as described elsewhere [26]. Wells were inoculated with 800 µL of *S. salivarius* 24SMB suspension and 200 µL of *S. oralis* 89a suspension were dispensed in the upper compartment of transwell inserts, and vice versa. Thereafter, mixed dual-species biofilms were also produced by inoculating 1 mL of a mixture of the two probiotic strains. In all the aforementioned experimental settings, *S. salivarius* and *S. oralis* were cultured in a 98:2 ratio (about 1.5×10^7 CFU/mL of *S. salivarius* and 3×10^5 CFU/mL of *S. oralis*), as that of the manufactured product. Mono-species biofilms of each strain were produced as positive controls, while medium alone was used as negative control. The experiment was performed in triplicate. Strains were incubated at 37 °C in proper conditions, and after 72 h the biofilm formation was evaluated.

Interference on biofilm formation

To investigate if soluble substances secreted by the probiotic bacteria *S. salivarius* 24SMB and *S. oralis* 89a could inhibit biofilm formation by the tested strains, co-cultures were performed with the use of transwell inserts, as described above. Wells were inoculated with 800 µL of the target bacterial species (1.5×10^7 CFU/mL) and 200 µL of a mixture of *S. salivarius* and *S. oralis* in a 98:2 ratio were inoculated in the transwell inserts (about 1.5×10^7 CFU/mL of *S. salivarius* and 3×10^5 CFU/mL of *S. oralis*). Thereafter, mixed species biofilms were also produced in order to evaluate if the biofilm formation by the selected pathogens requires a direct contact with the two probiotic strains to be inhibited. Mono-species biofilms of each strain were used as positive controls, while medium alone was used as negative control. The experiment was performed in triplicate for each strain. Plates were incubated at 37 °C in proper conditions. After 24, 48 and 72 h, transwell inserts and liquid medium were removed, and the amount of biofilm was evaluated by a spectrophotometric assay as described below.

Interference on pre-formed biofilm

To investigate whether the probiotic strains were able to break an existing biofilm down, biofilm of each target strain was grown for 72 h in proper conditions and then incubated in the presence of *S. salivarius* and *S. oralis* for an additional time (24, 48 and 72 h), as previously described. Mono-species biofilm of each strain was produced as positive control, while medium alone was used as negative control. The experiment was performed in triplicate for each tested strain. At each time point, the amount of biofilm was evaluated spectrophotometrically as described below, and expressed as percentage in respect to pre-treatment level.

Spectrophotometric assay

The amount of biofilm was quantified by means of the spectrophotometric assay developed by Christensen et al. [25], adjusting the volume of reagents for 24-well plates. Briefly, at the end of each incubation time, the culture medium was removed, and two washes with sterile saline were performed in order to remove non-adherent bacteria. After air-drying, each well was stained with 1 mL of 1% crystal violet solution (Merck, Darmstadt, Germany) for 10 min and the dye excess removed with three washes of sterile saline. Once dried, 1 mL of absolute ethanol was added to each well to solubilize the dye attached to the biofilm. An aliquot of the solubilized dye was finally transferred into a 96-wells plate for spectrophotometric reading which was performed at a wavelength of 595 nm using a microplate reader (Multiskan FC; Thermo Scientific, Milan, Italy).

Confocal laser scanning microscopy assay

The inhibition of biofilm formation was evaluated by confocal laser scanning microscopy (CLSM) assay. Specifically, biofilms were cultured on uncoated 10 mm diameter glass microscope coverslip (VWR International Srl, Milano, Italy) in 24-well plates for 72 h using the same set-up described for transwell experiments. After 72 h of incubation at proper conditions, biofilms were gently washed with sterile saline and stained with Filmtracer™ LIVE/DEAD™ Biofilm Viability Kit (Thermo Fisher Diagnostics SpA, Rodano, Italy), according to manufacturer's instructions. Briefly, the staining solution was prepared by adding 3 µL of SYTO9 and 3 µL of propidium iodide to 1 mL of filter-sterilized water. Biofilm samples were stained by incubation with 20 µL of staining solution for 15 min at room temperature in the dark. After incubation, samples were washed with sterile saline and examined with an upright TCS SP8 (Leica Microsystems CMS GmbH, Mannheim, Germany) using a 20× dry objective (HC PL FLUOTAR 20×/0.50 DRY) plus a 2× electronic zoom. A 488 nm laser line was used to excite SYTO9, while a 552 nm laser line was used to excite propidium iodide. Sequential optical sections of 1.27 µm were collected along the z-axis over the complete thickness of the sample. Images from at least three randomly selected areas were acquired for each coverslip. The obtained images were processed with Las X (Leica Microsystems CMS GmbH, Mannheim, Germany) and analyzed with Fiji software (Fiji, ImageJ, Wayne Rasband National Institutes of Health). The following parameters were evaluated: a) the overall volume to provide an estimation of the total biomass of the biofilm; b) the live/dead cells ratio; c) the substratum coverage, as the percentage of substrate area occupied by the biofilm.

Cell-free extract interference on biofilm formation

To investigate the nature of the inhibition of pathogens biofilm formation by *S. salivarius* 24SMB and *S. oralis* 89a, a cell-free extract (CFE) of the supernatant was obtained. Briefly, as described above, the probiotic strains were cultured in the upper compartment of the transwell, concomitantly with each of the tested bacterial species. After 24 h of incubation (48 h for *P. acnes*), the medium from both the well and the upper chamber of the transwell was collected in a 15 ml tube (Falcon®, Corning, New York, NY, USA), centrifuged for 10 min at 4200 rpm and filtered through a 0.2 μm filter (ClearLine®, Biosigma S.r.l., Cona, Italy). The resulting CFE was divided in three vials: one was not treated to assess the effect of CFE on bacterial biofilm formation; the second was neutralized to a pH value of 7.0 using NaOH 1 M; the third was heated at 100 °C for 10 min to assess the contribution of thermolabile molecules to biofilm inhibition.

To determine the activity of CFEs, biofilm formation assay was carried out on 96-well polystyrene plates (Biosigma S.r.l., Cona, Italy) by growing the pathogenic species in fresh BHI alone (for positive control) or adding ½ (*v*/v) or ¼ (v/v) of both treated and untreated CFE. Production of biofilm was then measured by spectrophotometric assay as described above.

Statistical analysis

Results were expressed as mean ± standard deviation and analysed for statistical significance with PRISM5 software (GraphPad, San Diego, CA, USA) using unpaired t test for CLSM assays, one-way analysis of variance (ANOVA) for the interaction between *S. salivarius* and *S. oralis* and the cell-free extract tests, two-way ANOVA the spectrophotometric assays. One-way ANOVA and two-way ANOVA were followed by Bonferroni post hoc correction. A *P*-value ≤0.05 was used as the significance level.

Results

Interaction between *S. salivarius* 24SMB and *S. oralis* 89a

The reciprocal interaction between the two probiotic strains led to an increase in biofilm production of both *S. salivarius* (21%) and *S. oralis* (24%), compared to biofilm produced when cultured separately (Fig. 1a and b). When the two species were put in direct contact (mixed) in dual-species biofilms, a significant increase of the biofilm formation was also observed, although the contribution of each strain could not be discriminated.

Interference on biofilm formation

Generally, the mixture of *S. salivarius* and *S. oralis* displayed an inhibitory activity against biofilm development of all tested bacteria, except for *S. pyogenes* whose biofilm formation was not significantly influenced by presence of the probiotic strains (Fig. 2). Biofilm production by staphylococci was strongly affected by *S. salivarius* and *S. oralis*: significant reductions were observed at all time points in both transwell (76–86% for *S. aureus* and 84–92% for *S. epidermidis*) and mixed biofilms (40–74% for *S. aureus* and 56–80% for *S. epidermidis*), compared to controls. Significant biofilm reductions were observed for *S. pneumoniae* (38–66%) and *P. acnes* (73–77%) after 48 h and 72 h of incubation in transwell experiments, while mixed co-cultures significantly inhibited *S. pneumoniae* biofilm production at 48 and 72 h (25–48%) and *P. acnes* at 72 h (44%). Finally, *S. salivarius* and *S. oralis* showed a significant inhibitory activity against *M. catarrhalis* at all time points in transwell experiments (44–88%) and at 24 h in mixed ones (57%), despite a sudden biofilm reduction in controls after 24 h might have masked the true effect of the two probiotic strains.

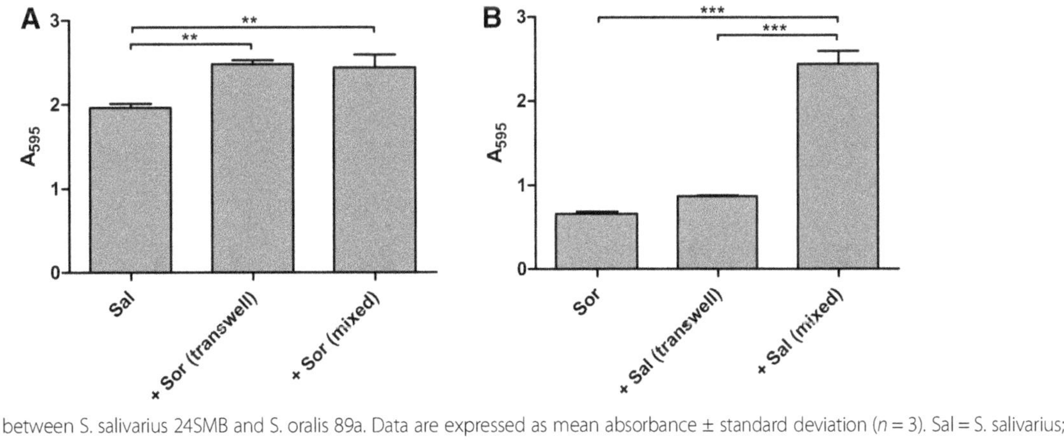

Fig. 1 Interaction between S. salivarius 24SMB and S. oralis 89a. Data are expressed as mean absorbance ± standard deviation (*n* = 3). Sal = S. salivarius; Sor = S. oralis; ** *P* ≤ 0.01; *** *P* ≤ 0.001. Panel A shows the effect of S. oralis 89a on S. salivarius 24SMB biofilm in indirect (transwell) and direct (mixed) contact. Panel B shows the effect of S. salivarius 24SMB on S. oralis 89a biofilm in indirect (transwell) and direct (mixed) contact

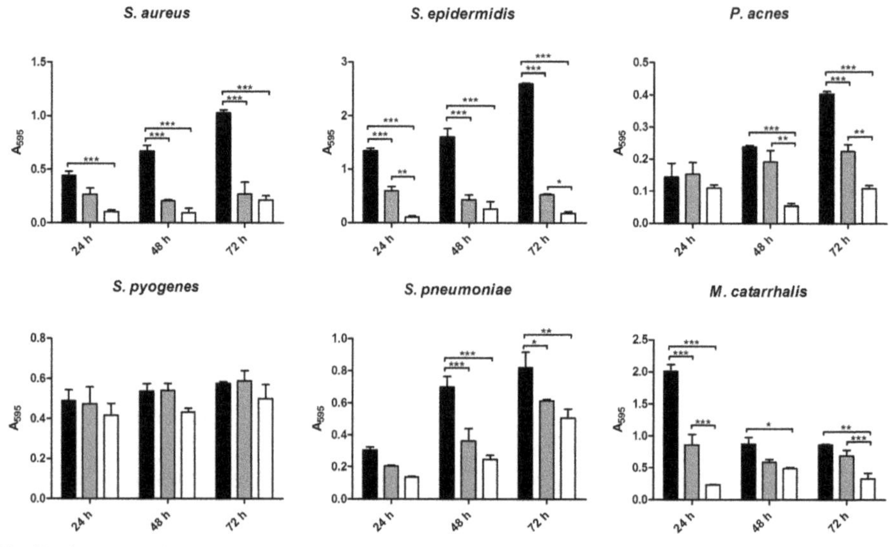

Fig. 2 Inhibition of biofilm formation during time. Data are expressed as mean absorbance ± standard deviation (n = 3). Black bars = controls; grey bars = mixed co-cultures; white bars = transwell co-cultures; * $P \leq 0.05$; ** $P \leq 0.01$; *** $P \leq 0.001$

In general, biofilm reduction was always higher in transwell experiments than in mixed ones, although such difference was not always statistically significant (Fig. 1).

Interference on pre-formed biofilm

The combination of *S. salivarius* and *S. oralis* was able to significantly disrupt the pre-formed biofilm of all tested bacteria. Conversely, *S. pyogenes* biofilm was only slightly affected by the probiotic strains (Fig. 3). After 24 h of incubation, almost the 50% of the mature biofilm of *S. aureus* was eradicated because of the presence of *S. salivarius* and *S. oralis* in both transwell and mixed experiments, and such inhibition was maintained during time. Similarly, *M. catarrhalis* biofilm was significantly reduced in experiments using the transwell system, with a constant reduction of about 50% at all the time points. On the other hand, the anti-biofilm activity of the probiotic strains against *S. epidermidis*, *P. acnes* and *S. pneumoniae* seemed to increase during time, showing the highest percentages of biofilm reduction at 72 h (64 and 68% for *S. epidermidis*, 46 and 47% for *P. acnes* and 55 and 60% for *S. pneumoniae* in transwell or mixed co-cultures, respectively).

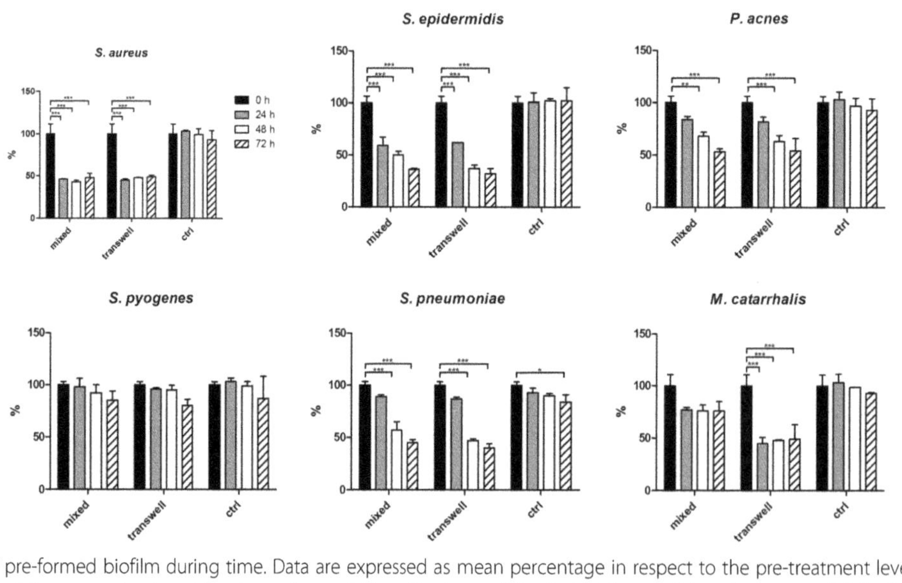

Fig. 3 Inhibition of pre-formed biofilm during time. Data are expressed as mean percentage in respect to the pre-treatment level ± standard deviation (n = 3). Black bars = pre-treatment level; grey bars = 24 h; white bars = 48 h; dashed bars = 72 h; ctrl = untreated; * $P \leq 0.05$; ** $P \leq 0.01$; *** $P \leq 0.001$

CLSM assay

The total biomass volume of samples incubated with *S. oralis* and *S. salivarius* in transwell experiments was significantly lower compared to control samples for all the tested strains (Fig. 4a). No differences in the live and dead cells ratio were found whit respect to treated and untreated biofilms (Fig. 4b). Substratum coverage was significantly lower for samples incubated with the probiotic strains than for control samples (Fig. 4c). As documented by CLSM images (Figs. 5 and 6), biofilms grown in presence of *S. oralis* and *S. salivarius* looked more scattered than control biofilms, especially those of *S. epidermidis* and *S. pneumoniae*.

CFE influence on biofilm formation

CFE had a significant inhibitory effect on all the tested strains with respect to the control biofilm growth, even if a general slight concentration-dependent effect was noticed (Fig. 7). All the other strains showed significant biofilm biomass reductions with all the formulations tested (45–50% and 41–51% for *S. aureus*, 49–77% for *M. catarrhalis*, 40–80% for *P. acnes*, 26–45% and 29–40% for *S. pneumoniae*, ½ and ¼ *v*/v respectively) with *S. epidermidis* being the most affected (78–86%). Differently, *S. pyogenes* was more recalcitrant to CFE addiction than the other tested species, with a significant reduction in the presence of higher amounts of CFE (CFE ½ v/v 35–49%). When CFEs were treated to neutralize the pH or heated at 100 °C to inactivate thermolabile molecules, a mild impairment of CFE activity was observed, but no significant differences were detected with respect to untreated CFEs (Fig. 7).

Discussion

Local administration of commensal probiotics as a sort of "bacteria-therapy", able to interfere with disease-associated disease is gaining increasing interest, finding applications in many fields [27].

Probiotics own different mechanisms that interfere with the activity of pathogenic bacteria, including: the production of antagonistic substances (e.g., bacteriocins, fatty acids, hydrogen peroxide and lactic acid), generation of environment conditions unfavorable for pathogens (e.g., competition for nutrients or pH alteration) and the competitive adhesion to human tissues preventing the colonization by harmful bacteria. Among bacterial species recently recognize as probiotic, *S. salivarius* 24SMB and *S. oralis* 89a isolated from the rhinopharynx of healthy children are suggestive strains of a healthy flora. *S. salivarius* 24SMB and *S. oralis* 89a are administered in a ratio of 98:2 by means of a nasal spray are present, with the aim of preventing ear, nose and throat diseases. The abundance of *S. salivarius* in the solution is due to its primary and predominant presence in the upper respiratory tract surfaces of humans and because its non-pathogenic behavior in healthy individuals [28]. In particular, the strain 24SMB was isolated in 2012 and selected as a promising probiotic due to the absence of virulence traits and antibiotic resistance genes and its ability to inhibit *S. pneumoniae* growth [21]. Santagati et al. demonstrated its safety and tolerability, and its capability to colonize the rhinopharynx when administrated as a nasal spray [22].

Conversely, *S. oralis* 89a was isolated from a recalcitrant healthy child during a tonsillitis outbreak and it was found to be able to inhibit the growth of group A

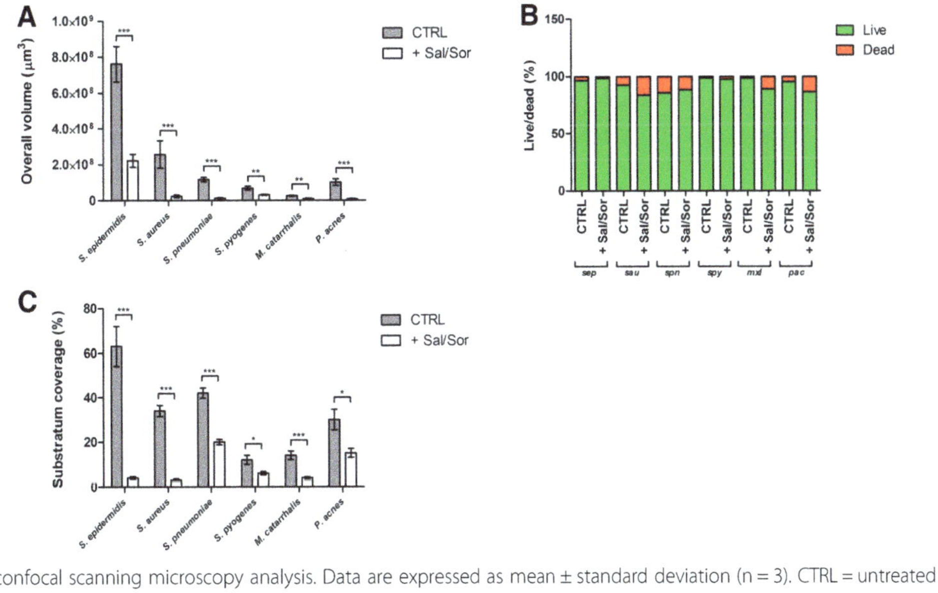

Fig. 4 Results of confocal scanning microscopy analysis. Data are expressed as mean ± standard deviation (n = 3). CTRL = untreated samples; + Sal/Sor = samples incubated with a mixture of *S. salivarius* and *S. oralis* by means of transwell inserts; sep = *S. epidermidis*; sau = *S. aureus*; spn = *S. pneumoniae*; spy = *S. pyogenes*; mxl = *M. catarrhalis*; pac = *P. acnes*; * P ≤ 0.05; ** P ≤ 0.01; *** P ≤ 0.001

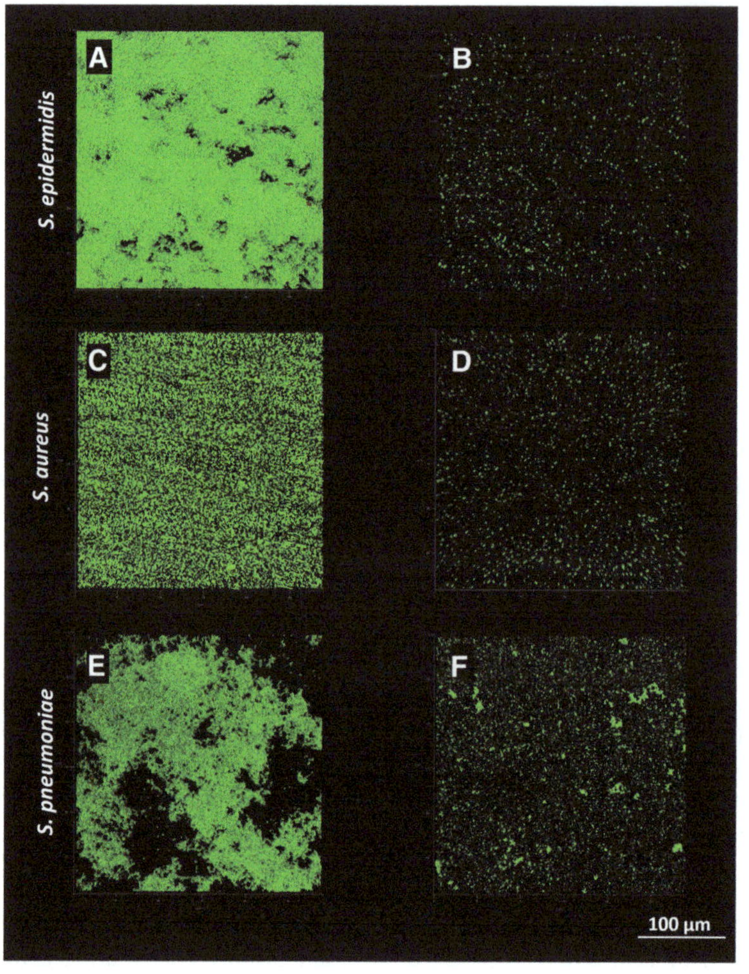

Fig. 5 Representative images of *S. epidermidis*, *S. aureus* and *S. pneumoniae* biofilms obtained by CSLM. Panels A, C and E show control biofilms, while panels B, D and F show biofilms co-cultured in presence of the probiotic strains by means of transwell inserts. Green = live cells; red = dead cells; 40× magnification

streptococci in vitro [29]. Since then, this strain has been used in in vitro and in vivo studies to evaluate its clinical effects on streptococcal tonsillitis and otitis media [19, 20, 30–32]. The whole genome of this strain was recently sequenced, identifying the gene encoding for the bacteriocin Colicin V and for tolerance to Colicin E2 [14].

As a preliminary step, the reciprocal interaction between *S. salivarius* 24SMB and *S. oralis* 89a was assessed. Using the transwell device, the two strains were physically separated by a membrane that permitted only the passage of diffusible molecules form one compartment to the other. In both cases, a significant increase in biofilm formation was observed, suggesting a possible positive synergistic effect between the two strains. Furthermore, when *S. salivarius* 24SMB and *S. oralis* 89a were simultaneously cultured in direct contact, the resulting biofilm appeared to be like the sum of the two strains grown individually. Unfortunately, the contribution of a single strains in mixed biofilms was not evaluated, being the used staining technique not species-specific, representing a limit of the study.

Then, the anti-biofilm activity resulting from the combination of *S. salivarius* 24SMB and *S. oralis* 89a against pathogens of the upper airways was investigated. In particular, the anti-biofilm activity was tested against *S. pneumoniae*, *S. pyogenes* and *M. catarrhalis* being the most common bacterial pathogens causing acute otitis media and bacterial pharyngotonsillitis [33, 34]. Moreover, the anti-biofilm effect was assessed on *S. aureus*, involved in 50% of recalcitrant chronic rhinosinusitis [35], and coagulase negative staphylococci and anaerobes, including *P. acnes* [36].

Biofilms are comprised of microorganisms enclosed in a hydrated self- produced polymeric matrix attached to a solid surface. They represent an important cause of chronic infectious diseases of the upper airways, including recurrent middle ear diseases, chronic rhinosinusitis and recurrent pharyngotonsillitis [2], but also teeth or in implant-associated infections. Biofilm-related infections

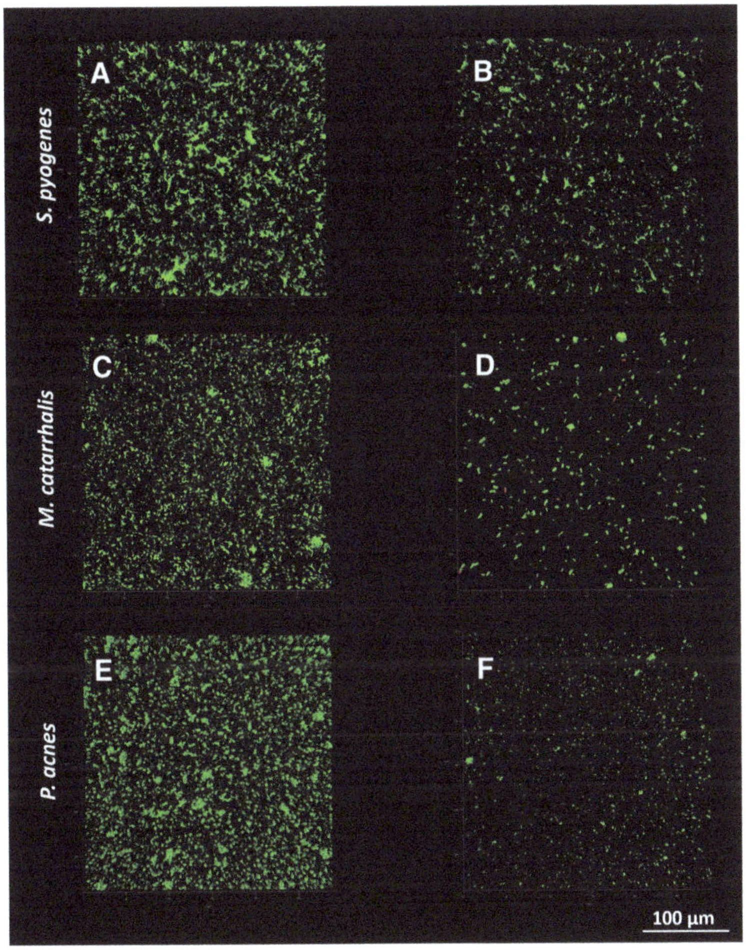

Fig. 6 Representative images of *S. pyogenes*, *M. catarrhalis* and *P. acnes* biofilms obtained by CLSM. Panels A, C and E show control biofilms, while panels B, D and F show biofilms co-cultured in presence of the probiotic strains by means of transwell inserts. Green = live cells; red = dead cells; 40× magnification

are often resistant to antibiotic therapy, posing serious concerns about the infection control. Frequent antibiotic intakes may have deleterious effects due to the depletion of the commensal microbiome and the subsequent colonization by microorganisms that are less susceptible to the prescribed antibiotics [37]. In this context, the use of probiotics able to disperse pathogens biofilm may be therapeutically beneficial and may offer a valid alternative or a coadjuvant treatment to conventional antimicrobials.

With the aim to test the aforementioned hypothesis, in the present study, co-culture experiments by means of the direct or indirect culture of the probiotic strains with the respiratory tract pathogens was performed. The combination of probiotics was able to both inhibit the biofilm development and to disperse the already established biofilms of all the tested pathogens with the exception of *S. pyogenes*. This behavior is not surprising; the inhibitory activity of *S. salivarius* 24SMB against *S. pyogenes* depends on the choice of the growth media [21]. Indeed, Santagati and co-workers described how *S. salivarius* was not able to inhibit *S. pyogenes* in Todd Hewitt broth supplemented with blood, while an increase in the inhibitory activity was observed on Columbia blood agar. In our experimental setting, the lack of activity against *S. pyogenes* could also be explained by the lack of supplementation of yeast extract, glucose or calcium salts in the growth medium, which are necessary supplement for an optimal production of bacteriocins [38, 39].

A more detailed investigation was carried out by CLSM analysis, which considered additional outcome variables as live/dead cells ratio and percentage of substratum coverage. Specifically, the total biomass volume was significantly lower when the tested pathogens were incubated with probiotics compared to that of controls. Differently to what observed in the spectrophotometric assay, the higher sensitivity of the CLSM analysis allowed to appreciate a significant biomass reduction also for *S. pyogenes*. Indeed, while the spectrophotometric assay allows the

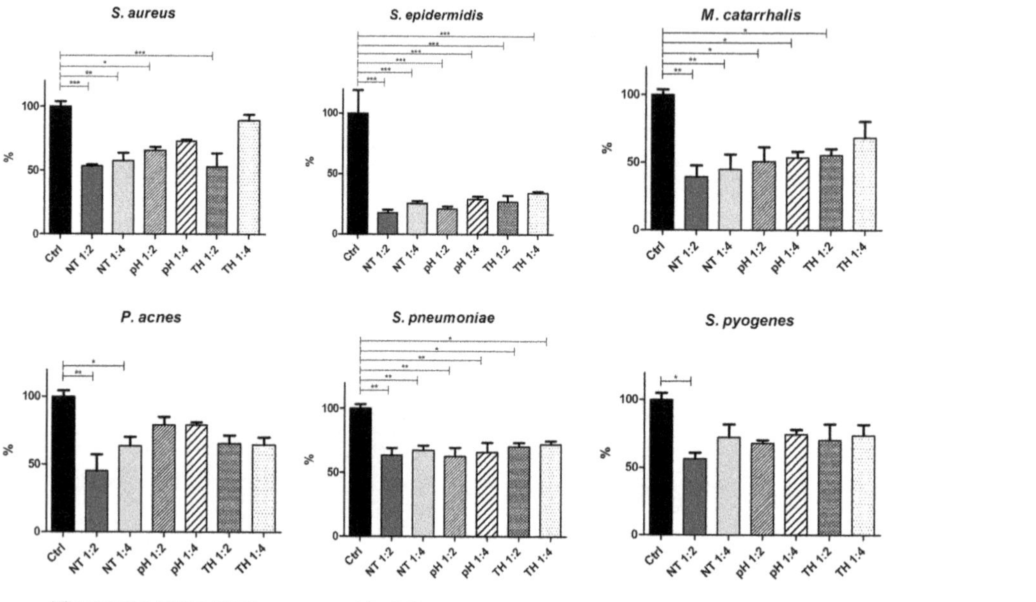

Fig. 7 Inhibition of biofilm formation by cell-free extracts. Data are expressed as mean percentage in respect to biofilm growth control in fresh BHI broth. Black bars = control; grey tone bars = untreated cell-free extract (NT); slanted lines bars = pH neutralized cell-free extract (pH); dotted bars = heat inactivated cell-free extract (TH). * P ≤ 0.05; ** P ≤ 0.01; *** P ≤ 0.001

semi-quantitative measurement of the air-dried biofilm biomass, CLSM gives the possibility to collect three-dimensional images of hydrated biological structures without fixation [40]. This non-destructive technique has radically transformed optical imaging in biology and microbiology, providing a useful tool for the examination of the structure of biofilms.

Concerning the live to dead cells ratio, no differences between treated and untreated samples were found, indicating a prevalent inhibitory effect rather than a potential bactericidal activity of the probiotic strains. On the contrary, substratum coverage was significantly lower in treated biofilms, with particular regard to that of *S. epidermidis* and *S. aureus*, which appeared more scattered than controls.

Recent studies shown that chemical interactions through secretion of molecules by different microbial species may affect spatial biofilm structure, regulating both its formation and dispersion [41–43]. Recently, Santagati et al. described the presence of a blpU-like bacteriocine cassette in the genome of *S. salivarius* 24SMB, which has been shown to mediate intra- and interspecies competition with inhibitory activity against *S. pyogenes* and *S. pneumoniae* and also to provide competitive advantage in colonization in vivo [15, 44]. However, no other genes responsible for production of bacteriocine (i.e. salivaricins, commonly produced by other *S. salivarius* strains) were identified throughout the genome [15]. Similarly, *S. oralis* 89a possess a locus for the production of a Colicin V, a proteolitically processed peptide antibiotic, which kills sensitive cells by disrupting membrane potential [45]. Interestingly, *S. oralis* 89a is characterized by the presence of *luxS* gene, responsible for the production of the quorum-sensing molecule AI-2, involved in cell-to-cell communication and able to influence the expression of virulence factors, motility and biofilm formation [46]. In particular, controlled concentrations of AI-2 are able to promote mutualistic biofilm formation and to influence structure and composition of other commensal streptococcal species biofilm [47, 48]. Unluckily, the genome sequence of *S. salivarius* 24SMB is not available in public databases and no information on the presence of quorum-sensing clusters involved in biofilm formation and regulation (e.g., Rgg transcriptional regulators family) are available.

Nonetheless, signaling is restricted only to those species with appropriate receptors, suggesting that other kind of unspecific interactions may play an important role in determining biofilm spatial structure [49]. For example, metabolic end products like lactic acid and hydrogen peroxide produced by streptococci,

can act with a broader spectrum by cause acid and oxidative stress, respectively. As expected, the presence of *S. salivarius* 24SMB and *S. oralis* 89a in the co-cultures slightly lowered the pH in all the cases except for *S. pyogenes* and *S. pneumoniae* (data shown in Additional file 1). Since the inhibitory activity was observed also for the two streptococci, it can be supposed that alteration in pH is not the only mechanism of action, but other specific interactions might occur.

Finally, a high reduction of biofilm biomass in transwell co-cultures was observed. This event might suggest that the anti-biofilm activity of the probiotic mixture is mediated by diffusible molecules secreted by the probiotic strains, rather than depending on a mechanism requiring physical contact. This was confirmed by supplementation of the cell-free extract to the medium, displaying an effect comparable to that observed in the transwell co-culture. In the attempt to elucidate the nature of the inhibition, the cell-free extracts were neutralized to a pH of 7.0, to evaluate the contribution of the acidic environment resulting from the streptococcal fermentation or were heated, to eliminate all the thermolabile secreted molecules. Even though, both the treatments did not completely impair the inhibitory effect of the cell-free extract, indicating a likely multifactorial and strain-specific strategy. Furthermore, the contribution to biofilm formation between pathogenic and probiotic strains in mixed species biofilms was not discriminated. Indeed, mixed biofilms were not analyzed by confocal microscopy, because of the lack of species-specific dyes able to differentiate the presence of different microbes. Stains able to discriminate among different bacteria should be used in future studies in order to investigate the role of probiotic strains in the biofilm production by pathogenic bacteria.

As the goal of the probiotics tested in this study is to create a barrier against pathogens, an interesting issue would be to investigate if pathogens are able to invade and establish within pre-existing probiotic biofilms.

Conclusions

In this preliminary study, we demonstrated the capability of *S. salivarius* and *S. oralis* to interfere with the biofilm formation capacity of the upper airways pathogens and disperse their pre-formed biofilms. The nature of inhibition seems to be multifactorial, involving both specific and unspecific mechanisms. However, additional studies are required to get further insights into the mechanisms underlying these interactions at molecular level.

Abbreviations

CLSM: Confocal laser scan microscopy; URTIs: Upper respiratory tract infections

Acknowledgements

Not applicable.

Funding

This work was supported by Consorzio Milano Ricerche (Milan, Italy). The sponsor was not involved in study design, in the collection, analysis and interpretation of data, the writing of the report nor in the decision to submit the article for publication.

Authors' contributions

AB, LD and MG conceived and designed the experiments. AB, RDG, MB and MT performed the experiments. AB, RDG, MB, MT and EDV analysed the data. AB prepared figures and graphs and wrote the manuscript. LD, EDV, MG revised the manuscript. All the authors read and approved the final manuscript.

Consent for publication

Not applicable.

Competing interests

The authors declare that the research was conducted in the absence of any commercial or financial relationships that could be construed as a potential conflict of interest.

Author details

[1]Laboratory of Clinical Chemistry and Microbiology, IRCCS Orthopedic Institute Galeazzi, Milan, Italy. [2]Department of Biomedical Sciences for Health, Laboratory of Clinical Microbiology, University of Milan, Milan, Italy. [3]Department of Basic Medical Science, Otolaryngology Unit, Neuroscience and Sensory Organs, University of Bari Aldo Moro, Bari, Italy.

References

1. Morris DP. Bacterial biofilm in upper respiratory tract infections. Curr Infect Dis Rep. 2007;9:186–92.
2. Nazzari E, Torretta S, Pignataro L, Marchisio P, Esposito S. Role of biofilm in children with recurrent upper respiratory tract infections. Eur J Clin Microbiol Infect Dis. 2015;34:421–9. https://doi.org/10.1007/s10096-014-2261-1.
3. Danielsen KA, Eskeland O, Fridrich-Aas K, Orszagh VC, Bachmann-Harildstad G, Burum-Auensen E. Bacterial biofilms in patients with chronic rhinosinusitis: a confocal scanning laser microscopy study. Rhinology. 2014; 52:150–5. https://doi.org/10.3109/00016489.2015.1092169.
4. Hall-Stoodley L, Costerton JW, Stoodley P. Bacterial biofilms: from the natural environment to infectious diseases. Nat Rev Microbiol. 2004;2:95–108. https://doi.org/10.1038/nrmicro821.
5. Hall-Stoodley L, Stoodley P. Evolving concepts in biofilm infections. Cell Microbiol. 2009;11:1034–43. https://doi.org/10.1038/nrmicro821.
6. Yaguchi T, Dwidar M, Byun CK, Leung B, Lee S, Cho YK, et al. Aqueous two-phase system-derived biofilms for bacterial interaction studies. Biomacromolecules. 2012;13:2655–61. https://doi.org/10.1021/bm300500y.
7. Wang Z, Xiang Q, Yang T, Li L, Yang J, Li H, et al. Autoinducer-2 of Streptococcus mitis as a target molecule to inhibit pathogenic multi-species biofilm formation *in vitro* and in an endotracheal intubation rat model. Front Microbiol. 2016;7:e88. https://doi.org/10.3389/fmicb.2016.00088.
8. Goers L, Freemont P, Polizzi KM. Co-culture systems and technologies: taking synthetic biology to the next level. J R Soc Interface. 2014;11. https://doi.org/10.1098/rsif.2014.0065.
9. Bernstein JM, Sagahtaheri-Altaie S, Dryja DM, Wactawski-Wende J. Bacterial interference in nasopharyngeal bacterial flora of otitis-prone and non-otitis-prone children. Acta Otorhinolaryngol. 1994;48:1–9.
10. Fujimori I, Hisamatsu K, Kikushima K, Goto R, Murakami Y, Yamada T. The nasopharyngeal bacterial flora in children with otitis media with effusion. Eur Arch Otorhinolaryngol. 1996;253:260–3.
11. FAO/WHO Expert Consultation. Health and Nutritional Properties of Probiotics in Food including Powder Milk with Live Lactic Acid Bacteria, 2001.
12. Carlsson J, Grahnen H, Jonsson G, Wikner S. Early establishment of Streptococcus salivarius in the mouth of infants. J Dent Res. 1970;49:415–8.
13. Kazor CE, Mitchell PM, Lee AM, Stokes LN, Loesche WJ, Dewhirst FE, et al. Diversity of bacterial populations on the tongue dorsa of patients with halitosis and healthy patients. J Clin Microbiol. 2003;41:558–63.
14. Sidjabat HE. Grahn Håkansson E, and Cervin ADraft genome sequence of the oral commensal Streptococcus oralis 89a with interference activity

against respiratory pathogens. Genome Announc. 2016;4:e01546. https://doi.org/10.1128/genomeA.01546-15.

15. Santagati M, Scillato M, Stefani S. Genetic organization of Streptococcus salivarius 24SMBc blp-like bacteriocin locus. Front Biosci (Schol Ed). 2018; 1(10):238–47.
16. Jimenez JC, Federle MJ. Quorum sensing in group A Streptococcus. Front Cell Infect Microbiol. 2014;12(4):127. https://doi.org/10.3389/fcimb.2014.00127.
17. Fiedler T, Riani C, Koczan D, Standar K, Kreikemeyer B, Podbielski A. Protective mechanisms of respiratory tract streptococci against Streptococcus pyogenes biofilm formation and epithelial cell infection. Appl Environ Microbiol. 2013;79:1265–76. https://doi.org/10.1128/AEM.03350-12.
18. Li J, Helmerhorst EJ, Leone CW, Troxler RF, Yaskell T, Haffajee AD, et al. Identification of early microbial colonizers in human dental biofilm. J Appl Microbiol. 2004;97:1311–8. https://doi.org/10.1111/j.1365-2672.2004.02420.x.
19. Roos K, Håkansson EG, Holm S. Effect of recolonisation with "interfering" alpha streptococci on recurrences of acute and secretory otitis media in children: randomised placebo-controlled trial. BMJ. 2001;322:210–2.
20. Skovbjerg S, Roos K, Holm SE, Grahn Håkansson E, Nowrouzian F, Ivarsson M, et al. Spray bacteriotherapy decreases middle ear fluid in children with secretory otitis media. Arch Dis Child. 2009;94:92–8. https://doi.org/10.1136/adc.2008.137414.
21. Santagati M, Scillato M, Patanè F, Aiello C, Stefani S. Bacteriocin-producing oral streptococci and inhibition of respiratory pathogens. FEMS Immunol Med Microbiol. 2012;65:23–31. https://doi.org/10.1111/j.1574-695X.2012.00928.x.
22. Santagati M, Scillato M, Muscaridola N, Metoldo V, La Mantia I, Stefani S. Colonization, safety, and tolerability study of the Streptococcus salivarius 24SMBc nasal spray for its application in upper respiratory tract infections. Eur J Clin Microbiol Infect Dis. 2015;34:2075–80. https://doi.org/10.1007/s10096-015-2454-2.
23. Marchisio P, Santagati M, Scillato M, Baggi E, Fattizzo M, Rosazza C, et al. Streptococcus salivarius 24SMB administered by nasal spray for the prevention of acute otitis media in otitis-prone children. Eur J Clin Microbiol Infect Dis. 2015;34:2377–83. https://doi.org/10.1007/s10096-015-2491-x.
24. Drago L, Vassena C, Saibene AM, Del Fabbro M, Felisati G. A case of coinfection in a chronic maxillary sinusitis of odontogenic origin: identification of Dialister pneumosintes. J Endod. 2013;39:1084–47. https://doi.org/10.1016/j.joen.2013.04.025.
25. Christensen GD, Simpson WA, Younger JJ, Baddour LM, Barrett FF, Melton DM, et al. Adherence of coagulase-negative staphylococci to plastic tissue culture plates: a quantitative model for the adherence of staphylococci to medical devices. J Clin Microbiol. 1985;22:996–1006.
26. Standar K, Kreikemeyer B, Redanz S, Münter WL, Laue M, Podbielski A. Setup of an *in vitro* test system for basic studies on biofilm behavior of mixed-species cultures with dental and periodontal pathogens. PLoS One. 2010;5:e13135. https://doi.org/10.1371/journal.pone.0013135.
27. Singh VP, Sharma J, Babu S. Rizwanulla, Singla a. role of probiotics in health and disease: a review. J Pak Med Assoc. 2013;63(2):253–7.
28. Wescombe PA, Heng NC, Burton JP, Chilcott CN, Tagg JR. Streptococcal bacteriocins and the case for Streptococcus salivarius as model oral probiotics. Future Microbiol. 2009;4:819–35. https://doi.org/10.2217/fmb.09.61.
29. Grahn E, Holm SE. Bacterial interference in the throat flora during a streptococcal tonsillitis outbreak in an apartment house area. Zentralbl Bakteriol Mikrobiologie Hyg. 1983;256:72–9.
30. Roos K, Grahn E, Lind L, Holm S. Treatment of recurrent streptococcal tonsillitis by recolonization with alpha-streptococci. Eur J Clin Microbiol Infect Dis. 1989;8:318–9.
31. Roos K, Grahn E, Holm SE, Johansson H, Lind L. Interfering alpha-streptococci as a protection against recurrent streptococcal tonsillitis in children. Int J Pediatr Otorhinolaryngol. 1993;25:141–8.
32. Rods K, Holm SE, Grahn-Håkansson E, Lagergren L. Recolonization with selected alpha-streptococci for prophylaxis of recurrent streptococcal pharyngotonsillitis - a randomized placebo-controlled multicenter study. Scand J Infect Dis. 1996;28:459–62.
33. Worrall G. Acute otitis media. Can Fam Physician. 2007;53:2147–8.
34. Murray RC, Chennupati SK. Chronic streptococcal and non streptococcal pharyngitis. Infect Disord Drug Targets. 2012;12:281–5.
35. Foreman A, Boase S, Psaltis A, Wormald PJ. Role of bacterial and fungal biofilms in chronic rhinosinusitis. Curr Allergy Asthma Rep. 2012;12:127–35.
36. Stressmann FA, Rogers GB, Chan SW, Howarth PH, Harries PG, Bruce KD, et al. Characterization of bacterial community diversity in chronic rhinosinusitis infections using novel culture-independent techniques. Am J Rhinol Allergy. 2011;25:e133ee140. https://doi.org/10.2500/ajra.2011.25.3628.
37. Liu CM, Soldanova K, Nordstrom L, Dwan MG, Moss OL, Contente-Cuomo TL, et al. Medical therapy reduces microbiota diversity and evenness in surgically recalcitrant chronic rhinosinusitis. Int Forum Allergy Rhinol. 2013;3:775–81. https://doi.org/10.1002/alr.21195.
38. Riley MA, Chavan MA. Bacteriocin: ecology and evolution. Berlin: Springer-Verlag; 2007.
39. Therdtatha P, Tandumrongpong C, Pilasombut K, Matsusaki H, Keawsompong S, Nitisinprasert S. Characterization of antimicrobial substance from lactobacillus salivarius KL-D4 and its application as biopreservative for creamy filling. Springerplus. 2016;5:e1060. https://doi.org/10.1186/s40064-016-2693-4.
40. Khajotia SS, Smart KH, Pilula M, Thompson DM. Concurrent quantification of cellular and extracellular components of biofilms. J Vis Exp. 2013;10:e50639. https://doi.org/10.3791/50639.
41. Davies DG, Marques CN. A fatty acid messenger is responsible for inducing dispersion in microbial biofilms. J Bacteriol. 2009;191:1393–403. https://doi.org/10.1128/JB.01214-08.
42. Iwase T, Uehara Y, Shinji H, Tajima A, Seo H, Takada K, et al. Staphylococcus epidermidis Esp inhibits Staphylococcus aureus biofilm formation and nasal colonization. Nature. 2010;465:346–9. https://doi.org/10.1038/nature09074.
43. Armbruster CE, Hong W, Pang B, Weimer KE, Juneau RA, Turner J, et al. Indirect pathogenicity of Haemophilus influenzae and Moraxella catarrhalis in polymicrobial otitis media occurs via interspecies quorum signaling. mBio. 2014;1:e00102. https://doi.org/10.1128/mBio.00102-10.
44. Dawid S, Roche AM, Weiser JN. The blp bacteriocins of Streptococcus pneumoniae mediate intraspecies competition both *in vitro* and *in vivo*. Infect Immun. 2007;75(1):443–51. https://doi.org/10.1128/IAI.01775-05.
45. Yang CC, Konisky J. Colicin V-treated Escherichia coli does not generate membrane potential. J Bacteriol. 1987;158(2):757–9.
46. Pereira CS, Thompson JA, Xavier KB. AI-2-mediated signalling in bacteria. FEMS Microbiol Rev. 2013;37(2):156–81. https://doi.org/10.1111/j.1574-6976.2012.00345.x.
47. Cuadra-Saenz G, Rao DL, Underwood AJ, Belapure SA, Campagna SR, Sun Z, et al. Autoinducer-2 influences interactions amongst pioneer colonizing streptococci in oral biofilms. Microbiology. 2012;158(Pt 7):1783–95. https://doi.org/10.1099/mic.0.057182-0.
48. Rickard AH, Palmer RJ Jr, Blehert DS, Campagna SR, Semmelhack MF, Egland PG, et al. Autoinducer 2: a concentration-dependent signal for mutualistic bacterial biofilm growth. Mol Microbiol. 2006;60(6):1446–56. https://doi.org/10.1111/j.1365-2958.2006.05202.x.
49. Stacy A, McNally L, Darch SE, Brown SP, Whiteley M. The biogeography of polymicrobial infection. Nat Rev Microbiol. 2016;14:93–105. https://doi.org/10.1038/nrmicro.2015.8.

21

Improving detection of tuberculosis among household contacts of index tuberculosis patients by an integrated approach in Myanmar

Kyaw Ko Ko Htet[1], Tippawan Liabsuetrakul[2*], Saw Thein[3], Edward B. McNeil[2] and Virasakdi Chongsuvivatwong[2]

Abstract

Background: Contact tracing for tuberculosis (TB) is a recommended measure to improve the case detection rate; however, actual implementation in Myanmar is limited and low detection rates have been reported. Household contacts of a known index TB case are at high risk of infection, thus a more strategic action for contact tracing is required to achieve the goal of the World Health Organization End TB Strategy. This study aimed to assess TB case detection rates among household contacts by an integrated approach and identify risk factors for TB.

Methods: A cross-sectional study was conducted in Mandalay City, Myanmar. Household contacts of index TB cases who had been receiving treatment for at least 3 months were prospectively investigated by an integrated approach which included modification of screening methods and active facilitation of screening investigations as follows. Initial chest x-ray (CXR) was performed for all contacts at the responsible facilities followed by sputum specimen collection for those aged ≥15 years and gene Xpert MTB/RIF examination. Transportation of all household contacts to health facilities and transportation of sputum samples for smear and gene Xpert MTB/RIF examination at centers were arranged by the research team to ensure that all household contacts received all investigations. Risk factors for TB among household contacts were identified by multiple logistic regression models.

Results: Of 174 household contacts, 115 were ≥ 15 years and 59 were < 15 years. The percentage of TB cases detected among the household contacts was 13.8%. There were 14 (12.2%) positive TB cases among the 115 contacts aged ≥15 years while 10 (16.9%) of those aged < 15 years had clinical signs and symptoms of TB with an abnormal CXR. Risk factors among household contacts for TB were being a caretaker of an index case, active and passive smoking, and drinking alcohol.

Conclusions: The integrated approach of TB contact tracing by special arrangement for CXR, sputum and gene Xpert MTB/RIF examination yielded a high TB detection rate in a high TB prevalence area. Logistic and financial administration is needed to strengthen contact tracing. Further research on high-risk household contacts should be considered for increasing TB detection rates.

Keywords: Tuberculosis, Screening, Case detection, Determinants, Contact tracing

* Correspondence: ltippawa@yahoo.com
[2]Epidemiology Unit, Faculty of Medicine, Prince of Songkla University, Hat Yai, Songkhla 90110, Thailand
Full list of author information is available at the end of the article

Background

Tuberculosis (TB) remains one of the top common infectious diseases, which is a global concern. The World Health Organization (WHO) estimated that two-fifths of new TB cases are undiagnosed and more country-specific actions are needed to identify these missing cases to achieve the global goal of ending the TB epidemic by 2035 [1]. Contact tracing among household family members is one of the active case-finding strategies that has been proposed to increase the case detection rate [2]. In 95 studies from low- and middle-income settings included in a systematic review, the prevalence of TB from household contact tracing varied from 2.1 to 10.1% [3, 4]. Efforts for early diagnosis of TB through effective case finding programs are needed to reduce the rate of TB transmission and to reduce the case detection gap.

Due to the limitations of current passive case-finding strategies and the global urgency to improve TB case-detection rates, WHO has called for more evidence on innovative ways of TB screening, especially from low-income countries. An integrated approach among individuals who are presumed to have TB but do not present to a health service (as commonly seen in the passive case finding approach), has gained interest to enhance the detection rate for early diagnosis and treatment of TB in high prevalence countries [5].

Myanmar is one of the 30 high TB burden countries with an estimated incidence of 365 TB cases per 100,000 population and a high death rate of 49 per 100,000 population in 2015 [1]. For contact investigations, WHO recommends the use of signs and symptoms consistent with TB followed by either acid-fast bacilli (AFB) smear or Chest X Ray (CXR) for contacts aged 10 years or above and less than 10 years, respectively [6]. However, the national guideline of the National Tuberculosis Programme (NTP), Myanmar has applied a diagnosis of TB for those aged < 15 years with signs and symptoms of TB based on CXR due to difficulty in performing the gastric lavage for sputum specimens. In addition, the community-based active case finding through community mobilization, symptom screening and referral, and contact tracing is recommended and the Gene Xpert Mycobacterium tuberculosis/Rifampicin (gene Xpert MTB/RIF examination) is performed in the contacts of multi-drug resistance TB, TB/HIV co-infected patients, TB defaulters and smear positive TB cases [7].

Although the policy of contact tracing has been adopted in Myanmar, there are still constraints and barriers to actually implement and improve TB case detection among household contacts. Therefore, this study aimed to assess TB case detection rates from an integrated approach using a modification of screening methods and active facilitation of screening investigations in Myanmar. Risk factors for TB among household contacts were also identified.

Methods

Study design and setting

A cross-sectional study was conducted in Mandalay City, Myanmar from September 2015 to February 2016. Mandalay City is a densely populated area located in the central region of Myanmar containing seven township health departments (THD). TB prevention and control is mainly based on a passive, not active, case finding strategy including screening of TB signs and symptoms followed by CXR among contacts aged < 15 years and sputum examination with CXR among household contacts aged ≥15 years. The community health personnel at each health facility of THD is responsible for TB screening and collection of sputum specimens. The heads of each household were informed about the importance of transporting the sputum samples to a health facility and ensuring that their household members have a CXR performed at a responsible health facility. CXR facilities are available at Mandalay General Hospital and THD in Amarapura Township, Mandalay City.

Study participants and methods

Index pulmonary TB patients who had been receiving treatment for at least 3 months under the NTP were identified. Temporary residents and those who lived alone or in a temple were excluded due to difficulty in identifying household contacts [8]. Those whose household contacts were not available for interview were also excluded. Sample size for household contacts was calculated based on the one-group precision formula. According to the previous prevalence of TB among household contacts of index TB cases estimated to be 0.13 [8], a type I error of 5% and a precision of 5%, at least 174 household contacts were required. With this sample size, we estimated that 60 index TB cases would be sufficient.

The integrated approach included active facilitation of screening investigations as follows. Initial CXR was performed for all contacts regardless of having signs and symptoms at the responsible facilities followed by sputum specimen collection and gene Xpert MTB/RIF examination for those aged ≥15 years as per the national guideline. For active facilitation of investigations in the initial research protocol, the contacts were encouraged to perform CXR at nearby health facilities and the sputum was collected and sent for further examination by the research team rather than the responsible THD personnel.

In the preparatory phase of the study, we observed that no contacts went to have a CXR by their own arrangement. Therefore, transportation to CXR health facilities for household contacts was arranged by the research team as follows. First, the research team drew a road map for transportation arrangement. Second, appointments were made at times that were convenient to the household contacts. Third, a passenger vehicle with a maximum capacity of 25 persons was organized to transport all contacts whose homes were on or near the same route to the nearby health facilities. Fourth, CXRs for all contacts was facilitated at health facilities and afterwards the contacts were taken back home. Facilitation of transportation for the household contacts to radiography facilities and the sputum specimens to examination facilities were considered as the key enablers of improving case detection rates of TB among household contacts. The assumption of this integrated approach is to enhance the feasibility of complete specimen capture and transport to diagnostic facilities.

Study sampling

The list of index TB cases receiving treatment for at least 3 months was obtained from the township TB register. From this list, the number of index TB cases was estimated and randomly selected using simple random sampling in order to obtain a sufficient number of household contacts. The research team then contacted the health staff to facilitate home visits of the sampled index TB cases. During these home visits, the inclusion and exclusion criteria of the index TB cases were considered. A second round of sampling of index TB cases was performed in order to achieve the required sample size.

Data collection

The index TB cases and their household contacts were then informed about the study including all investigations required and those who were willing to participate in the study were asked to sign a consent form independently and separately. The index TB cases and their respective household contacts were then interviewed for background and health-related characteristics by face-to-face interviews using a structured questionnaire.

A Garmin global positioning system (GPS) Colorado 300 device was used to record the distance of their location to health facilities [9]. The research team drew a road map and determined the closest responsible CXR facility based on the GPS and then arranged group transportation for the household contacts living in the same areas to the closest health facility. After the community health personnel in each assigned area collected the sputum specimen from household contacts, the research team transported the sputum specimens to the health facility for AFB or gene Xpert MTB/RIF examination. All of the above steps above were carried out prospectively. The results of all screening tests were interpreted by the responsible providers independently and blindingly.

Variables

The outcome variable was operationally defined as the positive TB detection of household contacts which was classified as one of the following conditions: (1) abnormal CXR suggestive of TB and the presence of any signs and symptoms of suspected TB among the household contacts aged < 15 years or along with positive sputum AFB or gene Xpert MTB/RIF assay among the household contacts aged ≥15 years, or (2) positive sputum with the presence of at least one AFB in at least one sputum sample among the household contacts aged ≥15 years. Contacts aged < 15 years without abnormal CXR finding were treated with antibiotics and observed for clinical response for at least two weeks according to the national guideline if they had one or more of the following symptoms: cough lasting 2 weeks or more, blood in sputum, fever lasting more than 2 weeks, weight loss and chest pain. The same treatment was given to the contacts aged ≥15 years who had abnormal CXR without confirmation with sputum AFB or gene Xpert MTB/RIF examinations.

Independent variables included background characteristics such as gender, age, ethnicity, education level, occupation, marital status, daily income, living alone in a separate room, number of persons living together, sharing a room with an index TB case and caretaker to index TB case, and health related risky characteristics such as active smoking status (never, former or current), smoking duration and intensity, passive smoking status, drinking status (never, former or current) and presence of any signs and symptoms of TB. Point coordinate data for location was collected as longitude and latitude to measure distance between patient's residences to the nearest CXR center.

Statistical analysis

All data were entered into EpiData and analyzed using R (2013 The R Foundation for Statistical Computing). The characteristics and information of index TB cases and their household contacts were presented descriptively using frequencies and percentages. The determinants of positive TB among household contacts were initially explored using univariate analysis and the variables having a p-value less than 0.2 were included in the initial multivariate logistic regression model. Variables having a p-value of < 0.05 were kept in the final model and considered as statistically significant.

Results

Of 308 index TB cases identified, 40 were included in the study together with 174 household contacts from two rounds of sampling. The diagram flow of study sampling is shown in Fig. 1. There were 34 index TB cases excluded due to living alone ($n = 2$), temporary resident ($n = 15$), and having no household contacts available ($n = 17$). The median duration of TB treatment was 4.1 months (Interquartile range - IQR: 3.2–4.8).

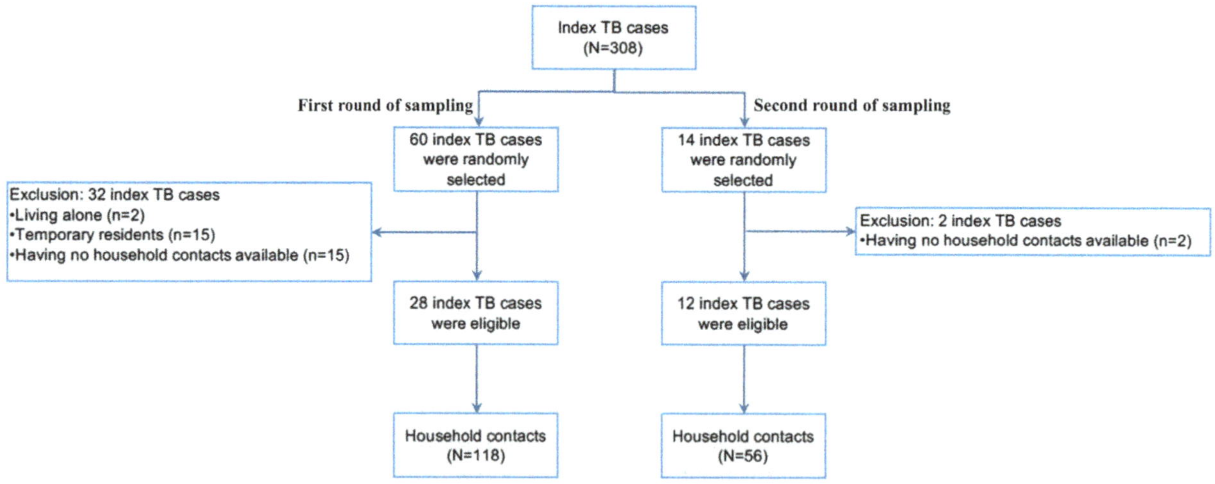

Fig. 1 Diagram flow of study sampling for index TB cases

Tables 1 and 2 present the background and health-related risk characteristics of the study index TB cases and household contacts, respectively. Males accounted for > 70% of index TB cases and 40% of household contacts. The mean ± standard deviation (SD) age was 34.6 ± 17.9 years for index TB cases and 28.9 ± 19 years for household contacts. Of the 174 contacts, 115 were aged ≥15 years (median age = 9, IQR 6–10) and 59 were aged < 15 years (median age = 38, IQR 29–50). Contacts aged under five years accounted for 4.6%. The average number of household contacts in a family was 4.0 (SD = 1.9, range 2–10). Among TB index cases, 30% were former or current smokers while the rate among household contacts was 18.4%. The prevalence of former or current drinking was 15% for both groups. Approximately 44% of contacts had signs and symptoms of TB.

Table 1 Background characteristics of index TB cases and household contacts

Variable	Index TB cases		Household contacts	
	(*n* = 40)		(*n* = 174)	
	n	(%)	n	(%)
Gender				
Male	29	(72.5)	71	(40.8)
Female	11	(27.5)	103	(59.2)
Age (years)				
< 15	7	(17.5)	59	(33.9)
≥15	33	(82.5)	115	(66.1)
Education				
None	15	(37.5)	57	(32.8)
Primary School	16	(40.0)	62	(35.6)
Middle School	3	(7.5)	38	(21.8)
High/Graduate School	6	(15.0)	17	(9.8)
Occupation				
Factory worker	12	(30.0)	47	(27.0)
Casual employee	12	(30.0)	37	(21.3)
Dependent/student	16	(40.0)	90	(51.7)
Marital Status				
Single	12	(30.0)	89	(51.1)
Married	28	(70.0)	85	(48.9)

TB tuberculosis

Table 2 Health related risky characteristics of index TB cases and household contacts

Variable	Index TB cases		Household contacts	
	(*n* = 40)		(*n* = 174)	
	n	(%)	n	(%)
Smoking status				
Never smoker	28	(70.0)	142	(81.6)
Former or current smoker	12	(30.0)	32	(18.4)
Number of cigarettes smoked per day among former or current smokers				
Mean (SD)	3.8	(1.0)	2.9	(1.9)
Duration of smoking (years) among former or current smokers				
< 20	6	(50.0)	20	(62.5)
≥ 20	6	(50.0)	12	(37.5)
Passive smoking status				
No	35	(87.5)	115	(66.1)
Yes	5	(12.5)	59	(33.9)
Drinking status				
Never drinker	34	(85.0)	149	(85.6)
Former or current drinker	6	(15.0)	25	(14.4)
Duration of drinking (years) among former or current drinkers				
Mean (SD)	9.6	(3.4)	6.3	(6.1)

TB tuberculosis, *SD* standard deviation

Of the 174 household contacts, abnormal CXR suggestive of TB was found in 27 contacts, of which 17 and 10 were aged ≥15 years and < 15 years, respectively. Among the 17 contacts aged ≥15 years with abnormal CXR, 9 were confirmed positive for TB by AFB, 5 by gene Xpert MTB/RIF examination, and 3 were negative, all of which were followed up by the responsible THD. The overall rate of positive TB detection among household contacts was 13.8%, of which 12.2% and 16.9% were detected among contacts aged ≥15 years ($n = 14/115$) and those aged < 15 years ($n = 10/59$), respectively. The distance from contacts' home to the responsible CXR facility at Amarapura township ranged from 1.1 to 9.7 km and at Mandalay General Hospital ranged from 2.9 to 17.5 km.

Table 3 shows results of the univariate analysis for identifying determinants of positive TB among household contacts. Significant factors were male gender, sharing a room with an index TB case, being a caretaker to an index TB case, current or passive smoker, and current or former drinker. Table 4 shows the results of the final multiple logistic regression model for predicting TB among household contacts. Significant risk factors were being caretaker of an index TB case, active smoker, passive smoker, and former or current drinker (Table 4).

Discussion

The integrated approach of TB contact tracing by special arrangement for CXR, sputum and Gene Xpert examination yielded a high rate of TB detection among household contacts in a high TB prevalence area. The determinants of positive TB among household contacts were being a caretaker of an index TB case, active and passive smoking, and former or current alcohol drinking. Without facilitation for transportation or a voluntary request that household contacts have a sputum test and CXR, the policy of household contact tracing is not feasible in Mandalay City.

The percentage of positive TB cases among household contacts in our study was higher than studies from China (3.8%) and Nepal (1.6%) [10, 11] and similar to studies from South Africa (13.8%) and India (10.1%) [3, 8]. The differences of case detection among household contacts can be explained by the use of comprehensive strategies to obtain the contacts, different measurement tools, or the nature of living styles in each country [12]. Apart from the National Tuberculosis Programme, Myanmar, international non-governmental organizations have also contributed to the activities of active case finding ranging from 15 to 52%, while the local non-governmental organizations contributed around 4 to 6% [13, 14]. Moreover, the integrated approach, which included three screening methods of diagnosis, namely CXR, sputum smear, and Xpert MTB/RIF, could have increased the rate of high TB case detection.

From previous studies, a low detection rate of 0.2 to 6.2% was found when TB signs and symptoms was used for initial screening [15], while high sensitivity of CXR to detect pulmonary TB was reported in both adults and children [16]. For the challenge of completing the investigations, active facilitation of contacts' transportation for CXR investigation and sputum examination introduced in our study could be helpful to overcome the financial hardship, especially on the indirect costs which was a common barrier for contact investigations [17]. One study in a community-based active TB care facility in Myanmar also revealed that transportation fees for sputum samples are inadequately covered by the NTP and are a probable barrier for improving TB case contribution [14]. This is consistent with the consideration of economic barriers and reducing the out-of-pocket expenses of TB patients and their contacts in the Global Fund to Fight AIDS, Tuberculosis and Malaria [18].

Being a caretaker of an index TB case has been shown to be a strong determinant of positive TB among contacts [19]. This may be explained by close exposure of infectious droplets from index cases without having proper protection [20]. The intensive education and practices on source control techniques, including cough etiquette and respiratory hygiene, spending time outside with good ventilation, and sleeping in separate rooms, have been shown to be important for preventing the spread of TB to household contacts [21]. Smoking and passive smoking can cause pathological changes in lung function and drinking alcohol can decrease the immune system's ability to fight infection [22]. Gender was found to be associated with positive TB [23]. Males are more likely to access a health center for confirming TB diagnosis where a passive case finding is used. In our study, we conducted active case finding and the gender ratio was balanced. Our results showed that gender was not a significant determinant for positive TB among contacts.

WHO has recently released chest radiography guidelines that recommend it as the preferred TB screening tool from the viewpoint of test accuracy, noting that it can be expensive and logistically challenging to use [24]. The findings of our integrated approach, which applied initial CXR with active facilitation of transport for contact investigations in both CXR and sputum examinations, will be useful to other similar resource-limited settings where TB is endemic. With this approach, a high TB detection rate among household contacts was assured as we conducted a prospectively active contact tracing study, thus reducing under-estimation of TB infection comparing to routine or passive case findings.

There were some limitations in this study. First, the exclusion of index TB cases if all of their household contacts were not available may have led to selection bias of the households with healthy contacts working out of the

Table 3 Comparison of background and health related characteristics among household contacts by TB status

Variable	TB status among household contacts				*P* value
	Negative		Positive		
	(*n* = 150)		(*n* = 24)		
	n	(%)	n	(%)	
Gender					0.003
Male	54	(36.0)	17	(66.7)	
Female	96	(64.0)	7	(33.3)	
Age (years)					0.53
< 15	49	(32.7)	10	(41.7)	
≥15	101	(67.3)	14	(58.3)	
Ethnicity					0.72
Burmese	135	(90.0)	21	(87.5)	
Others	15	(10.0)	3	(12.5)	
Education					0.24
≤ Primary	100	(66.7)	19	(79.2)	
> Primary	50	(33.3)	5	(20.8)	
Occupation					0.96
Factory worker	41	(27.3)	6	(25.0)	
Casual employee	32	(21.3)	5	(20.8)	
Dependent/student	77	(51.4)	13	(54.2)	
Marital status					0.73
Single	78	(52.0)	11	(45.8)	
Married	72	(48.0)	13	(54.2)	
Daily income (USD)					0.32
< 3	132	(88.0)	19	(79.2)	
≥ 3	18	(12.0)	5	(20.8)	
Living alone in separate room					0.76
No	128	(85.3)	20	(83.3)	
Yes	22	(14.7)	4	(16.7)	
Number of persons living together					0.601
≤ 3	87	(58.0)	12	(50.0)	
> 3	63	(42.0)	12	(50.0)	
Sharing room with a TB patient					0.002
No	87	(58.0)	5	(20.8)	
Yes	63	(42.0)	19	(79.2)	
Caretaker to index TB case					< 0.001
No	116	(77.3)	7	(29.2)	
Yes	34	(22.7)	17	(70.8)	
Smoking status					< 0.001
Never smoker	132	(88.0)	10	(41.7)	
Former or current smoker	18	(12.0)	14	(58.3)	
Number of cigarettes smoked per day among smokers					0.71
< 4	13	(72.2)	9	(64.3)	
≥ 4	5	(27.8)	5	(35.7)	
Duration of smoking (years) among smokers					1
< 20	11	(61.1)	9	(64.3)	
≥ 20	7	(38.9)	5	(35.7)	
Passive smoking status					0.003
No	106	(70.7)	9	(37.5)	
Yes	44	(29.3)	15	(62.5)	
Drinking status					< 0.001
Never drinker	138	(92.0)	11	(45.8)	
Former or current drinker	12	(8.0)	13	(54.2)	
Duration of drinking (years) (*n* = 25)					0.67
< 7	9	(76.9)	8	(58.3)	
≥ 7	3	(23.1)	5	(41.7)	
Signs and symptoms of TB					0.69
No	86	(57.3)	11	(45.8)	
Yes	64	(42.7)	13	(54.2)	

TB Tuberculosis, *USD* United States dollars

Table 4 Factors associated with positive TB among household contacts

Variable	Crude OR (95% CI)	Adjusted OR (95% CI)	*P* value[†]
Caretaker to index TB case			< 0.001
No	1	1	
Yes	8.3 (3.17–21.6)	10.4 (3.09–35.0)	
Active smoking status			0.044
Never smoker	1	1	
Former or current smoker	10.3 (3.97–26.5)	6.4 (1.42–28.5)	
Passive smoking status			0.017
No	1	1	
Yes	4.0 (1.64–9.9)	4.0 (1.28–12.7)	
Drinking status			0.015
Never drinker	1	1	
Former or current drinker	13.6 (5.02–36.8)	4.6 (1.02–20.8)	

[†]Likelihood ratio test
OR odds ratio, *CI* confidence interval, *TB* Tuberculosis

hometown. However, this was unavoidable and may not be relevant to the definition of household contacts. Second, both CXR and sputum testing could be collected only in contacts aged 15 years or more. Third, extra pulmonary TB and latent TB infections among contacts were not detected. Fourth, genotype matching was not performed, thus we could not ascertain whether or not the contacts were infected by the index TB cases living in the same household. Finally, active facilitation of transportation of household contacts for CXR and sputum investigation used in our study may not be generalized in real practice settings. However, this active facilitation of transportation can be considered in the strategic planning for other low-income countries where TB populations face financial difficulty in access to TB investigations and out-of-pocket transportation costs.

Conclusions

This study highlights a high rate of TB detection by an integrated approach. Household contacts who were caretakers of a TB patient, active and passive smokers, and former or current drinkers were high-risk groups. Transportation and financial relief should be considered and prioritized to strengthen the contact tracing strategy of the country. The appropriate amount of funding for TB prevention and control among household contacts needs to be determined.

Abbreviations

AFB: Acid-fast bacilli; CXR: Chest x-ray; Gene Xpert MTB/RIF: Gene Xpert Mycobacterium tuberculosis/Rifampicin; GPS: Global positioning system; IQR: Interquartile range; NTP: National Tuberculosis Programme; SD: Standard deviation; TB: Tuberculosis; THD: Township health departments; WHO: World Health Organization

Acknowledgements

This study was a part of the thesis of the Master degree in Epidemiology at Prince of Songkla University under the scholarship of Thailand's Education Hub for Southern Region of ASEAN countries. The authors wish to thank the study participants for their contribution to the research as well as the seven Township Medical Officers at Mandalay city and research officers and assistants from the Department of Medical Research (Pyin Oo Lwin branch). Our sincere thanks are directed to the authorities from the Ministry of Public Health, Myanmar and the Director General of Department of Medical Research for allowing us to conduct the study.

Funding

This work was supported by the Fogarty International Center-National Institutes of Health on the project "TB/MDR-TB Research Capacity Building in low- and middle-income countries in Southeast Asia". The funding agency had no involvement of design of the study, data collection and analysis, interpretation of data and in writing the manuscript.

Authors' contributions

Conception and Design: KKKH, TL, ST, VC. Data Collection: KKKH, ST. Data Analysis and interpretation: KKKH, TL, EM, VC. Manuscript drafting or critical review: KKKH, TL. Final approval of manuscript: KKKH, TL, ST, EM, VC.

Consent for publication

Not applicable.

Competing interests

The authors declare that they have no competing interests.

Author details

[1]Department of Medical Research (Pyin Oo Lwin Branch), Pyin Oo Lwin 100201, Myanmar. [2]Epidemiology Unit, Faculty of Medicine, Prince of Songkla University, Hat Yai, Songkhla 90110, Thailand. [3]Ministry of Health and Sports, National Tuberculosis Programme, Mandalay 100107, Myanmar.

References

1. World Health Organization. Global tuberculosis report 2016. Geneva: World Health Organization; 2016.
2. Rieder HL. Contacts of tuberculosis patients in high-incidence countries. Int J Tuberc Lung Dis. 2003;7(12 Suppl 3):S333–6.
3. Khaparde K, Jethani P, Dewan PK, Nair SA, Deshpande MR, Satyanarayana S, et al. Evaluation of TB case finding through systematic contact investigation, Chhattisgarh, India. Tuberculosis Research and Treatment. 2015;2015:1–5.
4. Fox GJ, Barry SE, Britton WJ, Marks GB. Contact investigation for tuberculosis: a systematic review and meta-analysis. Eur Respir J. 2013;41(1):140–56.
5. Kranzer K, Lawn SD, Meyer-Rath G, Vassall A, Raditlhalo E, Govindasamy D, et al. Feasibility, yield, and cost of active tuberculosis case finding linked to a Mobile HIV Service in Cape Town, South Africa: a cross-sectional study. PLoS Med. 2012;9(8):e1001281.
6. WHO. Recommendations for investigating contacts of persons with infectious tuberculosis in low- and middle-income countries. In: Geneva: WHO; 2012.
7. National tuberculosis program. Annual Report (2014). Myanmar: Ministry of Health; 2015.
8. Thind D, Charalambous S, Tongman A, Churchyard G, Grant AD. An evaluation of "Ribolola": a household tuberculosis contact tracing programme in north West Province, South Africa. Int J Tuberc Lung Dis. 2012;16(12):1643–8.
9. Phillips M, Hall T, Esmen N, Lynch R, Johnson D. Use of global positioning system technology to track subject's location during environmental exposure sampling. J Expo Anal Environ Epidemiol. 2001;11:207–15.
10. Xu C, Hu B. Prevalence of active pulmonary tuberculosis among household contacts of recently diagnosed pulmonary tuberculosis patients with positive sputum-smear. Zhonghua Liu Xing Bing Xue Za Zhi. 2008;29(7):693–5.
11. Gyawali N, Gurung R, Poudyal N, Amatya R, Niraula SR, Jha P, et al. Prevalence of tuberculosis in household contacts of sputum smears positive cases and associated demographic risk factors. Nepal Med Coll J. 2012;14(4):303–7.
12. Nishikiori N, Van Weezenbeek C. Target prioritization and strategy selection for active case-finding of pulmonary tuberculosis: a tool to support country-level project planning. BMC Public Health. 2013;13(1):97.
13. Soe KT, Saw S, Van Griensven J, Zhou S, Win L, Chinnakali P, et al. International non-governmental organizations' provision of community-based tuberculosis care for hard-to-reach populations in Myanmar, 2013–2014. Infect Dis Poverty. 2017;6(69) https://www.ncbi.nlm.nih.gov/pmc/articles/PMC5364576/ Accessed 23 Jun 2018.
14. Maung HMW, Saw S, Isaakidis P, Khogali M, Reid A, Hoa NB, et al. The contribution of a non-governmental organisation's community based tuberculosis care Programme to case finding in Myanmar: trend over time. Infect Dis Poverty. 2017;6(51) https://www.ncbi.nlm.nih.gov/pmc/articles/PMC5376678/ Accessed 23 Jun 2018.
15. Marks SM, Taylor Z, Qualls NL, Shrestha-Kuwahara RJ, Wilce MA, Nguyen CH. Outcomes of contact investigations of infectious tuberculosis patients. Am J Respir Crit Care Med. 2000;162(6):2033–8.
16. Den Boon S, White NW, Van Lill SWP, Borgdorff MW, Verver S, Lombard CJ, et al. An evaluation of symptom and chest radiographic screening in tuberculosis prevalence surveys. Int J Tuberc Lung Dis. 2006;10(8):876–82.

17. Morishita F, Yadav RP, Eang MT, Saint S, Nishikiori N. Mitigating financial burden of tuberculosis through active case finding targeting household and Neighbourhood contacts in Cambodia. PLoS One. 2016;11(9):e0162796.
18. Richter LM, Lönnroth K, Desmond C, Jackson R, Jaramillo E, Weil D. Economic support to patients in HIV and TB grants in rounds 7 and 10 from the global fund to fight AIDS, tuberculosis and malaria. PLoS One. 2014;9(1): e86225.
19. Elender F, Bentham G, Langford I. Tuberculosis mortality in England and Wales during 1982–1992: its association with poverty, ethnicity and AIDS. Soc Sci Med. 1998;46(6):673–81.
20. Guwatudde D, Nakakeeto M, Jones-Lopez EC, Maganda A, Chiunda A, Mugerwa RD, et al. Tuberculosis in household contacts of infectious cases in Kampala, Uganda. Am J Epidemiol. 2003;158(9):887–98.
21. Robert J, Affolabi D, Awokou F, Nolna D, Manouan BA, Acho YB, et al. Assessment of organizational measures to prevent nosocomial tuberculosis in health facilities of 4 sub-Saharan countries in 2010. Infect Control Hosp Epidemiol. 2013;34(2):190–5.
22. Van Zyl Smit RN, Pai M, Yew WW, Leung CC, Zumla A, Bateman ED, et al. Global lung health: the colliding epidemics of tuberculosis, tobacco smoking, HIV and COPD. Eur Respir J. 2010;35(1):27–33.
23. Onifade DA, Bayer AM, Montoya R, Haro M, Alva J, Franco J, et al. Gender-related factors influencing tuberculosis control in shantytowns: a qualitative study. BMC Public Health. 2010;10(1):381.
24. World Health Organization. Chest radiography in tuberculosis detection: summary of current WHO recommendations and guidance on programmatic approaches. Geneva: World Health Organization; 2016. http://www.who.int/iris/handle/10665/252424/ Accessed 23 Jun 2018.

22

Prevalence and associated factors of diabetes mellitus among tuberculosis patients in Hanoi, Vietnam

N. B. Hoa[1,2*], P. D. Phuc[3,4], N. T. Hien[3,4], V. Q. Hoa[1], P. H. Thuong[5], P. T. Anh[5] and N. V. Nhung[1,6]

Abstract

Background: Diabetes mellitus (DM) is recognized as an important comorbidity for the development of tuberculosis (TB). With the increase of DM burden globally, concerns have been raised about the emerging co-epidemics of DM and TB, especially in low- and middle-income countries.

Methods: A facility-based, cross-sectional study was carried out in all 30 district TB units in Hanoi, Vietnam. All eligible, diagnosed TB patients aged 15 years old or older were asked to provide consent and were screened for diabetes using fasting blood glucose (FBG). Pre-tested semi-structured questionnaires were used for collecting demographic data, lifestyle habits and clinical data. Identification of pre-diabetes or diabetes in TB patients was done in accordance to parameters set by the American Diabetes Association (2016).

Results: Of 870 eligible TB patients, 831 (95.5%) participated in the study. Of those, 241 (29%; 95%CI: 25.9–32.1%) were prediabetic and 114 (13.7%; 95%CI: 11.4–16.1%) were found to have DM. The risk of DM was higher in patients belonging to the age group 40–64 years (OR 6.09; 95%CI 2.81–13.2); or the age group 65 years or older (OR 2.65; 95%CI 1.65–4.25) or who have a family history of DM (OR 2.71; 95%CI 1.33–5.50).

Conclusions: This study demonstrated high prevalence of DM and prediabetes among TB patients in Hanoi, Vietnam. National Tuberculosis Programme needs to establish a systematic screening process for DM among TB patients.

Keywords: Tuberculosis (TB), diabetes mellitus (DM), prevalence, Risk factors, Vietnam

Background

Vietnam is a lower middle-income country and ranks 15th amongst the 30 highest Tuberculosis (TB) incidences globally [1]. The World Health Organization (WHO) estimated that there were 126,000 TB incidence cases in Viet Nam in 2016, which accounts for 123 cases per 100,000 population. The number of reported TB cases in Vietnam in 2016 was 106,527 TB cases [1]. The burden of Diabetes mellitus (DM) is increasing worldwide with the International Diabetes Federation (IDF) estimating that approxiately 425 million people are living with diabetes, amounting to 8.8% of the global population [2]. It was also estimated that approximately half of this population was unaware of their DM status in 2016 [2]. Low- and middle-income countries account for approximately 80% of the global DM burden, and more than 90% of the global TB burden [2].

DM is recognized as an important comorbidity for the development of TB, with those who have DM having a two to three times higher risk of developing TB than those without DM [3–5]. This leads to a higher prevalence rate of TB among DM patients; the rate of DM is also higher among TB patients than in general population [3]. People with TB and DM generally have a poorer response to TB treatments and increased the risk of relapse and death [3, 6, 7]. With the increase of DM burden globally, concerns have been raised about the emerging co-epidemics of DM and TB, especially in low- and middle-income countries.

* Correspondence: nguyenbinhhoatb@yahoo.com
[1]Vietnam National Lung Hospital, National Tuberculosis Programme Vietnam, 463 Hoang Hoa Tham street, Badinh District, Hanoi, Vietnam
[2]Centre for Operational Research, International Union Against Tuberculosis and Lung Disease, Paris, France
Full list of author information is available at the end of the article

In 2011, the WHO and the International Union Against Tuberculosis and Lung Disease (the UNION) recommended that TB patients should be routinely screened for DM [3]. The framework recommended all countries should be surveilling diabetes among TB patients [3]. Many studies conducted in different countries have shown the prevalence of DM among TB patients to be approximately 12–44% [8]. Currently, in Vietnam, there is no systematic screening for DM amongst TB patients and limited studies investigating the prevalence of DM amongst TB patients. One study conducted in the National Lung Hospital in 2006–2008 found the prevalence of DM among TB patients to be 8.8% [9].

Hanoi is the capital of Vietnam, has a high proportion of the total TB cases reported in the country. In 2016, Hanoi detected and reported 4382 TB cases, amounting to 59 cases per 100,000 population. This study aimed to identify the prevalence and some associated risk factors of DM amongst TB patients attending district TB units in Hanoi, Vietnam. The results will look to help to establish linkages between TB and DM and provide data to estimate the needs and requirements for DM care services among TB patients in Vietnam.

Methods

Setting and study population

This facility-based, cross-sectional study was conducted in all 30 districts of Hanoi where the total population was estimated at 7,328,400 in 2016. The study population included all TB patients aged over 15 years old, who had been diagnosed and enrolled for TB treatment from October to December of 2016.

The sample size was calculated based on the standard formula for estimating a single population:

$$n = \frac{Z^2_{1-\alpha/2} \cdot p \cdot (1-p)}{d^2} \times DE.$$

A previous study conducted in 2006–2008, at the National Lung Hospital in Hanoi, investigated the DM prevalence among 2867 newly diagnosed TB patients and discovered the DM prevalence to be 8.8% [9]. A similar DM prevalence was assumed for this study, with a 95% confidence interval and 20% relative precision. With a cluster sampling of 1.5 the sample size was calculated to be 740 participants. To account for an estimated non-participation rate of 15%, the final sample size required for this study was considered as 870 TB patients.

Sampling method

Patients who were aged 15 years or above and had been diagnosed with TB in any 30 districts of Hanoi were considered for the study. Participants were enrolled for TB treatment between October and December of 2016. Recruitment was continuous until the required sample size was met.

Data collection

All consenting participants were interviewed using pre-tested questionnaires to collect the patient's information. Questionnaires collected socio-demographic variables including age, sex, weight, height, education, occupation, marital status, average monthly income and HIV status. The questionnaires also collected information around lifestyle factors including smoking, drinking and exercise. The participant's disease profile and clinical records pertaining to TB and DM status were also collected. TB patients were asked about their DM status. If the TB patients were diagnosed with DM prior to the study, they were not further investigated for the DM, and the patients were requested to provide their most recent DM test results. If the TB patients were did not know or were unsure about their DM status, they were requested to undergo a fasting blood glucose (FBG) test, after the cessation of eating for at least 8 h.

Definition

TB patients' diagnosis and treatment outcomes were categorized following NTP's guidelines, which are in line with WHO's recommendations [10].

Patients with FBG levels ≥126 mg/dl (~ 7 mmol/l) were diagnosed as having DM. Patients with FBG levels between 100 and 126 mg/dl (5.6–6.9 mmol/l) were diagnosed as having impaired fasting glucose (IFG), or prediabetes, in line with guidance from the American Diabetes Association (ADA) [11].

Classification of socioeconomic status was determined following Vietnam Government criteria, issued by Prime Minister for the period 2016–2020 [12]. A "poor" household is one whose per capita income does not exceed 700,000 Vietnam Dong (VND) in rural area and 900,000 VND in urban area. Households are also classified as poor if their per capita income is between 700,000 – 1,000,000 VND in rural areas or 900,000-1,300,000 VND in urban areas when households have unfavourable outcomes in at least three of ten basic social service indicators (access to medical services, health insurance, education level of adults, school attendance of children, housing quality, average housing area per capital, residential water sources, hygienic latrines and toilets, telecom services, and assets to serve information access (TV, computer, radio, other). A "near-poor" household is one whose per capita income is between 700,000–1,000,000 VND or 900,000-1,300,000 VND in rural or urban areas, respectively, and have unfavourable outcomes in at least three of ten basic social service indicators A "medium" household is a household whose per capital income is between 1,000,000–1,500,000

VND in rural area and between 1,300,000-1,950,000 VND in urban area [12].

Statistical analysis

Data was entered into EpiData version 3.1 (EpiData Association, Odense, Denmark) and the analysis were carried out using Stata v.13 software (Stata Corporation, College Station, TX, USA). The main outcomes of the analysis were the number and proportion of TB patients with DM and prediabetes; data was then stratified by sex, age, education, occupation, marital status, residence, monthly incomes, socio-economic status and body mass index (BMI). The proportion of TB patients with DM and prediabetes was also stratified by lifestyle and other factors such as physical activity, smoking, drinking status, family history of DM, type of TB, treatment category and HIV status. Single proportion with 95% confidence interval (CI) was calculated. A Kruskal-Wallis test and Cuzick test were used for the nonparametric data and to test for trend across ordered groups. Odds ratio (OR) with 95% CI were used to describe association between groups. Multivariate logistic regression analysis was performed to calculate adjusted OR for analyzing the association of the related risk factors with the outcome variables.

Ethics approval

The study protocol was approved by the Institutional Review Board of the National Lung Hospital, Hanoi, Vietnam. Patients diagnosed with DM received appropriate treatment. Written informed consent was obtained from each participant prior to enrolment.

Results

A total of 851 eligible TB patients aged ≥15 years old were enrolled during the study period. 831 (97.7%) patients consented and were interviewed.

General characteristics

The socio-demographic characteristics of study's participants are presented in Table 1. Of 831 TB patients, 549 (66.1%) were males and 282 (33.9%) were females. The mean age of participants was 48.4 (standard deviation (SD): 18.2). More than half of the participants (531, 63.9%) had a secondary or high school education. The number of participants residing in urban areas was 401 (48.3%) and 468 (56.3%) had a monthly income less than 3,000,000 VND. The mean of BMI was 19.6 kg/m^2, (SD 3.0) with 34.8% patients was classified as underweight.

Prevalence of prediabetes and DM among TB patients

The overall prevalence of prediabetes and DM among TB patients and stratified by general characteristics are shown

Table 1 General characteristics of Tuberculosis patients enrolled for the study, Hanoi, Vietnam, 2016. ($n = 831$)

General characteristic	n	%
Total	831	*100.0*
Sex		
Male	549	*66.1*
Female	282	*33.9*
Age in years		
15–24	92	*11.1*
25–34	133	*16.0*
35–44	142	*17.1*
45–54	137	*16.5*
55–64	175	*21.1*
65 years and older	152	*18.3*
Mean age (SD)	48.4 *(18.2)*	
Education		
Primary and lower	143	*17.2*
Secondary; high school	531	*63.9*
Colleagues/University or higher	157	*18.9*
Occupation		
Unemployed	113	*13.6*
Farmer	259	*31.2*
Self-employed	49	*5.9*
Government employed/ Student; pupil / retired	410	*49.3*
Marital status		
Single	158	*19.0*
Married	629	*75.7*
Divorced / separated	44	*5.3*
Residence		
Rural	430	*51.7*
Urban	401	*48.3*
Monthly Income (VND)		
< 3,000,000 (~ 132.3 US$)	468	*56.3*
3,000,000 - 5,000,000 (~ 132.3–220.5 US$)	220	*26.5*
> 5,000,000 (~ 220.5 US$)	143	*17.2*
Socio-economic status		
Poor/ near-poor household	103	*12.4*
Medium household and above	728	*87.6*
BMI, kg/m2		
Underweight, < 18.5	289	*34.8*
Normal, 18.5–24.9	518	*62.3*
Overweight, > = 25	24	*2.9*
Mean (SD)	19.6 *(3.0)*	

**SD* Standard deviation; *VND* Vietnam dong; *BMI* Body mass index

Table 2 The prevalence of pre-diabetes and DM among TB patients, in Hanoi, Vietnam, 2016 ($n = 831$)

	Total TB patients evaluated for DM (n)	TB patients with pre-DM (n)	Prevalence of pre-DM (%; 95% CI)	*p* value*	TB patients with DM (n)	Prevalence of DM (%; 95% CI)	*p* value*
Total	**831**	**241**	**29.0 (25.9–32.1)**		**114**	**13.7 (11.4–16.1)**	
Sex				0.274			0.007
Male	549	166	30.2 (26.4–34.1)		88	16.0 (13.0–19.1)	
Female	282	75	26.6 (21.4–31.8)		26	9.2 (5.8–12.6)	
Age, years				**< 0.001**			**< 0.001**
15–24	92	19	20.7 (12.2–29.1)		5	5.4 (0.7–10.1)	
25–34	133	23	17.3 (10.8–23.8)		6	4.5 (0.9–8.1)	
35–44	142	37	26.1 (18.7–33.4)		16	11.3 (6.0–16.5)	
45–54	137	47	34.3 (26.3–42.4)		27	19.7 (13.0–26.5)	
55–64	175	61	34.9 (27.7–42.0)		33	18.9 (13.0–24.7)	
≥ 65	152	54	35.5 (27.8–43.2)		27	17.8 (11.6–23.9)	
Education				**0.002**			0.624
Primary or lower	143	49	34.3 (26.4–42.1)		19	13.3 (7.7–18.9)	
Secondary; high school	531	163	30.7 (26.8–34.6)		77	14.5 (11.5–17.5)	
Colleagues/University or higher	157	29	18.5 (12.3–24.6)		18	11.5 (6.4–16.5)	
Occupation				**0.002**			0.328
Unemployed	113	35	31.0 (22.3–39.6)		15	13.3 (6.9–19.6)	
Farmer	259	96	37.1 (31.1–43.0)		28	10.8 (7.0–14.6)	
Self-employed	49	15	30.6 (17.2–44.0)		9	18.4 (7.1–29.6)	
Government employed/ Student; pupil / retired	410	95	23.2 (19.1–27.3)		62	15.1 (11.6–18.6)	
Marital status				0.062			0.481
Single	158	34	21.5 (15.0–28.0)		17	10.8 (5.9–15.6)	
Married	629	192	30.5 (26.9–34.1)		91	14.5 (11.7–17.2)	
Divorced/separated	44	15	34.1 (19.5–48.7)		6	13.6 (3.1–24.2)	
Residence				0.084			0.107
Rural	430	136	31.6 (27.2–36.0)		51	11.9 (8.8–14.9)	
Urban	401	105	26.2 (21.9–30.5)		63	15.7 (12.1–19.3)	
Monthly income (VND)				**< 0.001**			0.636
< 3,000,000 (~ 132.3 US$)	468	153	32.7 (28.4–37.0)		60	12.8 (9.8–15.9)	
3,000,000 - 5,000,000 (~ 132.3–220.5 US$)	220	65	29.5 (23.5–35.6)		35	15.9 (11.0–20.8)	
> 5,000,000 (~ 220.5 US$)	143	23	16.1 (10.0–22.2)		19	13.3 (7.7–18.9)	
Socio-economic status				0.794			0.790
Poor/ near-poor household	103	31	30.1 (21.1–39.1)		15	14.6 (7.6–21.5)	
Medium household and above	728	210	28.8 (25.5–32.1)		99	13.6 (11.1–16.1)	
BMI, kg/m2				0.077			0.304
Underweight, < 18.5	289	94	32.5 (27.1–38.0)		38	13.1 (9.2–17.1)	
Normal, 18.5–24.9	518	142	27.4 (23.6–31.3)		69	13.3 (10.4–16.3)	
Overweight, > = 25	24	5	20.8 (3.3–38.4)		7	29.2 (9.6–48.8)	

TB Tuberculosis; *DM* Diabetes mellitus; *CI* Confidence interval; *SD* Standard deviation; *VND* Vietnam dong; *BMI* Body mass index
**p value by Kruskal-Wallis test and Cuzick test were used for the nonparametric data and to test for trend across ordered groups*

in Table 2. Of 831 TB patients, 241 (29%; 95% CI: 25.9–32.1%) were prediabetic and 114 (13.7%; 95% CI: 11.4–16.1%)) were found to have DM. The prevalence of DM was higher among males than females (16.0% vs 9.2%) and was shown to increase with age. The incidence of prediabetes was also higher among those in older age groups, those who had primary or lower education levels, those who worked as farmers and in those with a monthly income less than 3,000,000 VND.

Lifestyle factors

The proportion of DM among TB patients with a family history of DM was 29% (95% CI: 18.0–40.0%) higher than those who did not (12.4, 95% CI: 10.0–14.7%).

The level of pre-diabetes in TB patients who were currently smoking was 34.3% (95% CI: 25.2–43.4%) higher than those never smoked (26.3%; 95% CI: 22.4–33.1%). The proportion of prediabetes was also higher among TB patients with a family history of DM, with the

Table 3 The prevalence of pre-diabetes and DM among TB patients, stratified by lifestyles and risk factors, in Hanoi, Vietnam, 2016

	Total TB patients evaluated for DM (n)	TB patients with pre-DM (n)	Prevalence of pre-DM (%; 95% CI)	*p* value	TB patients with DM (n)	Prevalence of DM (%; 95% CI)	*p* value
Total	831	241	29.0 (25.9–32.1)		114	13.7 (11.4–16.1)	
Family history of DM				0.052			**< 0.001**
Yes	69	13	18.8 (9.4–28.3)		20	29.0 (18.0–40.0)	
No	762	228	29.9 (26.7–33.2)		94	12.4 (10.0–14.7)	
Physical activities				0.283			0.299
Yes	278	74	26.6 (21.4–31.8)		43	15.5 (11.2–19.7)	
No	553	167	30.2 (26.4–34.0)		71	12.8 (10.0–15.6)	
Frequently of physical activities				0.426			0.147
> 4 times per week	168	47	28.0 (21.1–34.8)		30	17.9 (12.0–23.7)	
1–4 times per week	63	16	25.4 (14.3–36.4)		9	14.3 (5.4–23.1)	
1–3 times per month	30	8	26.7 (9.9–43.5)		2	6.7 (0–16.1)	
< 1 time per month	17	3	17.6 (0.0–37.9)		2	11.8 (0–28.8)	
Smoker				**0.036**			0.116
Never smoker	510	134	26.3 (22.4–30.1)		61	12.0 (9.1–14.8)	
Ex-smoker	213	70	32.9 (26.5–39.2)		36	16.9 (11.8–22.0)	
Smoker	108	37	34.3 (25.2–43.4)		17	15.7 (8.8–22.7)	
Drinker				0.705			0.454
Drinker	374	106	28.3 (23.8–32.9)		55	14.7 (11.1–18.3)	
Non-drinker	457	135	29.5 (25.3–33.7)		59	12.9 (9.8–16.0)	
Type of TB				0.219			0.070
PTB - smear positive	391	122	31.2 (26.6–35.8)		60	15.3 (11.8–18.9)	
PTB - smear negative	271	68	25.1 (19.9–30.3)		40	14.8 (10.5–19.0)	
EPTB	169	51	30.2 (23.2–37.2)		14	8.3 (4.1–12.5)	
TB treatment category				0.138			0.815
New	713	200	28.1 (24.7–31.4)		97	13.6 (11.1–16.1)	
Previously treated	118	41	34.7 (26.0–43.5)		17	14.4 (8.0–20.8)	
HIV status				0.722			0.555
Positive	16	4	25.0 (1.2–48.8)		3	18.8 (10.1–40.2)	
Negative	815	237	29.1 (1.6–26.0)		111	13.6 (11.3–16.0)	

TB Tuberculosis; *PTB* Pulmonary Tuberculosis; *EPTB* Extra Pulmonary Tuberculosis; *DM* Diabetes mellitus;
CI confidence interval; *SD* Standard deviation; *VND* Vietnam dong; *BM* Body mass index
**p value by Kruskal-Wallis test and Cuzick test were used for the nonparametric data and to test for trend across ordered groups*

difference nearly reaching the statistical significance (p = 0.052). (Table 3).

Risk factors associated with DM

In the crude analysis, the associated factors for DM among TB patients were people aged '40 years or older', 'male' gender, 'family members with a history of DM', 'pulmonary TB cases' and a 'BMI > 25'. After adjusting for other factors in a logistic regression model, the associated factors for DM among TB patients found in this study were age ≥ 40 years and a family history of DM. (Table 4).

Additional yield of DM

Of the 831 screened TB patients, 114 (13.7%; 95% CI: 11.4–16.1%)) were found to have DM, of those, 50 (44%) were newly diagnosed as DM cases. The number of TB patients needed to be screened to diagnose a new DM case was 17, and the number of TB patients needed to carried-out blood testing to diagnose a new DM case was approximately 16. (Table 5).

Discussion

The prevalence of DM among TB patients in this study was 13.7% (95% CI: 11.4–16.1%), which is much higher than the estimated prevalence of DM among people aged 18–99 in the general population of Vietnam in 2016 (5.34%; 95% CI: 4.32–7.32%) [13]. The prevalence of DM amongst TB patients is also higher than in the previous study in 2006–2008, in Hanoi, Vietnam (8.8%) [9].

This study showed a 29% prevalence rate of prediabetes amongst TB cases in Hanoi. The prevalence of prediabetes among TB cases was slightly higher than study findings from India (24.5%) [14]; and much higher than study findings in Ethiopia (11.5%) [8]; China (7.8%) [15]; India (7%; 8.5%) [5, 16]. This finding may indicate an increased relatively higher prevalence of DM among TB patients in the future in Vietnam.

Table 4 Factors associated with DM among TB patients, in Hanoi, Vietnam, 2016 (n = 831)

Characteristics	OR (95% CI)	p value	aOR (95% CI)*	p value
Age (years)				
< 40	Reference			
40–64	3.56 (2.08–6.07)	< 0.001	6.09 (2.81–13.2)	< 0.001
≥ 65	3.42 (1.88–6.23)	< 0.001	2.65 (1.65–4.25)	< 0.001
Sex				
Female	Reference			
Male	1.74 (1.15–2.63)	0.007	1.62 (0.96–2.75)	0.071
Family history of DM				
No	Reference			
Yes	2.35 (1.55–3.56)	< 0.001	2.71 (1.33–5.50)	0.006
Type of TB				
Extra-pulmonary	Reference			
Smear negative	1.78 (1.00–3.17)	0.044	1.26 (0.83–1.91)	0.272
Smear positive	1.85 (1.07–3.22)	0.024	1.83 (0.86–3.93)	0.119
Smoker				
Never smoke	Reference			
Current smoker	1.32 (0.80–2.16)	0.283	0.75 (0.33–1.71)	0.494
Ex-smoker	1.41 (0.97–2.07)	0.076	0.58 (0.31–1.10)	0.094
BMI				
< 18.5	Reference			
18.5–24.9	1.01 (0.70–1.46)	0.945	1.03 (0.65–1.64)	0.885
> =25	2.22 (1.11–4.42)	0.032	2.27 (0.75–6.82)	0.146
Education				
Primary or lower	Reference			
Secondary; high school	1.09 (0.68–1.74)	0.712	1.07 (0.55–2.05)	0.850
Colleagues/University or higher	0.86 (0.47–1.58)	0.632	0.47 (0.12–1.84)	0.281

TB Tuberculosis; *DM* Diabetes mellitus; *OR* Odds ratio; *aOR* Adjusted odds ratio; *CI* Confidence interval; *BMI* Body mass index

**Adjusted for age; sex; residence; education; occupation; marital status; type of TB; family history of DM and BMI in Multivariate logistic regression*

Table 5 Number of patients needed to screen to find a new DM case among TB patients, in Hanoi, Vietnam, 2016. ($n = 831$)

Characteristic	Total TB patients evaluated for DM (n)	Number of patients with previous DM (n)	Number of newly diagnosed DM patients (n)	Additional yield (%)	Number needed to screen to diagnose a new case (n)
Total	831	64	50	43.9	17
Sex					
Male	549	49	39	44.3	14
Female	282	15	11	42.3	26
Age, years					
< 40	289	4	11	73.3	26
40–65	390	45	27	37.5	14
≥ 65	152	15	12	44.4	13
Family history of DM					
Yes	69	17	3	15.0	23
No	762	47	47	50.0	16
Type of TB					
PTB - smear positive	391	40	20	33.3	20
PTB - smear negative	271	21	19	47.5	14
EPTB	169	3	11	78.6	15
BMI, kg/m2					
Underweight, < 18.5	289	19	19	50.0	15
Normal, 18.5–24.9	518	38	31	44.9	17
Overweight, > = 25	24	7	0	0.0	

TB Tuberculosis; *PTB* Pulmonary Tuberculosis; *EPTB* Extra Pulmonary Tuberculosis; *DM* Diabetes mellitus; *BMI* Body mass index

The prevalence of DM among TB patients in this study (13.7%) is slightly lower than the global median DM prevalence among TB patients, estimated at 16% (IQR 9.0–25.3%) found by Mahteme et.al [17]. This systematic review had analysed 78 studies reporting DM prevalence among TB patients, representing 33 countries globally. The prevalence of DM amongst TB patients ranged from 1.9% in Cotonou-Benin to 45% in the Ebeye-Mashall Islands [18, 19]. Our study results are comparable with the overall median prevalence of DM among TB patients in Asia, estimated to be 17% (IQR 11.4–25.8%). The prevalence of DM among TB patients in Asia ranges from 5.1% in Salury-South India to 44% in Kerala-India. [5, 17, 20].

The associated risk factors for TBDM comorbidity including sex, age, family history of DM, pulmonary form of TB and positive sputum smear were found in many other studies [17]. In this study, all the above-mentioned factors were found to be associated factors in the bivariate analysis. However, after multivariate analysis, adjusted for other variables, only increasing age and family history of DM remained significant for factors associated with TBDM comorbidity.

Our study found that age was a significant risk factors for TB and DM comorbidity, a finding consistent with many other studies [8, 14, 17, 20, 21]. In our study, the risk of having DM was 6 times higher in the 40–65 age group when compared to those patients under 40 years old; the risk dropped to approximately 3 times higher in the age group 65 years old and older when compare to age groups of patients less than 40 years old. This may be explained by the link between increasing age and decreases in immune status, one risk factor for both TB and DM [8].

Having a family history of DM is known as a risk factor for DM [7, 12]. Our study also found the risk of DM is 2.7 times higher among TB patients who had a family history of DM. This finding was consistent with other studies conducted in Ethiopia, China, and India [8, 14, 17, 21].

Many studies have also reported a higher prevalence of DM and prevalence of prediabetes amongst males compared to females [6, 20]. In our study, male TB patients were also identified to have a higher risk of DM in the bivariate analysis. One reasons for this may be a higher frequency of habits such as smoking and drinking alcohol among men. However, the multivariate analysis could not show a significant association.

In this study, 17 TB cases were needed to be screened in order to diagnose one new DM case. This number is high compared to other studies in Ethiopia (20 cases) [8]; Gujarat-India (25 cases) [16]; and South, India (31 cases) [5]. Such a finding suggests that the implementation of a DM screening strategy for TB patients in Hanoi could be high-value.

This study also demonstrated that a high level of participation was possible for DM testing amongst TB patients in Hanoi, Vietnam. In 2011, in the collaboration framework, WHO and the UNION have recommended screening for DM among TB patients [3]. Given the high prevalence of DM, especially the high prevalence of prediabetes among TB patients, Vietnam NTP should collaborate with diabetes programme and establish a systematic screening process for DM among TB patients. This program would enable early diagnosis of DM to be made and reduce morbidity and mortality amongst TB patients.

This study has some limitations. As the study was conducted in an urban area, Hanoi city, the findings may not be representative of the entire country, particularly rural areas. Secondly, the study was only implemented among TB patients who were diagnosed and treated in NTP system, thus it may not be representative of TB patients diagnosed and treated in the private or non-NTP public sectors, or TB patients who have not been diagnosed. Thirdly, decisions on the diagnosis of DM were based on FBG only, this testing methodology may be less sensitive than glycosylated haemoglobin or oral glucose tolerance tests. Finally, this study used the standard cut-off points for BMI categories, it did not use cut-off points specific to Asian populations as recommended by the WHO.

Conclusions

In conclusion, this study illustrated the high prevalence of DM and prediabetes among TB patients in Hanoi, Vietnam. This was especially true for persons aged over 40 years old or who had a family history of DM. Given the high prevalence of DM, particularly the high prevalence of prediabetes among TB patients, this study recommends the Vietnam NTP need to collaborate with diabetes programme to establish a systematic screening process for DM amongst TB patients.

Abbreviations

ADA: The American Diabetes Association; BMI: Body Mass Index; CI: Confidence interval; DM: Diabetes Mellitus; EPTB: Extra Pulmonary Tuberculosis; FBG: Fasting blood glucose; IDF: International Diabetes Federation; IFG: Impaired fasting glucose; IQR: Interquartile range; NTP: National Tuberculosis Programme; OR: Odds Ratio; PTB: Pulmonary Tuberculosis;; SD: Standard Deviation; TB: Tuberculosis; UNION: The International Union Against Tuberculosis and Lung Disease; VND: Vietnam Dong; WHO: World Health Organization

Acknowledgements

We would like to thank the Vietnam NTP, Center for Public Health and Ecosystem Research, Hanoi University of Public Health; Institute of Environmental Health and Sustainable Development study team; and health staff of 30 DTUs in Hanoi and the patients for their kind cooperation and participation in the study.

We thank the Department for International Development (DFID), UK, for funding the Global Operational Research Fellowship Programme in which Nguyen Binh Hoa works as an operational research fellow. La Fondation Veuve Emile Metz-Tesch supported open access publications costs. The funders had no role in study design, data collection and analysis, decision to publish, or preparation of the manuscript.

Funding

Not applicable.

Authors' contributions

HNB, PDP, HVQ, HNT, TPH, APT and NVN contributed to develop the protocol and conducting the study. HNB, PDP and HNT analyzed and interpreted the patient data. NNV, HNB, HNT and PDP were a major contributor in writing the manuscript. All authors read and approved the final manuscript.

Consent for publication

Not applicable.

Competing interests

The authors declare that they have no competing interests.

Author details

[1]Vietnam National Lung Hospital, National Tuberculosis Programme Vietnam, 463 Hoang Hoa Tham street, Badinh District, Hanoi, Vietnam. [2]Centre for Operational Research, International Union Against Tuberculosis and Lung Disease, Paris, France. [3]Center for Public Health and Ecosystem Research, Hanoi University of Public Health, Hanoi, Vietnam. [4]Institute of Environmental Health and Sustainable Development, Hanoi, Vietnam. [5]Hanoi Lung Hospital, Hanoi, Vietnam. [6]Vietnam Association for Tuberculosis and Lung Disease, Hanoi, Vietnam.

References

1. World Health Organization. Global tuberculosis report 2017. World Health Organization Document. WHO/HTM/TB/2017. 2017;23:1–249.
2. International Diabetes Federation.Diabetes atlas. IDF. 8th edition. 2017. Available: http://www.diabetesatlas.org/resources/2017-atlas.html. Accessed 10 Jan 2018.
3. International Union Against Tuberculosis and Lung Disease, World Health Organization. Collaborative framework for care and control of tuberculosis and diabetes. World Health Organization Document. WHO/HTM/TB/2011. 2011;15:1–40.
4. Jeon CY, Murray MB. Diabetes mellitus increases the risk of active tuberculosis: a systematic review of 13 observational studies. PLoS Med. 2008;5(7):e152. https://doi.org/10.1371/journal.pmed.0050152.
5. Achanta S, Tekumalla RR, Jaju J, et al. Screening tuberculosis patients for diabetes in a tribal area in South India. Public Health Action. 2013;3(suppl 1).
6. Shidam UG, Roy G, Sahu SK, Kumar SV, Ananthanarayanan PH. Screening for diabetes among presumptive tuberculosis patients at a tertiary care Centre in Pondicherry, India. Int J Tuberc Lung Dis. 2015;19:1163–8.
7. Viney K, Cavanaugh J, Kienene T, et al. Tuberculosis and diabetes mellitus in the Republic of Kiribati: a case-control study. Tropical Med Int Health. 2015; 20:650–7.
8. Workneh MH, Bjune GA, Yimer SA. Prevalence and associated factors of diabetes mellitus among tuberculosis patients in South-Eastern Amhara region, Ethiopia: a cross sectional study. PLoS One. 2016;11:e0147621.
9. Thanh NP, Khue PM, Sy DN, et al. Diabète chez les nouveaux cas de tuberculose pulmonaire à Hanoï, Viet Nam. Bulletin de la Société de pathologie exotique. 2015;108(5):337–41.
10. World Health Organization. Definitions and reporting framework for tuberculosis-2013 revision. World Health Organization Document 2013. WHO/HTM/TB. 2013;2:1–40.
11. American Diabetes Association (2016), Diagnosing Diabetes and Learning About Prediabetes, accessed on 10 January 2018, from http://www.diabetes.org/diabetes-basics/diagnosis/.
12. Vietnam government. Decision No. 59/2015/QD-TTg dated November 19, 2015, promulgating multidimensional poverty levels applicable during 2016–2020. Accessed on 08 January 2018, from https://vanbanphapluat.co/decision-no-59-2015-qd-ttg-promulgating-multidimensional-poverty-levels-applicable.
13. International Diabetes Federation.Diabetes atlas. Diabetes by country. Country summary table (18-99 years). In: Available; 2017. http://www.diabetesatlas.org/resources/2017-atlas.html.

14. Viswanathan V, Kumpatla S, Aravindalochanan V, et al. Prevalence of diabetes and pre-diabetes and associated risk factors among tuberculosis patients in India. PLoS One. 2012;7(7):e41367. https://doi.org/10.1371/journal.pone.0041367.
15. Li L, Lin Y, Mi F, et al. Screening of patients with tuberculosis for diabetes mellitus in China. Tropical Med Int Health. 2012;17:1294–301.
16. Dave P, Shah A, Chauhan M, et al. Screening patients with tuberculosis for diabetes mellitus in Gujarat. India Public Health Action. 2013;3(suppl 1):S29–33.
17. Workneh MH, Bjune GA, Yimer SA. Prevalence and associated factors of tuberculosis and diabetes mellitus comorbidity: a systematic review. PLoS One. 2017;12:e0175925.
18. Ade S, Affolabi D, Agodokpessi G, et al. Low prevalence of diabetes mellitus in patients with tuberculosis in Cotonou, Benin. Public Health Action. 2015; 5:147–9.
19. Nasa JN, Brostrom R, Ram S, et al. Screening adult tuberculosis patients for diabetes mellitus in Ebeye. Republic of the Marshall Islands Public Health Action. 2014;4(Suppl 1):S50–2.
20. Balakrishnan S, Vijayan S, Nair S, et al. High diabetes prevalence among tuberculosis cases in Kerala, India. PLoS One. 2012;7:e46502.
21. Wang Q, Ma A, Han X, et al. Prevalence of type 2 diabetes among newly detected pulmonary tuberculosis patients in China: a community based cohort study. PLoS One. 2013;8(12):e82660. https://doi.org/10.1371/journal.pone.0082660.

Determinants of patient and health care services delays for tuberculosis diagnosis in Italy

Anna Maria Peri[1,2*], Davide Paolo Bernasconi[3], Nadia Galizzi[4], Alberto Matteelli[5], Luigi Codecasa[6], Vincenza Giorgio[7], Antonio Di Biagio[8], Fabio Franzetti[9], Antonella Cingolani[10], Andrea Gori[2] and Giuseppe Lapadula[1]

Abstract

Background: Prompt diagnosis of active tuberculosis (TB) has paramount importance to reduce TB morbidity and mortality and to prevent the spread of *Mycobacterium tuberculosis*. Few studies so far have assessed the diagnostic delay of TB and its risk factors in low-incidence countries.

Methods: We present a cross-sectional multicentre observational study enrolling all consecutive patients diagnosed with TB in seven referral centres in Italy. Information on demographic and clinical characteristics, health-seeking trajectories and patients' knowledge and awareness of TB were collected. Diagnostic delay was assessed as patient-related (time between symptoms onset and presentation to care) and healthcare-related (time between presentation to care and TB diagnosis). Factors associated with patient-related and healthcare-related delays in the highest tertile were explored using uni- and multivariate logistic regression analyses.

Results: We enrolled 137 patients, between June 2011 and May 2012. The median diagnostic delay was 66 days (Interquartile Range [IQR] 31–146). Patient-related and healthcare-related delay were 14.5 days (IQR 0–54) and 31 days (IQR: 7.25–85), respectively. Using multivariable analysis, patients living in Italy for < 5 years were more likely to have longer patient-related delay (> 3 weeks) than those living in Italy for > 5 years (Odds Ratio [OR] 3.47; 95% Confidence Interval [CI] 1.09–11.01). The most common self-reported reasons to delay presentation to care were the mild nature of symptoms (82%) and a good self-perceived health (76%). About a quarter (26%) of patients had wrong beliefs and little knowledge of TB, although this was not associated with longer diagnostic delay. Regarding healthcare-related delay, multivariate analysis showed that extra-pulmonary TB (OR 4.3; 95% CI 1.4–13.8) and first contact with general practitioner (OR 5.1; 95% CI 1.8–14.5) were both independently associated with higher risk of healthcare-related delay > 10 weeks.

Conclusions: In this study, TB was diagnosed with a remarkable delay, mainly attributable to the healthcare services. Delay was higher in patients with extra-pulmonary disease and in those first assessed by general practitioners. We suggest the need to improve knowledge and raise awareness about TB not only in the general population but also among medical providers. Furthermore, specific programs to improve access to care should be designed for recent immigrants, at significantly high risk of patient-related delay.

Keywords: Tuberculosis, Diagnostic delay, Access to care

* Correspondence: annamaria.peri@policlinico.mi.it
[1]Division of Infectious Diseases, "San Gerardo" Hospital, Via GB Pergolesi 33, Monza, Italy
[2]Infectious Diseases Unit, Fondazione IRCCS Ca' Granda, Ospedale Maggiore Policlinico, University of Milan, Milan, Italy
Full list of author information is available at the end of the article

Background

The delay in diagnosis of tuberculosis (TB) is one of the main factors contributing to the spread of *Mycobacterium tuberculosis* and preventing its elimination. Several studies reported a remarkable delay in TB diagnosis, often longer than 2 months. Both patients and healthcare-services can contribute to TB diagnostic delay, the former deferring their presentation to care and the latter missing the opportunity of a well-timed diagnosis. While most of the studies on this topic have been conducted in settings with limited resources and high TB incidence [1–11], substantial delays in TB diagnosis have been described also in high-resource settings [12–17]. A meta-analysis of the studies conducted between 1990 and 2008 showed that the mean diagnostic delay, including the proportion attributable to healthcare system, is not significantly different in constrained-resource and high-resource countries [18]. Determinants of TB diagnostic delay vary according to different studies and geographical contexts. Some studies reported that gender and age are associated with delayed TB diagnosis, with women and the elderly experiencing the highest delays [1, 4, 8, 11, 16, 17]. Social factors, such as unemployment, low income and low-grade education, have also been shown to influence time to TB diagnosis, particularly in low- and mid-resource settings [1, 7, 8, 11]. In addition, some studies from high-resource countries with low TB prevalence reported that TB diagnosis may require longer time in autochthonous patients than in immigrants [13, 15, 17]. In particular, in a study conducted in Norway, the delay attributable to healthcare services was significantly longer in patients born in Norway compared to patients born abroad. Of note, 86% of the 83 patients affected by TB included in the study were born abroad [13]. Similarly, an Italian survey from 2003 reported that a long delay attributable to healthcare services was significantly more frequent in Italians than in migrants while a long delay attributable to patients was significantly more frequent in recent migrants compared to Italians [15]. Also in UK, autochthonous patients had been demonstrated to have longer healthcare services delays than those born outside the UK [17].

Extra-pulmonary TB is often and universally reported as an important risk factor for diagnostic delay, because of its often non-specific signs and symptoms [14, 17]. This is true not only for high-incidence countries but also for low-incidence ones. Indeed, extra-pulmonary TB was associated with longer health care delay in Denmark, Norway and the UK [14, 15, 17].

With 4032 new cases diagnosed during the year 2016, incidence of TB in Italy has been estimated around 6.1 (5.3–7.1) per 100,000 population [19] with up to 50% of cases affecting migrants [20].

Country-specific assessment of TB diagnostic delay and identification of the determinants of such delay is essential to improve the access to care of patients with TB. Therefore, we performed a cross-sectional multicentre observational study, aimed at assessing patient- and healthcare-related delay in TB diagnosis in Italy and the risk factors associated with it.

Methods

Study design and setting

We conducted a cross-sectional multicentre observational study in seven referral centres for the diagnosis and treatment of TB in Italy, five in Northern Italy ("San Gerardo" Hospital, Monza; "Villa Marelli" Clinic, Milan; "Luigi Sacco" Hospital, Milan; "Spedali Civili" Hospital, Brescia, "San Martino" Hospital, Genova), one in Central Italy ("Policlinico Gemelli", Rome) and one in Southern Italy ("Fallacara" Hospital, Bari).

Participants

All consecutive adult patients (> 18 years old) diagnosed with TB between June 1st 2011 and May 30th 2012 were considered for enrolment. Patients with TB at any site (pulmonary and/or extra-pulmonary) were included. Patients whose clinical conditions interfered with their ability to comply with the study procedures or those who were unable to fill questionnaires because of lack of linguistic competence, as assessed by the investigators, were excluded.

The study protocol was approved by the Ethical Committees in all participant centres and was conducted according to Good Clinical Practice principles in agreement to the Declaration of Helsinki. All patients signed an informed consent before enrolment. The study protocol was registered under the US National Institute of Health ClinicalTrials.gov register, reference number: NCT01390987. Study start date: June 2011.

Variables and data measurement

Upon enrolment, the investigator recorded patients demographic, epidemiological and clinical data. The following demographic and epidemiological variables were collected: gender, age, nationality, year of arrival in Italy, school degree, occupation, annual income and housing condition. Clinical variables included: site of TB, symptoms at presentation, dates and results of TB diagnostic procedures, presence of comorbidities and risk factors for mycobacterial infections (i.e., congenital or acquired immunosuppressive conditions including HIV, cirrhosis, neoplasms, diabetes, chronic renal failure, recent incarceration, alcohol or drug abuse), family history of TB, previous history or exposure to TB.

Patients were asked to report the date of symptoms onset and the date and type of all the contacts with a physician or a medical care facility since then. Symptoms at TB presentation were explored with a self-administered questionnaire and their frequency was graded on a semi-quantitative scale ("never", "sometimes", "often", "very often"). Patients' beliefs on social impact of the disease and their knowledge about TB were also explored through a questionnaire, whose items were derived from a previous South African study and adapted to the Italian setting [21]. In particular, knowledge about multidrug resistant TB and correlation between TB and HIV were not explored, considering the low incidence of these conditions in our country. Eventually, patients were also asked to report the reasons that, in their opinion, had delayed their access to medical observation and to give suggestions about how to accelerate the access to care.

Bias

Results might be biased by the exclusion from enrolment of those patients not able to fill in the questionnaires because of linguistic barriers or particularly severe clinical conditions. Furthermore, recall bias should also be addressed, reflecting differences in the accuracy of the recollections retrieved by study participants.

Study size

Due to the observational nature of the study the size of the study sample was not formally calculated based on statistical power analysis.

Quantitative variables and statistical methods

Diagnostic delay was defined as the time between the onset of the symptoms and the date of the diagnosis of TB and further distinguished in patient-related and healthcare-related delay. Patient-related delay was defined as the time between the onset of symptoms of TB and the first time the patient sought medical care. Healthcare-related delay was defined as the time between the first presentation to care and the diagnosis of TB. Furthermore, treatment delay was defined as the time between diagnosis of TB and anti-TB treatment initiation.

Patients' characteristics were summarized using numbers (percentages) for categorical variables and median (Interquartile Range [IQR]) for numerical variables. Uni- and multivariable logistic regression models were used to assess the association between high patient-related delay (defined as >2nd tertile of the delay distribution) and the following factors: gender, age, nationality, years lived in Italy, housing conditions, school degree, occupation, annual income, risk factors for mycobacterial infections, site of infection, symptoms, healthcare structure of first assessment, reasons reported by patients as responsible of delaying access to care, beliefs and knowledge about TB. All factors considered in the univariable models were also included in the multivariable model except for housing conditions, school degree and occupation, which were excluded due to sparse data. Similar models were run to explore possible associations between high healthcare-related delay (defined as >2nd tertile of distribution) and the same factors (with the exclusion of patients' self-reported reasons for delaying access to care and their beliefs and knowledge about the disease) plus patient delay. Again, all factors considered in the univariable models were also included in the multivariable model, except for housing conditions, school degree and occupation. In order to exclude that the choice of a specific cut-off could have influenced the results, quantile regression was performed, considering healthcare- and patient-related delays as continuous variables (the same set of covariates included in the corresponding logistic models was used).

All presented P are two-sided with a $P < 0.05$ indicating conventional statistical significance. All analyses were performed using R software version 3.3.2.

Results

Among 163 patients evaluated for the study, 137 were enrolled. Reasons of exclusion from enrolment were: inability to sign the informed consent (8 patients), language barrier ($n = 5$), patient declined to participate to the study ($n = 8$), loss to follow up or death after the first visit ($n = 4$ and 1, respectively). Six patients returned blank questionnaires, thus information on symptoms, healthcare seeking pathway, knowledge and awareness of TB was available for 131/137 patients.

Patients characteristics

The median age at patient enrolment was 40 (IQR: 29–56) years. Most participants were male (87/137, 63%) and foreign-born (95/137, 69%). About half of the patients (70/137) reported to have no income or to earn < 10,000€ per year and 7% (10/137) were unemployed. Forty-three percent (57/132) of the patients attended school for ≤ 8 years. Exclusive extra-pulmonary TB involvement was diagnosed in about a third of the study participants (38/137). Diagnosis of TB was confirmed by positive cultures for *M.tuberculosis* in 82/137 cases (59.8%). Among the remaining patients, diagnosis was based on the presence of acid-fast bacilli at microscopy in 13/137 cases (9.5%), on positive molecular tests (*M.tuberculosis*-PCR) in 10/137 (7.3%), and on histology in 12/137 cases (8.8%). In the last 20/137 (14.6%) patients, a clinical diagnosis of TB was established defined as signs, symptoms and clinical history consistent with TB in association to clinical response to empirical treatment with anti-TB medication within 2 months of treatment initiation.

Complete patient characteristics are listed in Table 1.

Diagnostic delay

The median diagnostic delay was 66 days (IQR 31–146) since the onset of the symptoms. In particular, the median delay attributable to patients was 14.5 days (IQR 0–54), whilst the median healthcare-related delay was 31 days (IQR 7.25–85). Antimycobacterial treatment was initiated the same day of the diagnosis or the day after in most of patients (median therapeutic delay: 0 days, IQR: 0–3). Diagnostic delay was

Table 1 Characteristics of the 137 patients diagnosed with tuberculosis enrolled in the study

Characteristic	*N* = 137
Female gender	50 (36.5)
Age (median [IQR])	40 [29, 56]
Nationality	
Italian	42 (30.7)
African	31 (22.6)
South-American	17 (12.4)
Asian	27 (19.7)
Eastern European	20 (14.6)
Years lived in Italy (*N* = 95)	
<2	11 (11.6)
2–5	20 (21.0)
>5	49 (51.6)
Housing conditions	
Living with others	46 (33.6)
Living with family	71 (51.8)
Living alone	20 (14.6)
Have children	84 (61.3)
School degree	
Primary school degree	26 (19.0)
Secondary school degree	31 (22.6)
High school diploma	65 (47.4)
University degree	10 (7.3)
Occupation	
Unemployed	10 (7.3)
Employed/Retired	117 (85.4)
Student	10 (7.3)
Annual income	
No income	28 (20.4)
<10,000 €	42 (30.7)
10,000–30,000 € per year	42 (30.7)
>30,000 per year	6 (4.4)
HIV and other comorbidities	
HIV infection	10 (7.3)
Immunosuppressive therapies	5 (3.6)
Haematological diseases	2 (1.5)
Chronic kidney disease	2 (1.5)
Neoplasms	6 (4.4)
Cirrhosis	4 (2.9)
Diabetes	10 (7.3)
Social conditions	
Alcohol abuse	3 (2.2)
Drug abuse	2 (1.5)
Homelessness	3 (2.2)
Past imprisonment	5 (3.6)
History of potential exposure	
Family history	7 (5.1)
Professional exposure	3 (2.2)
Contact with TB patient	8 (5.8)
Site of involvement	
Extra-pulmonary	38 (27.7)
Pulmonary	78 (56.9)
Pulmonary and extra-pulmonary	20 (14.6)
Case Definition	
New Case	117 (85.4)
Relapse or previous failure	14 (10.2)
Diagnosis	
Culture	82 (59.8)
Microscopy	13 (9.5)
Molecular test	10 (7.3)
Histology	12 (8.8)
Clinical	20 (14.6)
Respiratory symptoms[a]	88 (67.2)
Healthcare structure of first assessment[a]	
General practitioner	55 (42.0)
Specialist consultation	25 (19.2)
Emergency Department	39 (29.8)
Other	11 (8.5)
Reasons for delay[a,b]	
Underestimation of symptoms	98 (74.8)
Fear of consequences	54 (41.2)
Barriers to healthcare access	49 (37.4)
Good TB knowledge[a]	80 (61.1)
Uncorrect beliefs about TB[a]	76 (58)

All results are presented as number of occurrences with percentages in brackets, unless otherwise specified

[a]Percentages calculated on the total of 131 patients who returned a filled questionnaire

Abbreviations: *HIV* human immunodeficiency virus, *IQR* inter-quartile range, *N/A* not applicable, *TB* tuberculosis

[b]"Underestimation of symptoms" includes the following self-reported reasons in the questionnaire: "symptoms did not seem to be important", "overall I felt well";

"Fear of consequences" includes the following self-reported reasons: "I was afraid of a positive result", "I was afraid I would be reported to the authorities", "I was afraid to lose my job", "I was afraid to be rejected by my friends", "My friends discouraged me"

"Barriers to healthcare access" includes the following self-reported reasons: "I did not have time to go to the doctor", "I did not know where to go", "I did not have money" significantly higher among subjects with extra-pulmonary than among those with pulmonary TB. This difference was mainly driven by a significant difference in healthcare-related delay (54 days [IQR 24–122] versus 17 days [IQR 3–63] among subjects with extra-pulmonary versus pulmonary TB, respectively; Mann-Whitney $p < 0.001$). Although also patient-related delay was higher among those with extra-pulmonary than among those with pulmonary TB, such difference did not reach statistical significance (27 days (IQR 0–58) versus 10 days (IQR 1–49); Mann-Whitney $p = 0.443$).

Notably, the median diagnostic delay did not statistically differ between Italian and foreign-born patients (68 days [IQR: 40–157] versus 65 days [IQR: 31–136], respectively; Mann-Whitney $p = 0.579$), nor it differed after stratification for site of infection. In detail, diagnostic delay of patients with pulmonary TB was, in median, 62 days (IQR 28–139) among Italians and 45 days (IQR 20–103) among foreign-born patients (Mann-Whitney $p = 0.278$). The median diagnostic delay of patients with extra-pulmonary TB was 94 days (IQR 54–276) among Italians versus 91 days (IQR 49–156) among foreign-born patients (Mann-Whitney $p = 0.659$).

There was no evidence of any statistically significant correlation between patient-related and healthcare-related delay (Spearman correlation index 0.17).

The most commonly reported reasons that led patients to procrastinate their presentation to care were the mild nature of the initial symptoms (108/131, 82%) and a good self-perceived health (99/131, 76%). A lower, but significant, proportion of patients, ranging from 17 to 32%, reported fear of the consequences of a diagnosis, fear to be reported to the authorities, lack of knowledge of the health system, time and economical constraints as additional barriers to the access to care. Figure 1 shows the complete results of the questionnaire aimed at assessing the reasons of delayed access to medical observation.

Knowledge and beliefs about tuberculosis

Almost two thirds of the patients (80/131, 61%) had a good knowledge about TB route of transmission, epidemiology and prognosis. In particular, 92% (120/131) of the patients were aware that TB is a communicable disease and is transmitted from person to person by direct contact, although only 82% (108/131) knew it spreads through airborne transmission. Whilst 6% (8/131) thought that TB is an untreatable disease, 94% (123/131) reported it could be cured with antibiotics. Most patients (127/131, 97%) were well aware of the risk of serious health consequences for those not taking treatment, but 18% (23/131) denied that untreated TB could lead to death. Of note, 15% (20/131) believed that TB only affects immigrants or people with pre-existing health problems.

A considerable number of study participants (28/131, 21%) had self-blame feelings, attributing the acquisition of TB to their own misbehaviour, while 27% (36/131) of the study population believed that they got TB due to wrong behaviours of other people. Eventually, 26% (34/131) of the patients reported that people affected by TB should be secluded from the society.

Risk factors for patient-related delay

Table 2 shows uni- and multivariable analyses investigating factors associated with a patient-related delay in the highest tertile (> 3 weeks). Using univariate analysis, no significant association was found between patient-related delay and age, gender, school degree, occupation, annual income, housing condition and nationality. Nonetheless, foreign-born patients living in Italy for < 5 years were more likely to present late to medical observation than Italians or foreign-born patients who had lived in Italy for ≥5 years (Odds Ratio [OR] 2.45; 95% Confidence Interval [CI] 1.03–5.87; $p = 0.043$). This result was confirmed in the multivariate analysis, after adjusting for possible confounders (Adjusted OR 3.47; 95% CI 1.09–11.01; $p = 0.035$). Moreover, using multivariable analysis, symptoms underestimation was also marginally associated with a higher patient-related delay (Adjusted OR 3.43; 95% CI 0.98–12.04; $p = 0.055$). Wrong knowledge and beliefs on TB, on the contrary, were not significantly associated with a delayed presentation to care.

Sensitivity analysis using quantile regression (full results shown in Additional file 1: Table S1) yielded to only slightly different results, suggesting older age (difference of the medians 0.05; 95% CI 0.03–0.09; $p = 0.019$) to be a possible additional factor associated with longer patient-related delay.

Risk factors for healthcare-related delay

Table 3 shows the results of uni- and multivariable analyses assessing factors associated with healthcare-related delay in the highest tertile (> 10 weeks). Using univariate analysis, the following factors were significantly associated with a healthcare-related delay: absence of respiratory symptoms (OR 2.57; 95% CI 1.19–5.55; $p = 0.016$), first assessment performed by the general practitioner (OR 5.95; 95% CI 2.66–13.31; $p < 0.001$) and extra-pulmonary TB (OR 4.09; 95% CI 1.82–9.22; $p = 0.001$). Using multivariate analysis, first assessment by the general practitioner was confirmed to be independently associated with a higher risk of diagnostic delay attributable to the healthcare system (Adjusted OR 5.09; 95% CI 1.78–14.54; $p = 0.002$). Extra-pulmonary involvement (Adjusted OR 4.34; 95% CI 1.36–13.81; $p = 0.013$) and absence of respiratory symptoms (OR 3.29; 95% CI 1.18–9.23; $p = 0.023$) were also confirmed to be two additional independent predictors of healthcare-related delay, although these two variables were explored in two separated multivariate models, in order to avoid multicollinearity.

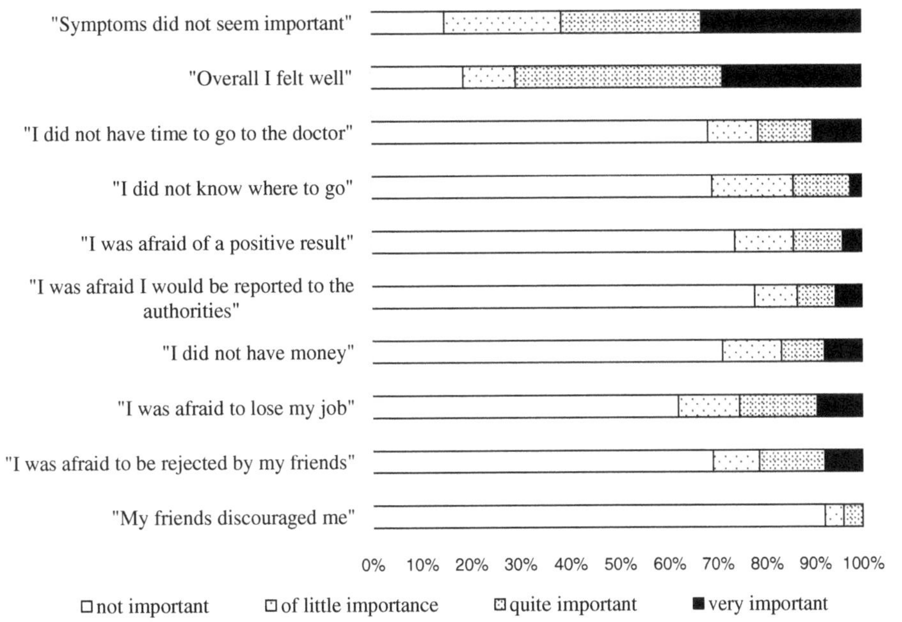

Fig. 1 Self-reported reasons for delayed access to care

No association was found between healthcare-related delay and other explored covariates, including patient nationality, demographic and social characteristics.

Using quantile regression (Additional file 1: Table S2), first assessment by General Practitioner (difference of the medians 6.45; 95% CI 4.23–9.51; $p < 0.001$), extra-pulmonary involvement (difference of the medians 5.51; 95% CI 2.25–10.52; $p < 0.001$) and absence of respiratory symptoms (difference of the medians 2.53; 95% CI 1.08–10.40; $p = 0.001$) were confirmed to be associated with longer healthcare-related delay.

Health seeking pathways

Overall, the median number of medical consultation or contacts with an healthcare facility before diagnosis was 2 (IQR 1–3). Figure 2 shows the pathways followed by the patients, from the first time they presented to a healthcare provider up to the diagnosis. The health-seeking pathways are distinguished according to the first healthcare provider the patients consulted (general practitioner, emergency department or specialist consultant). Patients that initially sought medical care from their general practitioner consulted an average of 2.8 healthcare providers before the diagnosis, patients evaluated in a hospital-based Emergency Department had a mean of 1.8 consultations before receiving the correct diagnosis, whereas patients that were first evaluated by a specialist consultant in outpatient clinics were diagnosed after a mean of 1.4 consultations. Suspect of tuberculosis was raised after the first contact in 46% (18/39) of patients presenting to an emergency departments, in 60% (15/25) of those attending a specialist consultation and in 11% (6/55) of the patients evaluated by the general practitioner.

Discussion

Herein we report a cross-sectional observational study assessing the diagnostic delay in the diagnosis of tuberculosis in seven TB referral centres in Italy. A considerable latency between symptom onset, clinical presentation and TB diagnosis was observed. In most of the patients, the diagnostic delay was longer than 2 months and about a quarter of the population was diagnosed after > 5 months since the onset of the symptoms. Our results are consistent with those from previous studies [5, 8, 12–18] and confirm that unacceptable diagnostic delays still exist, in high-resource as well as in resource-constrained settings. In our study, the diagnostic delay attributable to healthcare services was about two-times longer than that attributable to patients (in median, 31 versus 14 days, respectively). Although this finding is similar to a previous regional survey conducted in Italy [15], several other studies conducted in high-resource settings showed patients and healthcare service to be equally responsible for the overall diagnostic delay of TB [12–14, 16, 22, 23]. Possible explanations for this apparent discrepancy might depend on the proportion of elderly and foreign-born patients in the general population and on differences between healthcare systems, in particular in their arrangements for migrants, translating into variable access to care.

We found that native and non-native patients had similar time of presentation to care. Nonetheless, when we distinguished patients according to the time of their

Table 2 Univariate and multivariate regression analysis assessing risk factors for patient diagnostic delay > 3 weeks

Factors	Univariate analysis OR (95% CI)	Multivariate analysis OR (95% CI)
Age (years)	*1 (0.98; 1.02)*	*1.03 (1; 1.06)*
Female gender	1.52 (0.74; 3.13)	1.72 (0.68; 4.39)
Nationality		
Italian	1	1
African	1.66 (0.61;4.50)	2.91 (0.62; 13.60)
South-American	1.25 (0.39;4.01)	1.54 (0.33; 7.15)
Asian	1.79 (0.65;4.90)	1.48 (0.33; 6.56)
Eastern European	1.98 (0.65;6.04)	3.19 (0.64; 15.76)
Living in Italy for < 5 years	*2.46 (1.03;5.87)*	*3.47 (1.09; 11.01)*
Annual income		
≥10,000 €	1	1
<10,000 €	0.930 (0.43;2)	1.21 (0.47; 3.14)
No source of income	1.89 (0.64;5.58)	2.84 (0.53; 15.24)
Housing conditions		
Living with others	1	
Living with family	1.14 (0.53;2.47)	
Living alone	0.47 (0.14;1.54)	
School degree		
University degree	1	
Primary/secondary school degree	1.50 (0.38;5.88)	
High school diploma	1.00 (0.26;3.92)	
Occupation		
Unemployed	1	
Employed/Retired	0.82 (0.20;3.44)	
Student	0.50 (0.07;3.55)	
Comorbidities	0.79 (0.34;1.80)	0.95 (0.33; 2.70)
Social conditions	1.61 (0.41;6.30)	1.50 (0.27; 8.25)
History of potential exposure	0.68 (0.30;1.54)	0.61 (0.22; 1.71)
Extra-pulmonary TB	1.36 (0.63;2.94)	1.43 (0.51; 4.03)
Absence of respiratory symptoms[a]	0.96 (0.46;2.03)	1.38 (0.53; 3.61)[a]
First assessment by General Practitioner	0.93 (0.45;1.88)	0.63 (0.24; 1.64)
Reasons for delay[b]		
Underestimation of symptoms	1.47 (0.65;3.34)	3.43 (0.98; 12.04)
Fear of consequences	0.87 (0.43;1.77)	1.01 (0.34; 2.98)
Barriers to healthcare access	1.02 (0.50;2.10)	1.35 (0.49; 3.74)
Bad TB knowledge	1.17 (0.57;2.40)	1.23 (0.48; 3.19)
Uncorrect beliefs about TB	0.78 (0.38;1.57)	0.59 (0.23; 1.51)

Statistically significant results are shown in italics
[a]assessed in a separate multivariable model not including extra-pulmonary TB
Abbreviations: *OR* Odd Ratio, *CI* Confidence Interval, *TB* Tuberculosis
[b]For details of self-reported reasons for delay see Table 1

first arrival in Italy, those who lived in Italy for < 5 years had considerable higher risk of late presentation to care than long-term and permanent residents. This suggests that recently immigrated subjects experience significant difficulties in accessing to Health Services, possibly because of bureaucratic, legal and economical barriers,

Table 3 Univariate and multivariate regression analysis assessing risk factors for healthcare system diagnostic delay > 10 weeks

Factors	Univariate analysis OR (95% CI)	Multivariate analysis OR (95% CI)
Age (years)	1.00 (0.98;1.02)	1 (0.96; 1.03)
Female gender	1.60 (0.75;3.38)	1.90 (0.65; 5.55)
Nationality		
Italian	1	1
African	1.43 (0.52;3.93)	0.63 (0.11; 3.57)
South-American	0.45 (0.11;1.83)	0.20 (0.03; 1.35)
Asian	1.43 (0.52;3.93)	1.09 (0.23; 5.12)
Eastern European	0.55 (0.15;2.00)	0.58 (0.10; 3.38)
Living in Italy for < 5 years	1.09 (0.45;2.64)	1.00 (0.28; 3.65)
Annual income		
≥ 10,000 €	1	1
< 10,000 €	1.99 (0.89;4.45)	1.78 (0.60; 5.27)
No source of income	1.30 (0.43;3.97)	1.74 (0.39; 7.73)
Housing conditions		
Living with others	1	
Living with family	1.14 (0.51;2.55)	
Living alone	0.38 (0.09;1.51)	
School degree		
University degree	1	
Primary/secondary school degree	1.90 (0.37;9.82)	
High school diploma	2.10 (0.41;10.79)	
Occupation		
Unemployed	1	
Employed/Retired	3.55 (0.42;29.88)	
Student	3.50 (0.28;43.16)	
Comorbidities	0.57 (0.22;1.45)	0.58 (0.17; 2.04)
Social conditions	0.24 (0.03;2.02)	0.70 (0.07; 7.41)
History of potential exposure	0.50 (0.20;1.28)	0.67 (0.20; 2.27)
Extra-pulmonary TB	*4.09 (1.82;9.22)*	*4.34 (1.36; 13.81)*
Absence of respiratory symptoms	*2.57 (1.19;5.55)*	*3.29 (1.17; 9.23)*[a]
First assessment by the General Practitioner	*5.95 (2.66;13.31)*	*5.09 (1.78; 14.54)*
Patient delay (per week longer)	1.00 (0.99;1.02)	0.99 (0.97; 1.01)

Statistically significant results are shown in italics
[a]assessed in a separate multivariable model not including extra-pulmonary TB
Abbreviations: *OR* Odd Ratio, *CI* Confidence Interval, *TB* Tuberculosis

which were, indeed, reported by 12–18% of the patients. By converse, foreign-born patients who had settled in Italy for ≥5 years behaved similarly to native Italians. Given the fact that recent immigrants are also those with the highest risk of TB reactivation/reinfection, specific screening program, targeted information campaigns and social inclusion programs could be beneficial for these patients. Symptoms underestimation was the most common reason leading patients not to seek early medical care and, in multivariate model, it was associated with a > 3-fold increased risk of high patient-related delay. In this respect, promoting an adequate knowledge about TB risk and its clinical presentation is advisable.

We did not find any significant association between other socioeconomic determinants (such as level of education, employment status, annual income or family condition) and delayed presentation to care or health care-related delay. Despite the fact that the association between social disadvantage and TB has been well documented, this finding is not completely surprising because

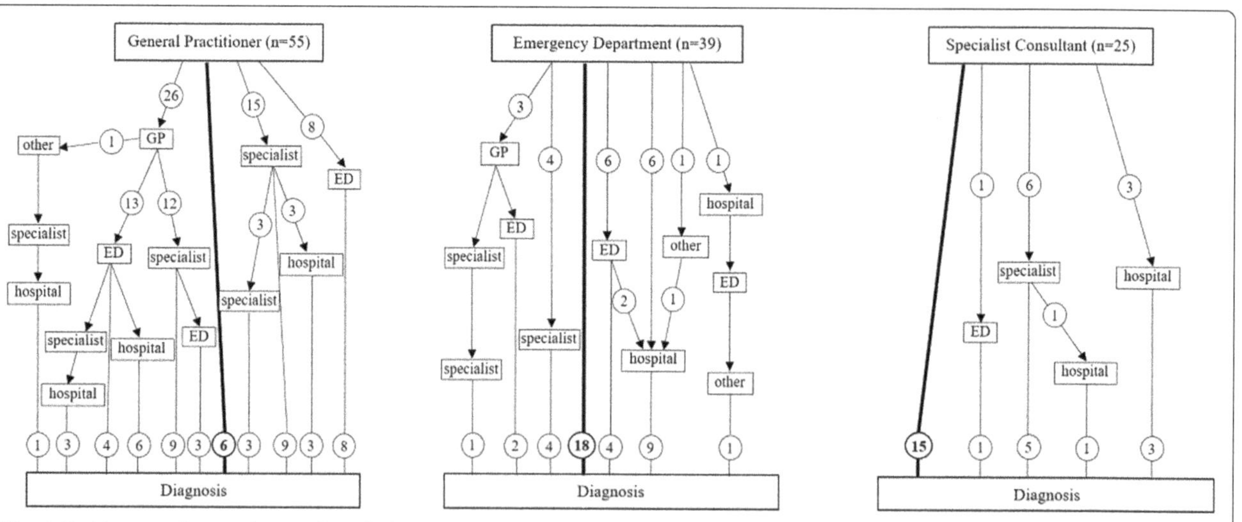

Fig. 2 Healthcare seeking pathways of enrolled patients according to the first medical provider consulted. Numbers in circles refer to patients assessed by different medical providers before diagnosis of tuberculosis. Abbreviations: ED, emergency department; GP, general practitioner

no single measure of socioeconomic status can capture all the aspects of social vulnerabilities and health inequalities that determine delayed diagnosis.

Healthcare related delay was, in our study, the main contributor to total TB diagnostic delay. Consistently with other studies [13, 14, 16, 17], extra-pulmonary TB involvement and lack of respiratory symptoms were associated with longer diagnostic delays. Unspecific symptoms, unusual clinical presentations and difficulties in obtaining specimens for the diagnosis are all likely explanation for this finding and reflect the challenges faced by clinicians during TB diagnosis. It is unrealistic to believe that, particularly in low-incidence countries, all TB can get to a prompt and rapid diagnosis and, from an epidemiological point of view, delays in extra-pulmonary TB diagnosis can look less important than delaying the diagnosis of other communicable forms of TB. Nonetheless, extra-pulmonary TB is often clinically severe and life-threatening and diagnostic delays can be associated with disease progression and a bad prognosis. Before a definite diagnosis is determined, a certain index of suspicion for TB disease should be maintained in patients with compatible symptoms and/or epidemiological risk factors, even when other diagnoses are deemed more likely.

Health-seeking pathways had high influence on diagnostic delay, with a major role played by the first health care provider consulted by patients. Patients initially assessed by the general practitioner experienced longer healthcare-related delay and needed a higher number of contacts with the healthcare system before diagnosis, than those who had direct access to the hospital or consulted a specialist. Various reasons may explain this difference. First, Italy is a low-incidence country and TB rates have steadily reduced in the last 50 years. In such setting, the ability of general practitioner to recognize and diagnose a disease that they rarely see is likely to have reduced over time. As a matter of fact, TB diagnostic delay in healthcare structures has been previously demonstrated to be inversely proportional to the number of cases annually diagnosed by the health-care structures themselves [24]. It is not surprising, therefore, that specialist physicians play an important role in case detection, nowadays. Nonetheless, more than 40% of the patients, in our study, referred to the general practitioner, in the first instance. Informative campaigns and continuous education programs on TB for general practitioners are therefore highly warranted and likely to have an impact on diagnostic delay. Another possible explanation for the health-seeking pathway impact on healthcare-related delay is that symptoms of patients presenting to the emergency department could be more severe or specific than those of patients who contacted their general practitioner, thus facilitating a more prompt diagnosis. Lastly, patients presenting to the emergency department or specialist consultation could also be those more likely to be perceived at risk for TB, because undocumented migrants and other marginalized patients could have easy and free access to hospital care and to TB facilities, but not to primary care.

Results from the present survey add new and important information about TB diagnostic delay in a low-incidence country. Some limitations of the study should be, however, acknowledged. In particular, the small sample size (about 10% of the TB cases notified every year in Italy), the exclusion from enrolment of patients due to language barriers and inability to sign informed consent and the heterogeneous geographical distribution of the TB referral centres included in the study may limit its generalizability. Nonetheless, it should be noted that the preponderance of centres located in large urban areas of Northern Italy included in our study reflects the higher burden of TB in these areas. Moreover, two important reference centres, one in Central and one in Southern Italy, were also involved. Another limitation of the study is the lack of previous validation of the questionnaire on knowledge and beliefs of the patients, which was indeed derived and adapted from a questionnaire previously validated in a different context [21], but not further validated on our population. On the other hand, despite the previously discussed recall bias, the use of specifically designed questionnaires is an invaluable strength of this research, because it allowed to collect precise data on patients' socio-economic conditions, path of access to the healthcare services and patients' beliefs and opinions. Finally, consensus about what duration between onset of TB symptoms and diagnosis is considered as delay is lacking in the literature and to this extent quantiles were used in our analysis. Nonetheless, the principle "the later, the worse" is certainly reasonable at least for highly contagious forms of TB.

Conclusions

In conclusion, our study showed that TB diagnostic delay is common. Recently immigrated patients are those most at risk for a delayed presentation to care, whereas those with extra-pulmonary disease have lower chances of being diagnosed early after presentation for care. In addition, patient evaluated, in the first instance, by primary care physicians are more likely to delay the diagnosis and to need repeat consultations before TB is suspected. Since delaying TB diagnosis can have severe implications for patients health as well as for TB transmission, informative campaigns for patients and continuous education programs for physicians are highly warranted.

Abbreviations

TB: Tuberculosis

Acknowledgements

Not applicable.

Funding

No funding was received to perform this study.

Authors' contributions

GL conceived and designed the study. AMP contributed to analysis and interpretation of data and wrote the manuscript under the supervision of GL who revised it for important intellectual content. DB performed the statistical analysis. GL, NG, AM, LC, VG, ADB, FF, AC and AG contributed to patients' enrolment from their centres and to data collection. All authors contributed to revising the manuscript and approved its final version for publication. All authors also agreed to be accountable for all aspects of the work.

Ethics approval and consent to participate

The study protocol was approved by the Ethical Committees in all participant centres, in particular: Ethical Committee of "San Gerardo" Hospital, Monza, Ethical Committee of "Villa Marelli" Clinic, Milan, Ethical Committee of "Luigi Sacco" Hospital, Milan, Ethical Committee of "Spedali Civili" Hospital, Brescia, Ethical Committee of "San Martino" Hospital, Genova, Ethical Committee of "Policlinico Gemelli", Rome the Ethical Committee of "Fallacara" Hospital, Bari.
The study was conducted according to Good Clinical Practice principles in agreement to the Declaration of Helsinki. All patients signed an informed consent before enrolment.
The study protocol was registered under the US National Institute of Health ClinicalTrials.gov register, reference number: NCT01390987. Study start date: June 2011.

Consent for publication

Not applicable.

Competing interests

The authors declare that they have no competing interests.

Author details

[1]Division of Infectious Diseases, "San Gerardo" Hospital, Via GB Pergolesi 33, Monza, Italy. [2]Infectious Diseases Unit, Fondazione IRCCS Ca' Granda, Ospedale Maggiore Policlinico, University of Milan, Milan, Italy. [3]Centre of Biostatistics for Clinical Epidemiology, School of Medicine and Surgery, University of Milano-Bicocca, Milan, Italy. [4]"San Raffaele" Hospital, "Vita-Salute" University, Milan, Italy. [5]Department of Infectious and Tropical Diseases, WHO Collaborating Centre for TB/HIV and TB elimination, University of Brescia, Brescia, Italy. [6]Regional TB Reference Centre, "Villa Marelli" Institute, Niguarda Hospital, Milan, Italy. [7]"L. Fallacara" Hospital, Triggiano, BA, Italy. [8]Infectious Diseases Department, IRCCS AOU San Martino-IST, Genova, Italy. [9]"L. Sacco" Hospital, University of Milan, Milan, Italy. [10]Policlinico "Gemelli", "Sacro Cuore" Catholic University, Rome, Italy.

References

1. Ndeikoundam Ngangro N, Chauvin P, Halley des Fontaines V. Determinants of tuberculosis diagnosis delay in limited resources countries. Rev Epidemiol Sante Publique. 2012;60(1):47–57.
2. Finnie RK, Khoza LB, van den Borne B, et al. Factors associated with patient and health care system delay in diagnosis and treatment for TB in sub-Saharan African countries with high burdens of TB and HIV. Tropical Med Int Health. 2011;16(4):394–411.
3. Bogale S, Diro E, Shiferaw AM, et al. Factors associated with the length of delay with tuberculosis diagnosis and treatment among adult tuberculosis patients attending at public health facilities in Gondar town, northwest, Ethiopia. BMC Infect Dis. 2017;17(1):145.
4. Ben Amar J, Hassairi M, Ben Salah N, et al. Pulmonary tuberculosis: diagnostic delay in Tunisia. Med Mal Infect. 2016;46(2):79–86.
5. Mistry N, Rangan S, Dholakia Y, et al. Durations and delays in care seeking, diagnosis and treatment initiation in uncomplicated pulmonary tuberculosis patients in Mumbai, India. PLoS One. 2016;11(3):e0152287.
6. Das D, Dwibedi B. Delay in diagnosis among pulmonary tuberculosis patients of Rayagada District, Odisha, India. Int J Mycobacteriol. 2016;5(Suppl 1):S172–S3.
7. Mahato RK, Laohasiriwong W, Vaeteewootacharn K, et al. Major delays in the diagnosis and Management of Tuberculosis Patients in Nepal. J Clin Diagn Res. 2015;9(10):LC05–9.
8. Machado AC, Steffen RE, Oxlade O, et al. Factors associated with delayed diagnosis of pulmonary tuberculosis in the state of Rio de Janeiro, Brazil. J Bras Pneumol. 2011;37(4):512–20.
9. Sasaki NS, Santos ML, Vendramini SH, et al. Delays in tuberculosis suspicion and diagnosis and related factors. Rev Bras Epidemiol. 2015;18(4):809–23.
10. Rodríguez DA, Verdonck K, Bissell K, et al. Monitoring delays in diagnosis of pulmonary tuberculosis in eight cities in Colombia. Rev Panam Salud Publica. 2016;39(1):12–8.

11. Cai J, Wang X, Ma A, et al. Factors associated with patient and provider delays for tuberculosis diagnosis and treatment in Asia: a systematic review and meta-analysis. PLoS One. 2015;10(3):e0120088.
12. Tattevin P, Che D, Fraisse P, et al. Factors associated with patient and health care system delay in the diagnosis of tuberculosis in France. Int J Tuberc Lung Dis. 2012;16(4):510–5.
13. Farah MG, Rygh JH, Steen TW, et al. Patient and health care system delays in the start of tuberculosis treatment in Norway. BMC Infect Dis. 2006;6:33.
14. Leutscher P, Madsen G, Erlandsen M, et al. Demographic and clinical characteristics in relation to patient and health system delays in a tuberculosis low-incidence country. Scand J Infect Dis. 2012;44(1):29–36.
15. Gagliotti C, Resi D, Moro ML. Delay in the treatment of pulmonary TB in a changing demographic scenario. Int J Tuberc Lung Dis. 2006;10(3):305–9.
16. Sultan H, Haroon S, Syed N. Delay and completion of tuberculosis treatment: a cross-sectional study in the west midlands, UK. J Public Health (Oxf). 2013;35(1):12–20.
17. Saldana L, Abid M, McCarthy N, et al. Factors affecting delay in initiation of treatment of tuberculosis in the Thames Valley, UK. Public Health. 2013;127(2):171–7.
18. Sreeramareddy CT, Panduru KV, Menten J, et al. Time delays in diagnosis of pulmonary tuberculosis: a systematic review of literature. BMC Infect Dis. 2009;9:91.
19. TB burden estimates, notifications and treatment outcomes for individual countries and territories, WHO regions and the world. http://www.who.int/tb/publications/global_report/gtbr2017_annex4.pdf?ua=1. Accessed 10 Jan 2018.
20. La tubercolosi in Italia, rapporto 2008. http://www.salute.gov.it/imgs/C_17_pubblicazioni_1472_allegato.pdf. Accessed 10 Jan 2018.
21. Cramm JM, Finkenflügel HJ, Møller V, et al. TB treatment initiation and adherence in a south African community influenced more by perceptions than by knowledge of tuberculosis. BMC Public Health. 2010;10:72.
22. Sherman LF, Fujiwara PI, Cook SV, et al. Patient and health care system delays in the diagnosis and treatment of tuberculosis. Int J Tuberc Lung Dis. 1999;3(12):1088–95.
23. Ward J, Siskind V, Konstantinos A. Patient and health care system delays in Queensland tuberculosis patients, 1985-1998. Int J Tuberc Lung Dis. 2001; 5(11):1021–7.
24. Greenaway C, Menzies D, Fanning A, et al. Delay in diagnosis among hospitalized patients with active tuberculosis--predictors and outcomes. Am J Respir Crit Care Med. 2002;165(7):927–33.

Characterization of *Mycobacterium tuberculosis* strains in Beijing, China: drug susceptibility phenotypes and Beijing genotype family transmission

Yi Liu, Xuxia Zhang, Yuqing Zhang, Yong Sun, Cong Yao, Wei Wang and Chuanyou Li*

Abstract

Background: The most prevalent strains of *Mycobacterium tuberculosis* (*M.tb*) in Beijing belong to the Beijing genotype family. The influence of Beijing genotype prevalence on the development of drug resistance, and the association of infection with Beijing genotype *M.tb* with population characteristics, in Beijing, however, are still unclear.

Methods: In this retrospective study, 1189 isolates were subjected to drug susceptibility testing (DST) and molecular epidemiological analysis, and differences in the percentage of drug resistance between Beijing and non-Beijing genotype strains were compared. The association between the occurrence of drug resistance and the prevalence of Beijing genotype *M.tb* was analyzed using statistical methods.

Results: The Beijing genotype family was the dominant genotype (83.3%) among the 1189 *M.tb* isolates. Beijing genotype *M.tb* strains were more likely to spread among males [$p = 0.018$, OR (95% CI):1.127(1.004–1.264)] and people in the 45–64 age group [$p = 0.016$, OR (95% CI): 1.438 (1.027–2.015)]. On the contrary, non-Beijing genotype *M.tb* strains were more probably disseminated among the over 65 [$p = 0.005$, OR (95% CI): 0.653 (0.474–0.9)] and non-resident population [$p = 0.035$, OR (95% CI):1.185(0.985–1.427)]. DST results showed that 849 (71.4%) strains were fully sensitive to first-line drugs, while 340 (28.6%) strains were resistant to at least one drug, and 9% (107/1189) were MDR-TB. The frequency of INH-resistance among Beijing genotype strains was significantly lower than that among non-Beijing genotype strains ($p = 0.032$). In addition, the Beijing genotype family readily formed clusters.

Conclusions: Our findings indicate that male and middle-aged people were more probably be infected by Beijing genotype *M.tb*, older people and non-residents were more probably be infected by non-Beijing genotype *M.tb*. The high percentage of resistance to INH occurring in non-Beijing genotype strains suggested that non-Beijing genotype strains should be given much more interest in Beijing.

Keywords: *Mycobacterium tuberculosis*, Beijing genotype, Prevalence, Drug resistance, Association

* Correspondence: lichuanyou6688@hotmail.com
Department of Bacteriology and Immunology, Beijing Key Laboratory on Drug-Resistant Tuberculosis Research, Beijing Tuberculosis and Thoracic Tumor Research Institute/Beijing Chest Hospital, Capital Medical University, Beijing 101149, China

Background

Tuberculosis (TB) is an infectious disease and a significant global public health problem [1, 2]. There were an estimated 10.1 million incident TB cases worldwide in 2017 [3], of which about 6.4 million were notified. Of these, there were an estimated 558,000 cases of multidrug-resistant TB (MDR-TB) and rifampicin resistant TB (RR-TB) [3]. China is one of the 30 high TB burden countries. Although the TB incidence rate and the case fatality ratio have fallen, TB continues to be a public health problem in China [3]. TB is also a public health problem in Beijing, the capital of the People's Republic of China [4]. There is a need for more studies to clarify the association between drug resistance and genotype diversity in Beijing, in particular to, investigate the relationship between drug resistance and Beijing genotype family strains.

Molecular biology tools have been used extensively to determine the genotypic diversity of *M.tb* strains, and have played an important role in TB control and understanding TB epidemiology over the last few decades [5–7]. Spoligotyping and Variable number of tandem repeat (VNTR) are considered to be powerful tools for differentiating the *M.tb* complex into various genotypes [8, 9].While there are many different *M.tb* genotypes, *M.tb* Beijing genotype strains have attracted global attention because of their wide geographical distribution [10]. Beijing genotype strains were first described by van Soolingen et al. in 1995, and were named after Beijing as they were isolated there [11]. Later, the Beijing genotype was also detected in other regions of the world, especially in East Asia [12–14]. Beijing genotype strains are generally considered to be correlated with community outbreaks of TB [15], escaping from the protective effect of the BCG vaccine [16], efficient dissemination or increased virulence [17], and an increased risk on the occurrence of drug resistance [18, 19].

It is very important to have a clearer understanding of the association between the prevalence of Beijing genotype *M.tb* and resistance to anti-TB drugs. Studies to date have not come to consistent conclusions. While some studies have suggested that development of drug resistance in *M.tb* is associated with its genotype [8, 20], drug resistance more likely occurring among Beijing genotype strains [19, 21, 22], and that Beijing genotype strains are more probably develop MDR-TB [23] and be clustered [24], different results have been obtained in different cities and regions [7, 25]. It would appear that the conclusion drawn from a particular study depends upon the project setting considered, the types of drugs considered and the geographical distribution of strains [26].

Beijing is confronting public health issues in the prevention and control of TB [4, 27]. The association between the prevalence of Beijing genotype strains and their drug resistance status in Beijing is unclear. Studies to date have been hindered by many problems, including the fact that the *M.tb* strains chosen were not sufficiently representative, or the number of strains included in was relatively low [21, 22, 28]. It is thus necessary to clarify the situation, particularly considering the high prevalence of tuberculosis and the inconsistent conclusions obtained from different regions and laboratories.

To clarify if there is an association between the Beijing genotype and resistance to anti-TB drugs, we investigated drug susceptibility patterns in Beijing genotype and non-Beijing genotype strains of *M.tb* strains in Beijing, comparing differences in patterns of drug resistance, and analyzing the relationship between genotype patterns and DST results. This study provides important insight into the association between Beijing genotype family strains and resistance to first-line anti-TB drugs in Beijing.

Methods

Description of isolated strains

The 1189 *M.tb* strains analyzed in this study were obtained from pulmonary TB patients, whose sputum was culture-positive for *M.tb.* Strains were collected in 2009 from all districts of Beijing and delivered to the Beijing Tuberculosis and Thoracic Tumor Research Institute [4]. Protocols used in this study were approved by the Ethics Committee of the Beijing Tuberculosis and Thoracic Tumor Research Institute. Patients were included once they signed an informed consent form.

Spoligotyping

Spoligotyping was performed using the standard protocol [29], and was used to identify the genotype of TB strains according to direct repeat (DR) locus as described previously [4]. Both typical Beijing and Beijing-like genotypes were considered to belong to the Beijing genotype. A commercially available kit (SPOLIGOTYPING KIT, Isogen Bioscience BV, Maarssen, The Netherlands) was used according to the manufacturer's instructions. The membrane was detected with a chemiluminescence system, using ECL detection liquid (Amersham, Buckinghamshire, United Kingdom) and X-OMAT film (Kodak, Rochester, NY, US) [4].

VNTR typing

Primers used for amplification of the seven MIRU loci (MIRU-10, 16, 20,23,31,39 and 40), two QUB loci (QUB-11b and QUB-4156C) and three Mtub loci (Mtub04, Mtub21, Mtub24) are listed in Additional file 1: Table S2. VNTR typing was carried out as described previously [4].

Drug susceptibility testing

Drug susceptibility testing (DST) of the *M.tb* strains to four first-line anti-TB drugs (Isonazid, Rifampin, Ethambutol, and Streptomycin) was performed using the proportion method, as recommended by WHO/IUATLD [30]. Concentrations of drugs in L-J media were as follows: isoniazid (INH) 0.2 μg/mL, rifampin (RFP) 40 μg/mL, ethambutol (EMB) 2 μg/mL and streptomycin (SM) 4 μg/mL [22]. Strains were considered resistant to drugs when the growth rate exceeded 1% compared to the control strain [9]. H37Rv strain was used as a control strain and was tested each batch of DST. Strains which showed resistance to isoniazid and rifampin were defined as MDR-TB. All drugs were purchased from Sigma-Aldrich (St. Louis, MO).

Data management

Spoligotyping data and VNTR data were analyzed using BioNumerics software (Version 5.0, Applied-Maths, Sint-Martens-Latem, Belgium) [9]. All spoligotyping data were compared with the SITVIT_WEB database (http://www.pasteur-guadeloupe.fr:8081/SITVIT_ONLINE/) [31]. The Hunter-Gaston discriminatory index (HGDI) of each genotyping method was calculated according to the previously published article [32]. The percentage clustering was calculated as $(n_c\text{-}C)/N$, where N is the total number of isolates, C is the number of clusters, and n_c is the total number of clustered isolates [27, 33].

Statistical analysis

Statistical calculations were performed in SPSS 21 software. Chi-square or Fisher's exact probability tests were used to compare the proportions of different groups [9]. A *p*-value less than 0.05 was considered statistically significant. Odd ratios (ORs) and 95% confidence intervals (CI) were calculated to measure the association between genotype and DST results [27].

Results

The characteristics of studied population

Basic information of the 1189 individual *M.tb* strains collected from Beijing were analyzed (Fig. 1). All isolates investigated in this study were classified according to patient's age and gender (Table 1). The study population included 819 men (76.9%) and 370 women (23.1%), with a median age of 35 (range from 13 to 92) years, of whom 651 were Beijing residents and 538 were non-residents (Table 1). These data suggest that the resident population and non-resident population made an equal contribution to TB prevalence in the population studied.

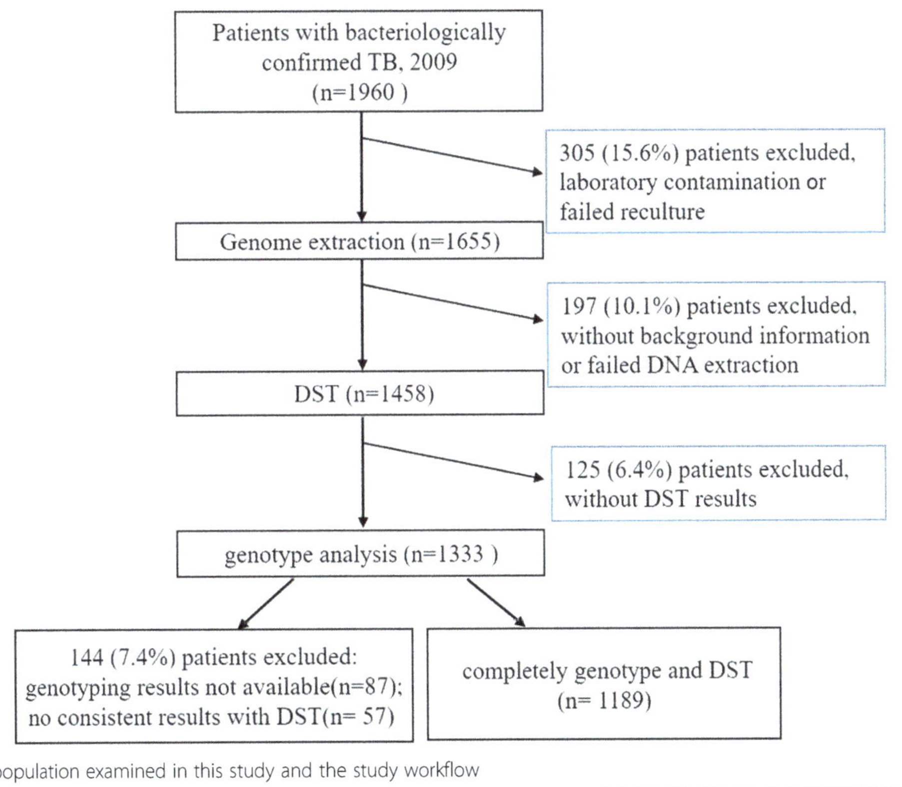

Fig. 1 The study population examined in this study and the study workflow

Table 1 The background information of 1189 patients

Characteristic	Variable	Number of reported cases	Beijing family (%)	Non-Beijing Family (%)	OR (95% CI)	*p* value
All		1189	990	199		
Sex	Male	819	695(70.2)	124(62.3)	1.127(1.004–1.264)	0.018
	Female	370	295(29.8)	75(37.7)		
Age groups, years	< 25	296	242(24.5)	54(27.1)	0.901(0.7–1.16)	0.237
	25–44	462	389(39.3)	73(36.7)	1.071(0.878–1.306)	0.272
	45–64	261	229(23.1)	32(16.1)	1.438(1.027–2.015)	0.016
	≥65	170	130(23.1)	40(20.1)	0.653(0.474–0.9)	0.005
History of TB	New cases	1065	885(89.4)	180(90.5)	0.981(0.909–1.063)	0.383
	Treatment	124	105(10.6)	19(9.5)	1.111(0.698–1.767)	
Registered residence	Residence	651	530(53.5)	121(60.8)	0.880(0.776–0.998)	0.035
	Non-residence	538	460(46.5)	78(39.2)	1.185(0.985–1.427)	

p value indicates whether there is a significant difference between Beijing family and non-Beijing family in sex, age, household, and history of TB. ($p < 0.05$ represents a statistically significant difference)

The genotyping structure of *M.tb* strains

To investigate the genotype of the prevalent strains, the 1189 individual *M.tb* strains were analyzed by spoligotyping and VNTR methods. Of these strains, Beijing genotype families accounted for 83.3% (990/1189) (94.7% were belonged to typical Beijing families and 5.3% were belonged to atypical Beijing families), non-Beijing genotype families accounted for 16.7% (199/1189) (Additional file 2: Table S1). The non-Beijing genotype family mainly included the T1 (SIT53), T2 (SIT52) and MANU2 (SIT54) families et al. Furthermore, a newly discovered genotype cluster included forty-two (3.5%) *M.tb* strains.

Allelic diversity among the 1189 strains was calculated for each VNTR locus using the HGDI (Additional file 1: Table S2). Beijing genotype strains showed a significantly higher clustering rate than the non-Beijing genotype strains after cluster analysis, no matter using spoligotyping or VNTR genotyping data (Table 2).

Association with infection by Beijing genotype strains

There were almost three times as many men as women in the study population (ratio = 2.21; 819/370), and Beijing genotype family strains showed higher prevalence in men (ratio = 2.36; 695/295; $p = 0.018$) (Table 1). We found that Beijing genotype *M.tb* strains were more probably be isolated from men [$p = 0.018$, OR (95%CI):1.127(1.004–1.264)]and people in the 45–64 age group [$p = 0.016$, OR (95% CI): 1.438 (1.027–2.015)]. These results suggest that being male or middle aged is associated with infection by Beijing genotype strains. Conversely, non-Beijing genotype *M.tb* strains were more probably be isolated from people who are older than 65 [$p = 0.005$, OR (95%CI): 0.653 (0.474–0.9)] or non-resident [$p = 0.035$, OR (95%CI): 1.185(0.985–1.427)], indicating that being older or non-resident is associated with infection by non-Beijing genotype strains.

Different association factors were obtained when data from the pan-susceptible TB and drug resistant TB groups were analyzed separately (Table 3). In all the pan-susceptible TB groups, males [$p = 0.035$, OR (95%CI): 1.127(0.980–1.295)] and those aged 45–64 [$p = 0.021$, OR (95%CI): 1.556(1.001–2.419)] were more probably be infected with Beijing genotype strains, consistent with the results above. In all the drug resistant TB groups, results showed that the over 65 s [$p < 0.001$,

Table 2 Comparison of clustered and individual strains between the Beijing and non-Beijing family

Genotyping	Genotype	Beijing family($n = 990$)	Non-Beijing family($n = 199$)	*p* value
Spoligotyping	Individual strains, n	10	58	
	Clustered strains, n	980	141	< 0.001
	Clusters, n	11	22	
	Clustering rate, %	98.9	70.8	
VNTR	Individual strains, n	765	181	
	Clustered strains, n	225	18	< 0.001
	Clusters, n	68	8	
	Clustering rate, %	22.7	9	

($p < 0.05$ represents a statistically significant difference)

Table 3 The General demographic characteristics difference of Beijing genotype family and non-Beijing family patients among the Pan-susceptible TB and any drug resistant TB

Characteristic	Category	Pan-susceptible TB					Any drug resistant TB				
		Number of reported cases	Beijing family (%)	Non-Beijing family (%)	OR (95% CI)	*p* value	Number of reported cases	Beijing family (%)	Non-Beijing family (%)	OR (95% CI)	*p* value
All		849	710	139			340	280	60		
sex	Male	581	495(69.7)	86(61.9)	1.127(0.980–1.295)	0.035	238	200(71.4)	38(63.3)	1.128(0.918–1.386)	0.107
	Female	268	215(30.3)	53(38.1)			102	80(28.6)	22(36.7)		
Age, years	< 25	226	182(25.6)	44(31.7)	0.810(0.615–1.066)	0.071	70	60(21.4)	10(16.7)	1.286(0.7–2.363)	0.242
		318	266(37.5)	52(37.4)	1.001(0.792–1.267)	0.445	144	123(43.9)	21(35)	1.255(0.868–1.816)	0.125
	25–44										
	45–64	170	151(21.3)	19(13.7)	1.556(1.001–2.419)	0.021	91	78(27.9)	13(21.7)	1.286(0.767–2.156)	0.211
	≥65	135	111(15.6)	24(17.3)	0.905(0.606–1.354)	0.315	35	19(6.8)	16(26.7)	0.254(0.139–0.465)	< 0.001
History TB	New cases	800	667(94)	133(95.7)	0.982(0.943–1.022)	0.216	265	218(77.9)	47(78.3)	0.994(0.858–1.151)	0.544
	Retreated case	49	43(6)	6(4.3)	1.403(0.609–3.232)		75	62(22.2)	13(21.7)	1.022(0.602–1.734)	
registered residence	Residence	467	389(54.8)	78(56.1)	0.976(0.831–1.147) 1.030(0.840–1.264)	0.424	184	141(50.4)	43(71.7)	0.703(0.577–0.856) 1.752(1.152–2.665)	0.002
	Non-residence	382	321(45.2)	61(43.9)			156	139(49.7)	17(28.3)		

p value indicates whether there is a significant difference between Beijing family and non-Beijing family
($p < 0.05$ represents a statistically significant difference)

OR (95%CI): 0.254(0.139–0.465)] and non-residents [p = 0.002, OR (95%CI): 0.703(0.577–0.856)] were more probably be infected with non-Beijing genotype strains, indicating that being older and non-resident are association factors for infection with the non-Beijing genotype.

Difference in drug resistance patterns

DST experiments were carried out on the 1189 strains to investigate the drug-resistance profile of prevalent strains. Results showed that 849 isolates (71.4%) were sensitive to the four first-line anti-TB drugs and 340 isolates (38.6%) were resistant to at least one of the drugs. The percentage of overall drug resistance (resistance to any anti-TB drug) was 38.6%, and that of MDR-TB was 9%. 82.4% (280/340) of the drug resistant *M.tb* strains belonged to the Beijing genotype family. The percentage of strains resistant to INH/ RFP/SM/EMB among Beijing genotype family strains (16.3%/10%/18.7%/13%, respectively) was lower than that among non-Beijing strains (22.1%/10.1%/20.6%/16.1%, respectively).

In this study, the percentage of drug resistance among new TB cases was significantly lower than that in patients undergoing retreatment (Additional file 3: Table S3), suggesting the possibility that improper use of antibiotics, and/or poor treatment compliance among TB patients, may have led to an increase in the occurrence of drug resistance. We compared the percentage of drug resistant strains between Beijing and non-Beijing genotype family strains; the only difference observed was that the percentage of INH-resistance in Beijing genotype strains was significantly lower than that in non-Beijing genotype family strains [16.3% vs 22.1%, OR (95% CI): 0.736(0.547–0.989), $p = 0.032$] (Table 4). We also looked for differences between new ($n = 1065$) and retreated TB cases ($n = 124$) group (Table 4); a similar result was observed [12.4% vs 17.2%, OR (95% CI): 0.722(0.501–1.040), $p = 0.042$] in the new cases group (Table 4). However, statistical analysis did not reveal any difference in these characteristics between Beijing family and non-Beijing family in retreatment TB cases. Our study has revealed a relatively high prevalence of MDR-TB in Beijing, but does not indicate any significant association between MDR-TB and the Beijing genotype family.

Discussion

As far as we know, this is a large-scale study to assess the prevalence of the Beijing genotype *M.tb* strains in Beijing and their association with drug resistance. The Beijing genotype family of *M.tb* is one of the most successful lineages in the present global tuberculosis epidemic. In order to understand how drug-resistant TB develops and to find better ways to control TB, it is essential to understand the molecular epidemiology of *M.tb*. Prior to this study, however, the prevalence of Beijing strains and their drug resistance status in Beijing, the city after which they were named, was unclear.

To examine these problems, we made use of strain collection containing 1189 isolates from a previous project in Beijing [4]. We described the detailed population structure of both Beijing and non-Beijing genotype strains, and investigated the association between the prevalence of Beijing genotype strains of *M.tb* and drug resistance in Beijing.

It has often been found that the prevalence of TB is higher in men than in women [32]. Consistent with results of previous studies [21, 34], we found that men are more probably be infected by *M.tb;* in the pan-susceptible group, men were more probably be infected by Beijing genotype *M.tb* strains (Table 3). As this the result may be affected by the gender ratio in the local population [31], we examined the overall gender ratio in Beijing. As the gender ratio in Beijing was 1.07 to1 (male: female) in 2010 [35], it is likely that the reason for the difference observed is due to differences in susceptibility to *M.tb* among local populations.

With the exception of gender, age was an association factor for infection by the Beijing genotype. A previous study demonstrated that younger patients (aged under 25 years) were likely to be infected with the Beijing genotype [21]. However, we did not observe such a tendency. Instead, we observed that individuals in the middle-aged group were more probably be infected with Beijing genotype strains of *M.tb*, and elderly people were more probably be infected with non-Beijing genotype strains. These results may reflect the possibility that middle-aged and older population groups in Beijing may have different social networks and work situations, suggesting that the population of different region could confront different risks. Further research is required to clarify this hypothesis. Except for age, we found that the non-resident population was more probably be infected by non-Beijing genotype strains of *M.tb*. Non-residents tend to live in areas of Beijing where the population density is high and work in crowded public environments. Non-Beijing genotype *M.tb* strains probably likely spread more readily in these districts.

Research on molecular epidemiology has greatly improved our understanding of TB prevalence. A study from Shanghai has also suggested that Beijing genotype strains are associated with recent transmission of TB and are more probably be clustered [36] [24]. Consistent with this finding, we found that Beijing genotype strains in the study population were significantly associated with clustering, suggesting recent transmission mechanisms are likely significantly different from those of non-Beijing genotype strains. Moreover, VNTR method separated the *M.tb* Beijing genotype strains into much more branches and much smaller clusters, suggesting

Table 4 The difference of drug susceptibility between Beijing genotype family and non-Beijing genotype family when considered first-line drug resistance ($n = 1189$)

Characteristic	Category	Total					New cases					Retreated cases				
		Number of reported cases	Beijing family (%)	Non-Beijing family (%)	OR (95% CI)	*p* value	Number of reported cases	Beijing family (%)	Non-Beijing family (%)	OR (95% CI)	*p* value	Number of reported cases	Beijing family (%)	Non-Beijing family (%)	OR (95% CI)	*p* value
All		1189	990	199			1065	885	180			124	105	19		
DST profile	Pansusceptible	849	710(71.7)	139(69.9)	1.027 (0.930–1.134)	0.325	800	667(75.4)	133(73.9)	1.020(0.928–1.121)	0.348	49	43(41)	6(31.6)	1.297 (0.644–2.613)	0.221
	INH	205	161(16.3)	44(22.1)	0.736 (0.547–0.989)	0.032	141	110(12.4)	31(17.2)	0.722(0.501–1.040)	0.042	64	51(48.6)	7(36.9)	1.318 (0.709–2.453)	0.173
	RIF	119	99(10)	20(10.1)	0.995 (0.631–1.569)	0.534	64	53(6)	11(6.1)	0.980(0.522–1.839)	0.475	55	46(43.8)	9(47.4)	0.925 (0.549–1.557)	0.337
	SM	226	185(18.7)	41(20.6)	0.907 (0.670–1.227)	0.295	176	143(16.2)	33(18.3)	0.881(0.625–1.242)	0.237	50	42(40)	8(42.1)	0.950 (0.534–1.692)	0.431
	EMB	161	129(13)	32(16.1)	0.810 (0.568–1.157)	0.151	117	92(10.4)	25(13.9)	0.748(0.496–1.130)	0.086	44	37(35.2)	7(36.9)	0.956 (0.503–1.820)	0.447
	MDR	107	88(8.9)	19(9.6)	0.931 (0.581–1.492)	0.427	58	48(5.4)	10(5.6)	0.976(0.503–1.893)	0.473	49	40(38.1)	9(47.4)	0.804 (0.472–1.370)	0.224

INH Isoniazid, *LFP* Rifampicin; *SM* Streptomycin; *EMB* Ethambutol; *MDR* multi-drug resistance
p value indicates whether there is a significant difference between Beijing family and non-Beijing family ($p < 0.05$ represents a statistically significant difference)

that it possessed a higher discriminatory power than the spoligotyping method [27].

Evidence has shown that drug resistance in *M.tb* is more probably occur among Beijing genotype strains [19, 21, 22]. However, the nature of the association found between drug resistance and the Beijing genotype has varied between studies, [7, 25]. When we analyzed the percentage of drug resistant strains in different genotypes, results indicated that there was an association between the occurrence of INH resistance and the prevalence of non-Beijing genotype strains. In regard to MDR-TB, some studies have suggested that Beijing genotype strains are more probably develop MDR-TB [23]. Here, however, our data did not support this hypothesis. Our data also revealed a relatively high prevalence of MDR-TB in Beijing, but did not show a significant difference in the percentage of MDR-TB between Beijing and non-Beijing genotypes, suggesting that there is no significant association between the occurrence of MDR-TB and the prevalence of Beijing genotype strains.

According to previous reports and this study, the association between the occurrence of drug-resistance and the prevalence of Beijing genotype strains is variable [19–21]. Possible explanations for the variability include: 1) the number and percentage of Beijing genotype strains included in a study influences the results [36, 37]; 2) variation in the frequency of strains with different drug resistance patterns is influenced by differences in treatment regimens and tuberculosis control programs in different regions [38], as well as characteristics of the host population, socioeconomic factors, or any combination of these factors [39]; and 3) the uneven geographical distribution of the Beijing genotype will also influence the association [40, 41]. Further detailed studies on the association are needed.

While our results are important, this study has some limitations. The association between genotypic diversity and drug resistance is a very complex problem, and research that bears additional factors and underlying reasons in mind is required [37]. Although no selection bias was detected in the demographic characteristics of our study population, there is a higher incidence of serious TB cases in this region, which may have led to an overestimation of drug-resistant TB. In addition, we used traditional Spoligotyping and VNTR methods; better methods may be available used in the future to identify and analyze the Beijing genotype. With developments in science and technology, whole genome sequencing (WGS) can provide greater precision than traditional genotyping for studying the recent transmission of *M.tb* [38]. Nevertheless, spoligotyping and VNTR are still valuable tools for identifying genotypes and performing cluster analysis [39–42]. Each technique has its own advantages and disadvantages and we will combine classical genotyping, WGS, and epidemiological investigations in future studies.

Conclusions

In summary, our results suggest that male and middle-aged patients in the study population were more probably infected by Beijing genotype *M.tb* strains, and elderly patients and non-residents were more likely to be infected by non-Beijing genotype *M.tb*. The Beijing genotype was prevalent in this study population, and Beijing genotype strains readily formed clusters. Our data also indicates that there is a higher percentage of INH-resistant in the middle of non-Beijing genotype family than that among Beijing genotype family *M.tb* strains in Beijing. This study provides important insights into the prevalence of *M.tb* strains in Beijing.

Abbreviations

CI: Confidence intervals; DST: Drug susceptibility testing; EMB: Ethambutol; HGDI: Hunter-Gaston discriminatory index; INH: Isoniazid; *M.tb*: *Mycobacterium tuberculosis*; MDR: Multidrug-resistant; ORs: Odd ratios; RFP: Rifampin; SM: Streptomycin; TB: Tuberculosis; VNTR: Variable number of tandem repeat; WHO: World Health Organization; XDR: Extremely drug-resistant

Acknowledgements

We are grateful to Dr. Yu Pang for performing the BioNumerics analysis, and to Dr. Chongguang Yang for helping with setting up software. We thank Dr. Joy Fleming for editing the English of the manuscript.

Funding

This work was supported by the Capital's Funds for Health Improvement and Research (grant# No. CFH2018-1-1041) and Beijing Municipal Administration of Hospitals' Ascent Plan (grant# No. DFL20151501). The funders had no role in the study design, data collection and analysis, decision to publish, or preparation of the manuscript.

Authors' contributions

YL: conception, design, strain collection, DNA extraction and genotyping, statistical analysis, drafting and revising the manuscript. XXZ: strain collection, DNA extraction and genotyping. YQZ: DNA extraction and genotyping. YS: DNA extraction and genotyping. CY: strain collection, DNA extraction. WW: DNA extraction. CYL: conception, design, critical revision of the manuscript. All authors read and approved the final manuscript.

Consent for publication

Not applicable.

Competing interests

The authors declare that they have no competing financial interests.

References

1. An Yansheng ZL. Tu Dehua: impact of immigration on epidemic of tuberculosis in Beijing. The Journal of The Chinese Antituberculosis Association. 2004;26(6):319–23.
2. Lixing Z. Trends of tuberculosis incidence in Beijing. The Journal of The Chinese Antituberculosis Association. 2003;25(4):204–8.
3. WHO. Global tuberculosis report 2018. Geneva: WHO; 2018.
4. Liu Y, Tian M, Wang X, Wei R, Xing Q, Ma T, Jiang X, Li W, Zhang Z, Xue Y, et al. Genotypic diversity analysis of Mycobacterium tuberculosis strains collected from Beijing in 2009, using spoligotyping and VNTR typing. PLoS One. 2014;9(9):e106787.
5. Barnes PF, Cave MD. Molecular epidemiology of tuberculosis. N Engl J Med. 2003;349(12):1149–56.
6. Singhal P, Dixit P, Singh P, Jaiswal I, Singh M, Jain A. A study on pre-XDR & XDR tuberculosis & their prevalent genotypes in clinical isolates of Mycobacterium tuberculosis in North India. Indian J Med Res. 2016;143(3): 341–7.
7. Yuan L, Huang Y, Mi LG, Li YX, Liu PZ, Zhang J, Liang HY, Li F, Li H, Zhang SQ, et al. There is no correlation between sublineages and drug resistance of Mycobacterium tuberculosis Beijing/W lineage clinical isolates in Xinjiang, China. Epidemiol Infect. 2015;143(1):141–9.
8. Singh J, Sankar MM, Kumar P, Couvin D, Rastogi N, Singh S, Indian TBDN. Genetic diversity and drug susceptibility profile of Mycobacterium tuberculosis isolated from different regions of India. J Infect. 2015;71(2):207–19.
9. Li Y, Cao X, Li S, Wang H, Wei J, Liu P, Wang J, Zhang Z, Gao H, Li M, et al. Characterization of Mycobacterium tuberculosis isolates from Hebei, China: genotypes and drug susceptibility phenotypes. *BMC infectious diseases.* 2016;16:107.
10. Yang C, Luo T, Shen X, Wu J, Gan M, Xu P, Wu Z, Lin S, Tian J, Liu Q, et al. Transmission of multidrug-resistant Mycobacterium tuberculosis in Shanghai, China: a retrospective observational study using whole-genome sequencing and epidemiological investigation. Lancet Infect Dis. 2017;17(3): 275–84.
11. van Soolingen D, Qian L, de Haas PE, Douglas JT, Traore H, Portaels F, Qing HZ, Enkhsaikan D, Nymadawa P, van Embden JD. Predominance of a single genotype of Mycobacterium tuberculosis in countries of East Asia. J Clin Microbiol. 1995;33(12):3234–8.
12. Bifani PJ, Mathema B, Kurepina NE, Kreiswirth BN. Global dissemination of the Mycobacterium tuberculosis W-Beijing family strains. Trends Microbiol. 2002;10(1):45–52.
13. Luo T, Comas I, Luo D, Lu B, Wu J, Wei L, Yang C, Liu Q, Gan M, Sun G, et al. Southern east Asian origin and coexpansion of Mycobacterium tuberculosis Beijing family with Han Chinese. Proc Natl Acad Sci U S A. 2015;112(26): 8136–41.
14. Shitikov E, Kolchenko S, Mokrousov I, Bespyatykh J, Ischenko D, Ilina E, Govorun V. Evolutionary pathway analysis and unified classification of east Asian lineage of Mycobacterium tuberculosis. Sci Rep. 2017;7(1):9227.
15. Li D, Dong CB, Cui JY, Nakajima C, Zhang CL, Pan XL, Sun GX, Dai EY, Suzuki Y, Zhuang M, et al. Dominant modern sublineages and a new modern sublineage of Mycobacterium tuberculosis Beijing family clinical isolates in Heilongjiang Province, China. Infect Genet Evol. 2014;27:294–9.
16. Grode L, Seiler P, Baumann S, Hess J, Brinkmann V, Nasser Eddine A, Mann P, Goosmann C, Bandermann S, Smith D, et al. Increased vaccine efficacy against tuberculosis of recombinant Mycobacterium bovis bacille Calmette-Guerin mutants that secrete listeriolysin. J Clin Invest. 2005;115(9):2472–9.
17. Lopez B, Aguilar D, Orozco H, Burger M, Espitia C, Ritacco V, Barrera L, Kremer K, Hernandez-Pando R, Huygen K, et al. A marked difference in pathogenesis and immune response induced by different Mycobacterium tuberculosis genotypes. Clin Exp Immunol. 2003;133(1):30–7.
18. Ebrahimi-Rad M, Bifani P, Martin C, Kremer K, Samper S, Rauzier J, Kreiswirth B, Blazquez J, Jouan M, van Soolingen D, et al. Mutations in putative mutator genes of Mycobacterium tuberculosis strains of the W-Beijing family. Emerg Infect Dis. 2003;9(7):838–45.
19. European Concerted Action on New Generation Genetic M, Techniques for the E. Control of T: Beijing/W genotype Mycobacterium tuberculosis and drug resistance. *Emerging infectious diseases.* 2006;12(5):736–43.
20. Maeda S, Hang NT, Lien LT, Thuong PH, Hung NV, Hoang NP, Cuong VC, Hijikata M, Sakurada S, Keicho N. Mycobacterium tuberculosis strains spreading in Hanoi, Vietnam: Beijing sublineages, genotypes, drug susceptibility patterns, and host factors. Tuberculosis. 2014;94(6):649–56.
21. Pang Y, Song Y, Xia H, Zhou Y, Zhao B, Zhao Y. Risk factors and clinical phenotypes of Beijing genotype strains in tuberculosis patients in China. BMC Infect Dis. 2012;12:354.
22. Pang Y, Zhou Y, Zhao B, Liu G, Jiang G, Xia H, Song Y, Shang Y, Wang S, Zhao YL. Spoligotyping and drug resistance analysis of Mycobacterium tuberculosis strains from national survey in China. PLoS One. 2012;7(3): e32976.
23. Zhou Y, van den Hof S, Wang S, Pang Y, Zhao B, Xia H, Anthony R, Ou X, Li Q, Zheng Y, et al. Association between genotype and drug resistance profiles of Mycobacterium tuberculosis strains circulating in China in a national drug resistance survey. PLoS One. 2017;12(3):e0174197.
24. Zhang Z, Lu J, Liu M, Wang Y, Qu G, Li H, Wang J, Pang Y, Liu C, Zhao Y. Genotyping and molecular characteristics of multidrug-resistant Mycobacterium tuberculosis isolates from China. J Infect. 2015;70(4):335–45.
25. Yang C, Luo T, Sun G, Qiao K, DeRiemer K, Mei J, Gao Q. Mycobacterium tuberculosis Beijing strains favor transmission but not drug resistance in China. Clin Infect Dis. 2012;55(9):1179–87.
26. Guo YL, Liu Y, Wang SM, Li CY, Jiang GL, Shi GL, Song CX. Genotyping and drug resistance patterns of Mycobacterium tuberculosis strains in five provinces of China. Int J Tuberc Lung Dis. 2011;15(6):789–94.
27. Liu Y, Jiang X, Li W, Zhang X, Wang W, Li C. The study on the association between Beijing genotype family and drug susceptibility phenotypes of Mycobacterium tuberculosis in Beijing. Sci Rep. 2017;7(1):15076.
28. Wan K, Liu J, Hauck Y, Zhang Y, Zhao X, Liu Z, Lu B, Dong H, Jiang Y, Kremer K, et al. Investigation on Mycobacterium tuberculosis diversity in China and the origin of the Beijing clade. PLoS One. 2011;6(12):e29190.
29. Kamerbeek J, Schouls L, Kolk A, van Agterveld M, van Soolingen D, Kuijper S, Bunschoten A, Molhuizen H, Shaw R, Goyal M, et al. Simultaneous detection and strain differentiation of Mycobacterium tuberculosis for diagnosis and epidemiology. J Clin Microbiol. 1997;35(4):907–14.
30. Anti-tuberculosis drug resistance in the world [www.who.int/tb/publications/2008/drs_report4_26feb08.pdf].
31. Demay C, Liens B, Burguiere T, Hill V, Couvin D, Millet J, Mokrousov I, Sola C, Zozio T, Rastogi N. SITVITWEB--a publicly available international multimarker database for studying Mycobacterium tuberculosis genetic diversity and molecular epidemiology. Infect Genet Evol. 2012;12(4):755–66.
32. Hunter PR, Gaston MA. Numerical index of the discriminatory ability of typing systems: an application of Simpson's index of diversity. J Clin Microbiol. 1988;26(11):2465–6.
33. Small PM, Hopewell PC, Singh SP, Paz A, Parsonnet J, Ruston DC, Schecter GF, Daley CL, Schoolnik GK. The epidemiology of tuberculosis in San Francisco. A population-based study using conventional and molecular methods. N Engl J Med. 1994;330(24):1703–9.
34. Pang Y, Zhang Z, Wang Y, Wang S, Song Y, Zhao B, Zhou Y, Ou X, Li Q, Xia H, et al. Genotyping and Prevalence of Pyrazinamide- and Moxifloxacin-Resistant Tuberculosis in China, 2000 to 2010. Antimicrob Agents Chemother. 2017;61(2):e02170–16.
35. Main data bulletin of the sixth national population census of Beijing in 2010. [http://www.stats.gov.cn/tjsj/tjgb/rkpcgb/dfrkpcgb/201202/t20120228_30381.html].
36. Yang C, Luo T, Sun G, Qiao K, Sun G, DeRiemer K, Mei J, Gao Q. Mycobacterium tuberculosis Beijing strains favor transmission but not drug resistance in China. Clin Infect Dis. 2012;55(9):1179–87.
37. Hong EP, Go MJ, Kim HL, Park JW. Risk prediction of pulmonary tuberculosis using genetic and conventional risk factors in adult Korean population. PLoS One. 2017;12(3):e0174642.
38. Allix-Beguec C, Wahl C, Hanekom M, Nikolayevskyy V, Drobniewski F, Maeda S, Campos-Herrero I, Mokrousov I, Niemann S, Kontsevaya I, et al. Proposal of a consensus set of hypervariable mycobacterial interspersed repetitive-unit-variable-number tandem-repeat loci for subtyping of Mycobacterium tuberculosis Beijing isolates. J Clin Microbiol. 2014;52(1):164–72.
39. Pan XL, Zhang CL, Nakajima C, Fu J, Shao CX, Zhao LN, Cui JY, Jiao N, Fan CL, Suzuki Y, et al. A quantitative and efficient approach to select MIRU-VNTR loci based on accumulation of the percentage differences of strains for discriminating divergent Mycobacterium tuberculosis sublineages. Emerg Microbes Infect. 2017;6(7):e68.
40. Guthrie JL, Kong C, Roth D, Jorgensen D, Rodrigues M, Tang P, Thejoe M, Elwood K, Cook VJ, Johnston J, et al. Universal genotyping for tuberculosis prevention programs: a five-year comparison with on-request genotyping. J Clin Microbiol. 2018;56(5):e01778–17.

Clinical features and outcomes of abdominal tuberculosis in southeastern Korea

Jin-Kyu Cho[1†], Young Min Choi[2†], Sang Soo Lee[2,3,4*], Hye Kyong Park[4], Ra Ri Cha[2,4], Wan Soo Kim[2,4], Jin Joo Kim[2,4], Jae Min Lee[2,3,4], Hong Jun Kim[2,3], Chang Yoon Ha[2,3], Hyun Jin Kim[2,3,4], Tae Hyo Kim[2,3], Woon Tae Jung[2,3] and Ok Jae Lee[2,3]

Abstract

Background: Abdominal tuberculosis (TB) is an uncommon form of infection with *Mycobacterium tuberculosis* in Korea. In this study, we aimed to highlight the clinical features, diagnostic methods, and outcomes of abdominal TB over 12 years in Southeastern Korea.

Methods: A total of 139 patients diagnosed as having abdominal TB who received anti-TB medication from January 2005 to June 2016 were reviewed. Among them, 69 patients (49.6%) had luminal TB, 28 (20.1%) had peritoneal TB, 7 (5.0%) had nodal TB, 23 (16.5%) had visceral TB, and 12 (8.6%) had mixed TB.

Results: The most frequent symptoms were abdominal pain (34.5%) and abdominal distension (21.0%). Diagnosis of abdominal TB was confirmed using microbiologic and/or histologic methods in 76 patients (confirmed diagnosis) , while the remaining 63 patients were diagnosed based on clinical presentation and radiologic imaging (clinical diagnosis). According to diagnostic method, frequency of clinical diagnosis was highest in patients with luminal (50.7%) or peritoneal (64.3%) TB, while frequency of microscopic diagnosis was highest in patients with visceral TB (68.2%), and frequency of histologic diagnosis was highest in patients with nodal TB (85.2%). Interestingly, most patients, except those with nodal TB, showed a good response to anti-TB agents, with 84.2% showing a complete response. The mortality rate was only 1.4% in the present study.

Conclusions: Most patients responded very well to anti-TB therapy, and surgery was required in only a minority of cases of suspected abdominal TB.

Keywords: Tuberculosis, Abdomen, Extra-pulmonary, Luminal, Peritoneal

Background

Abdominal tuberculosis (TB) is defined as infection of the gastrointestinal tract, peritoneum, abdominal solid organs, and/or abdominal lymphatics with *Mycobacterium tuberculosis* [1]. Abdominal TB constitutes approximately 12% of extrapulmonary TB cases and 1 to 3% of total TB cases [1, 2]. Abdominal TB is one of the most common forms of extrapulmonary TB [3]. Abdominal TB is relatively rare, but it is recognized that abdominal TB is increasing in both developing and developed countries [4–8]. Abdominal TB accounts for approximately 4% of all TB cases in Korea [9]. Diagnosis of abdominal TB is often overlooked and delayed due to lack of specific symptoms and no specific diagnostic test. A high index of suspicion is necessary for early diagnosis of abdominal TB; however, it remains a considerable diagnostic dilemma and can mimic many other diseases, such as Crohn's disease, abdominal lymphoma, and malignancy of the abdominal organs.

Abdominal TB can usually be classified into 4 forms: luminal, peritoneal, nodal, and visceral involving the

* Correspondence: 3939lee@naver.com
†Jin-Kyu Cho and Young Min Choi contributed equally to this work.
[2]Department of Internal Medicine, Gyeongsang National University School of Medicine and Gyeongsang National University Hospital, 15, Jinju-daero 816 beon-gil, Jinju-si, Gyeongnam 52727, Republic of Korea
[3]Institute of Health Sciences, Gyeongsang National University, Jinju, Republic of Korea
Full list of author information is available at the end of the article

intra-abdominal solid organs [10]. The most common forms are luminal (ileocecal area) and peritoneal [11]. The modes of infection of abdominal TB include swallowing infected sputum, ingestion of bacilli from infected milk products or meat, hematogenous spread from a lung focus, spread via lymphatics from infected lymph nodes, and contiguous spread from adjacent organs [12]. The clinical presentation of abdominal TB depends on the site of infection. Abdominal pain, diarrhea, bleeding from the luminal tract, intestinal obstruction, fever, and weight loss are frequent features of intestinal TB; ascites and abdominal distension are common manifestations of peritoneal TB [8]. Diagnosis of abdominal TB may also vary depending on the site of infection [13]. Colonoscopy is useful in patients suspected of having intestinal TB, while laparoscopy and biopsy are more useful in peritoneal TB; although ascitic fluid analysis is more accessible, its acid-fast bacilli (AFB) culture has a low sensitivity.

The aim of the present study was to evaluate the clinical features, diagnostic methods, and outcomes of abdominal TB, including luminal, peritoneal, nodal, visceral, and mixed TB.

Methods

Study populations

Between January 2005 and June 2016, a total of 139 consecutive adult patients aged > 18 years diagnosed as having abdominal TB began treatment with anti-TB drugs at Gyeongsang National University Hospital, located on the southeast coast of Korea. Age, sex, body mass index, alcohol consumption, history of TB, history of malignancy, TB infection site, date of anti-TB drug prescription, regimen of anti-TB drugs, laboratory data, underlying disease, clinical features, diagnostic method, and clinical outcome were reviewed. The present study was approved by the Institutional Review Board of the Gyeongsang National University Hospital.

Definitions and classification

Abdominal TB was defined as infection of the luminal tract, peritoneum, intra-abdominal lymph nodes, and/or intra-abdominal solid-organs with *M. tuberculosis*. Diagnosis of abdominal TB was based on: (1) positive AFB smear or culture from ascites, urine, or biopsy specimen (microbiologic diagnosis); (2) demonstration of caseating granulomas on biopsy specimen (histologic diagnosis); (3) typical presentation and good response to anti-TB agents (clinical diagnosis); or (4) high index of suspicion in susceptible patients and good response to anti-TB agents (clinical diagnosis). When peritoneal TB could not be diagnosed by biopsy, the high ascitic adenosine deaminase (> 33 IU/L) criteria was used for clinical diagnosis. Confirmed diagnosis was defined as microbiologic or histologic evidence of *M. tuberculosis* [14].

Patients were classified into 5 groups according to site of TB infection: (1) luminal, (2) peritoneal, (3) nodal, (4) visceral, and (5) mixed. Luminal TB was further divided into esophageal, gastric, duodenal, jejunal, ileocecal, and colorectal. Peritoneal TB was divided into 3 types [10, 15]: (1) the wet ascitic type was associated with large amounts of free or loculated ascites; (2) the fixed fibrotic type was associated with involvement of the omentum and mesentery and was characterized by presence of bowel loop entanglement; and (3) the dry plastic type was characterized by peritoneal and mesenteric thickening with caseous nodules and presence of adhesions. To avoid confusion, we classified peritonal TB into two types, the wet and dry type (fixed fibrotic and dry plastic type). Nodal TB was divided into mesenteric, porta hepatitis, celiac axis, peripancreatic, and combined. Visceral TB was divided into hepatic, splenic, genitourinary, adrenal, and combined.

Clinical outcomes

Abdominal TB outcomes were classified as follows [16]: (1) complete response: resolution of symptoms, disappearance of AFB on smear or culture, disappearance of tuberculous granulomas, and disappearance or healing of active tuberculous lesions on relook colonoscopy; (2) partial response: resolution of symptoms and partial disappearance of tuberculous lesions at end of treatment; (3) no response: persistence of symptoms, persistence of AFB on smear or culture, persistence of tuberculous granulomas, and persistence of active tuberculous lesions on relook colonoscopy at end of treatment; (4) lost to follow up: treatment interrupted for ≥2 consecutive months; (5) death: death from any cause during treatment; (6) recurrence: colonoscopic or radiologic documentation of recurrent lesions after a complete response had been achieved; and (7) transfer out: transferred to another reporting and recording unit.

Statistical analysis

All analyses were performed using PASW version 18 (SPSS Inc., Chicago, IL, USA). Continuous variables were expressed as median (interquartile range). Intergroup differences in quantitative data were measured using the Mann-Whitney *U* test, while the Fisher exact test was used for qualitative data. All analyses were 2-sided and a P value of < 0.05 was considered statistically significant.

Results

Patient characteristics

A total of 139 patients (72 male, 51.8%) with a median age of 47.0 years were diagnosed has having abdominal

TB. Among them, 69 patients (49.6%) were diagnosed with luminal TB, 28 (20.1%) with peritoneal TB, 7 (5.0%) with nodal TB, 23 (16.5%) with visceral TB, and 12 (8.6%) with mixed TB (Fig. 1). The ileocecum (67.1%) was the most frequently involved site in patients with luminal TB. Wet ascitic type (75.7%) was the most common type in patients with peritoneal TB. Genitourinary tract (69.0%) and porta hepatitis (35.7%) were the most frequently involved sites in patients with visceral and nodal TB, respectively (Table 1). The demographic characteristics of the patients are presented in Table 2. There were no significant differences in sex, body mass index, chronic hepatitis B, HIV infection, alcohol consumption, liver cirrhosis, end-stage renal disease, history of malignancy, history of TB, or anemia at diagnosis among the 5 study groups. The mixed TB group was significantly younger (median age, 32.0 years) than the other 4 groups. The rate of history of TB was significantly higher in the visceral TB group (21.7%) than in the peritoneal TB group (0%).

Abdominal pain was the most common symptom (34.5%; Table 3). Incidence of abdominal distension was significantly higher in the peritoneal TB group than in the other 4 groups. However, there were no significant differences in the frequencies of other symptoms among the 5 study groups.

Diagnostic methods

In the 139 patients with abdominal TB, diagnosis was confirmed microbiologically in 51 patients (37.0%) and histologically in 59 patients (42.8%). Confirmed diagnosis was achieved in 76 patients (54.7%), while the remaining 63 patients (45.3%) were diagnosed clinically (Table 4). The frequency of microbiologic diagnosis (AFB smear or culture) was significantly higher in the visceral TB group (68.2%) than in the luminal (33.3%) and peritoneal (25.0%) TB groups. The frequency of histologic diagnosis (caseating granulomas on biopsy specimen) was significantly higher in the nodal TB group (85.7%) than in the luminal (39.1%) and peritoneal (28.6%) TB groups. The frequency of clinical diagnosis was significantly higher in the peritoneal TB group (64.3%) than in the nodal (14.3%) and visceral (13.6%) TB groups.

Surgery was performed in 21 patients (15.1%) and provided a good diagnostic yield in 90.4% (19/21). Among them, 10 underwent surgery for diagnosis of suspected abdominal TB, and 11 for management of numerous complications, such as intussusception, abscess, perforation, obstruction, and hemorrhage. The frequency of surgery was higher in the nodal (42.9%) and visceral (43.5%) TB groups than in the luminal (2.9%) and peritoneal (14.3%) TB groups. Percutaneous biopsy was performed in 16 patients (11.5%); endoscopy or

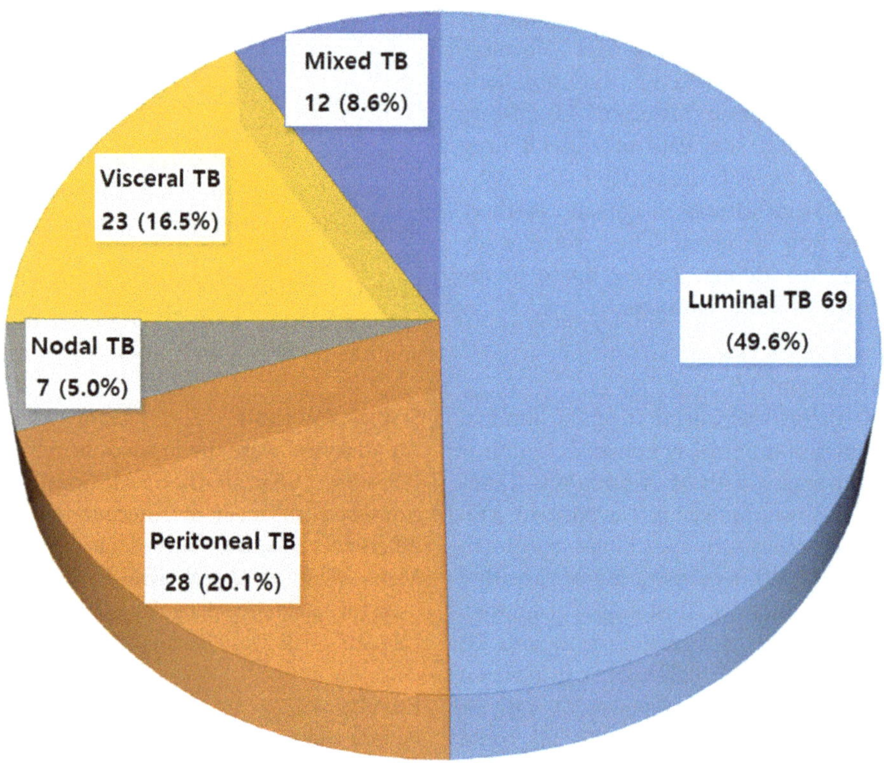

Fig. 1 Sites of abdominal tuberculosis (TB)

Table 1 Site of involvement in abdominal tuberculosis ($n = 139$)

Site	N (%)
Luminal TB	
Esophageal	3 (3.9%)
Stomach	0 (0%)
Duodenal	3 (3.9%)
Jejunal	7 (9.2%)
Ileocecal	51 (67.1%)
Colorectal	12 (15.8%)
Peritoneal TB	
Wet ascitic type	28 (75.7%)
Dry ascitic type	9 (24.3%)
Nodal TB	
Mesenteric	2 (14.3%)
Porta hepatis	5 (35.7%)
Along the celiac axis	1 (7.1%)
Peripancreatic	2 (14.3%)
Retroperitoneal	1 (7.1%)
Combined	3 (21.4%)
Visceral TB	
Hepatic	3 (10.3%)
Splenic	4 (13.8%)
Genitourinary	20 (69.0%)
Adrenal	1 (3.4%)
Combined	1 (3.4%)
Mixed TB	
Luminal and peritoneal	4 (33.3%)
Luminal and nodal	1 (8.3%)
Luminal and peritoneal, and nodal	2 (16.7%)
Peritoneal and visceral	2 (16.7%)
Nodal and visceral	2 (16.7%)
Peritoneal and visceral, and nodal	1 (8.3%)

TB: tuberculosis
Data are presented as the median (interquartile range) for continuous data and percentages for categorical data

colonoscopy was performed in 70 patients (50.4%). Ascitic diagnosis through paracentesis was achieved in 33 patients (23.7%). Among them, a positive yield for AFB culture was observed in only 8 patients (24.2%). Diagnostic yield for confirmed diagnosis from surgery, percutaneous biopsy, endoscopy/colonoscopy, and paracentesis was 90.4, 81.3, 48.6, and 24.2%, respectively.

Treatment outcomes

Of the 139 patients who underwent anti-TB treatment, 117 (84.2%) showed a complete response, 1 (0.7%) showed a partial response, 2 (1.4%) showed no response, 12 (8.6%) were lost to follow-up, 3 (2.2%) had recurrence, and 3 (2.2%) transferred out (Table 5). The frequency of complete response was significantly lower in the nodal TB group than in the other 4 study groups. Only 2 patients (1.4%) died during anti-TB therapy. One patient was positive for HIV and multidrug-resistant abdominal TB involving the liver, spleen, and genitourinary tract. The major cause of death in this patient was concomitant TB meningitis. Another non-HIV-positive patient died due to intestinal obstruction with sepsis.

Twenty-one patients (15.2%) had adverse effects due to anti-TB agents, and 9 (6.5%) developed drug-induced liver injury. The median duration of anti-TB treatment was 194 days; 131 patients were treated with first-line anti-TB agents, while 8 received second-line anti-TB agents. Figure 2 shows an overall decrease of approximately 60% in number of TB cases in southeastern Korea in the period 2005–2008 to 2013–2016.

Discussion

In the current study, we described the distribution of abdominal TB at a tertiary hospital in southeastern Korea. The most frequent site of abdominal TB was the luminal tract (49.6%) followed by the peritoneum (20.1%), solid viscera (16.5%), mixed organs (8.6%), and lymph nodes (5.0%). The most common presentation was abdominal pain (34.5%), whereas abdominal distension was a unique presentation in patients with peritoneal TB. According to diagnostic method, the frequency of clinical diagnosis was highest in the luminal and peritoneal TB groups, while the frequency of microscopic diagnosis was highest in the visceral TB group, and the frequency of histologic diagnosis was highest in the nodal TB group. Interestingly, 117 patients (84.2%) showed a complete response and the mortality rate was only 1.4%.

Abdominal TB poses a considerable diagnostic challenge due to the lack of specific symptoms and pathognomonic findings. Moreover, no single diagnostic method is sufficient for diagnosis. Based on our findings, colonoscopy and paracentesis may be useful in cases of luminal and peritoneal TB, where mucosal or peritoneal lesions are accessible. However, colonoscopy and peritoneal fluid analysis have a low diagnostic yield for confirmed diagnosis of abdominal TB (49.2 and 22.2%, respectively). Therefore, the majority of luminal and peritoneal TB cases were diagnosed based on clinical response to anti-TB agents and radiologic findings. Among these, laparotomy was performed in only 2 and 4 patients in the luminal and peritoneal TB groups, respectively. Peritoneal fluid analysis is the most useful nonoperative diagnostic method for peritoneal TB. High ascitic adenosine deaminase activity level (> 33 IU/L) and low serum ascitic albumin gradient (< 1.1) have a sensitivity of 97% and specificity of 100% [17]. Therefore, laparoscopy could be used to rule out other

Table 2 Demographic characteristics of 139 patients with abdominal tuberculosis

Characteristic	All patients ($n = 139$)	Luminal TB ($n = 69$)	Peritoneal TB ($n = 28$)	Nodal TB ($n = 7$)	Visceral TB ($n = 23$)	Mixed TB ($n = 12$)
Age	47.0 (32.0–58.0)	48.0 (38.5–58.5)	52.5 (27.3–63.0)	53.0 (27.0–57.0)	46.0 (33.0–56.0)	32.0 (25.5–45.8) [d, g, j]
Male sex	72 (51.8%)	36 (52.2%)	18 (64.3%)	3 (42.9%)	9 (39.1%)	6 (50%)
BMI (m/kg2)	21.80 (19.56–24.53)	21.3 (19.6–24.1)	21.6 (19.3–24.5)	23.7 (20.1–27.8)	20.1 (22.8–25.3)	20.8 (18.0–22.8)
Chronic hepatitis B	10 (7.2%)	5 (7.2%)	2 (7.1%)	0 (0%)	2 (8.7%)	1 (8.3%)
Chronic hepatitis C	3 (2.2%)	1 (1.4%)	0 (0%)	2 (28.6%) [b, e, h]	0 (0%)	0 (0%)
HIV-infection	2 (1.4%)	0 (0%)	0 (0%)	0 (0%)	1 (4.3%)	1 (8.3%)
Alcohol > 40 g/day	16 (11.5%)	6 (8.7%)	6 (21.4%)	0 (0%)	2 (8.7%)	2 (16.7%)
Cirrhosis	3 (2.2%)	2 (2.9%)	0 (0%)	0 (0%)	0 (0%)	1 (8.3%)
Diabetes	9 (6.5%)	3 (4.3%)	3 (10.7%)	1 (14.3%)	2 (8.7%)	0 (0%)
ESRD or CAPD	8 (5.8%)	3 (4.3%)	3 (10.7%)	1 (14.3%)	1 (4.3%)	0 (0%)
History of malignancy	7 (5.0%)	3 (4.3%)	2 (7.1%)	0 (0%)	2 (8.7%)	0 (0%)
History of TB	13 (9.4%)	7 (10.1%)	0 (0%)	1 (14.3%)	5 (21.7%) [f]	0 (0%)
Anemia at diagnosis	46 (33.1%)	21 (30.4%)	11 (39.3%)	3 (42.9%)	5 (21.7%)	6 (50.0%)
Leukocytosis at diagnosis	30 (21.6%)	16 (23.2%)	3 (10.7%)	3 (42.9%)	3 (13.0%)	5 (41.7%) [g]

HIV: human immunodeficiency virus; ESRD: end-stage renal disease; CAPD: continuous ambulatory peritoneal dialysiData are presented as the median (interquartile range) for continuous data and percentages for categorical data
Defined as hemoglobin of 12 g/dl
Defined as a white blood cell count of 10,000/mm3
[a]: $P < 0.05$ Luminal TB vs. Peritoneal TB, [b]: $P < 0.05$ Luminal TB vs. Nodal TB, [c]: $P < 0.05$ Luminal TB vs. Visceral TB, [d]: $P < 0.05$ Luminal TB vs. Mixed TB, [e]: $P < 0.05$ Peritoneal TB vs. Nodal TB, [f]: $P < 0.05$ Peritoneal TB vs. Visceral TB, [g]: $P < 0.05$ Peritoneal TB vs. Mixed TB, [h]: $P < 0.05$ Nodal TB vs. Visceral TB, [i]: $P < 0.05$ Nodal TB vs. Mixed TB, [j]: $P < 0.05$ Visceral TB vs. Mixed TB

intra-abdominal malignancies and to minimize any possible diagnostic delay in these groups. On the other hand, diagnosis of nodal TB was confirmed from surgical procedures or percutaneous biopsy in 6 patients (confirmed diagnosis), while 1 patient was diagnosed based on clinical response to anti-TB agents and computed tomography imaging (clinical diagnosis). Diagnosis of visceral TB was confirmed from surgical procedures or percutaneous biopsy in 13 patients, and from urine AFB in 7 patients (confirmed diagnosis), while 3 patients were diagnosed based on clinical response to anti-TB agents and computed tomography imaging (clinical diagnosis). Although

Table 3 Clinical features in 139 patients with abdominal tuberculosis

Characteristic	All patients ($n = 139$)	Luminal TB ($n = 69$)	Peritoneal TB ($n = 28$)	Nodal TB ($n = 7$)	Visceral TB ($n = 23$)	Mixed TB ($n = 12$)
Abdominal pain	48 (34.5%)	23 (33.3%)	7 (25.0%)	3 (42.9%)	9 (39.1%)	6 (50.0%)
Fever	16 (11.5%)	5 (7.2%)	6 (21.4%)	0 (0%)	3 (13.0%)	2 (16.7%)
Anorexia	9 (6.5%)	6 (8.7%)	1 (3.6%)	1 (14.3%)	0 (0%)	1 (8.3%)
Body weight loss	5 (3.6%)	4 (5.8%)	1 (3.6%)	0 (0%)	0 (0%)	0 (0%)
Abdominal distension	29 (21.0%)	2 (2.9%)	22 (78.6%) [a, e, f, g]	0 (0%)	0 (0%)	5 (41.7%) [d, j]
Bloody stool	11 (7.9%)	10 (14.5%)	0 (0%)	0 (0%)	1 (4.3%)	0 (0%)
Dyspnea	2 (1.4%)	0 (0%)	1 (3.6%)	0 (0%)	1 (4.3%)	0 (0%)
Diarrhea	6 (4.3%)	5 (7.2%)	0 (0%)	0 (0%)	0 (0%)	1 (8.3%)
Hematuria	1 (0.7%)	0 (0%)	0 (0%)	0 (0%)	1 (4.3%)	0 (0%)
Dysuria	2 (1.4%)	0 (0%)	0 (0%)	0 (0%)	2 (8.7%)	0 (0%)
Palpable mass	3 (2.2%)	1 (1.4%)	0 (0%)	1 (14.3%)	1 (4.3%)	0 (0%)
Scrotal swelling	1 (0.7%)	0 (0%)	0 (0%)	0 (0%)	1 (4.3%)	0 (0%)
Jaundice	1 (0.7%)	0 (0%)	0 (0%)	1 (14.3%)	0 (0%)	0 (0%)
No symptom	31 (22.3%)	23 (33.3%) [a, d]	1 (3.6%)	2 (28.6%)	5 (21.7%)	0 (0%)

Data are presented as the median (interquartile range) for continuous data and percentages for categorical data
[a]: $P < 0.05$ Luminal TB vs. Peritoneal TB, [b]: $P < 0.05$ Luminal TB vs. Nodal TB, [c]: $P < 0.05$ Luminal TB vs. Visceral TB, [d]: $P < 0.05$ Luminal TB vs. Mixed TB, [e]: $P < 0.05$ Peritoneal TB vs. Nodal TB, [f]: $P < 0.05$ Peritoneal TB vs. Visceral TB, [g]: $P < 0.05$ Peritoneal TB vs. Mixed TB, [h]: $P < 0.05$ Nodal TB vs. Visceral TB, [i]: $P < 0.05$ Nodal TB vs. Mixed TB, [j]: $P < 0.05$ Visceral TB vs. Mixed TB

Table 4 Diagnostic method in 139 patients with abdominal tuberculosis

Characteristic	All patients ($n = 139$)	Luminal TB ($n = 69$)	Peritoneal TB ($n = 28$)	Nodal TB ($n = 7$)	Visceral TB ($n = 23$)	Mixed TB ($n = 12$)
Microbiologic diagnosis	51 (37.0%)	23 (33.3%)	7 (25.0%)	2 (28.6%)	15 (68.2%) [c, f]	4 (33.3%)
Histological diagnosis	59 (42.8%)	27 (39.1%)	8 (28.6%)	6 (85.7%) [b, e]	12 (54.5%)	6 (50.0%)
Clinical diagnosis	63 (45.3%)	35 (50.7%) [c]	18 (64.3%) [e, f]	1 (14.3%)	3 (13.6%)	6 (50.0%) [j]
Operation	21 (15.1%)	2 (2.9%)	4 (14.3%)	3 (42.9%) [b]	10 (43.5%) [c, f]	2 (16.7%)
*Confirmed diagnosis by operation	19 (90.4%)	2 (100%)	4 (100%)	3 (100%)	9 (90%)	1 (50%)
Percutaneous biopsy group	16 (11.5%)	0 (0%) [a, b, c, d]	6 (21.4%)	3 (42.9%)	3 (13.0%)	4 (33.3%)
*Confirmed diagnosis by percutaneous biopsy	13 (81.3%)	0/0	4 (66.7%)	2 (66.7%)	3 (100%)	4 (100%)
Endoscopy or colonoscopy	70 (50.4%)	65 (94.2%) [a, b, c, d]	0 (0%)	0 (0%)	0 (0%)	4 (33.3%) [g, j]
*Confirmed diagnosis by endoscopy or colonoscopy	34 (48.6%)	32 (49.2%)	0 (0%)	0 (0%)	0 (0%)	1 (25%)
Paracentesis	33	0	27 (96.4%) [a, e, f, g]	0	0	6 (50.0%) [g, j]
*Confirmed diagnosis by paracentesis	8 (24.2%)	0 (0%)	6 (21.4%) [a,f]	0 (0%)	0 (0%)	2 (33.3%) [d]

Data are presented as the median (interquartile range) for continuous data and percentages for categorical data
*A Confirmed diagnosis was defined as microbiologic or histological diagnosis
[a]: $P < 0.05$ Luminal TB vs. Peritoneal TB, [b]: $P < 0.05$ Luminal TB vs. Nodal TB, [c]: $P < 0.05$ Luminal TB vs. Visceral TB, [d]: $P < 0.05$ Luminal TB vs. Mixed TB, [e]: $P < 0.05$ Peritoneal TB vs. Nodal TB, [f]: $P < 0.05$ Peritoneal TB vs. Visceral TB, [g]: $P < 0.05$ Peritoneal TB vs. Mixed TB, [h]: $P < 0.05$ Nodal TB vs. Visceral TB, [i]: $P < 0.05$ Nodal TB vs. Mixed TB, [j]: $P < 0.05$ Visceral TB vs. Mixed TB

nodal and visceral TB are mainly treatable medically, surgery is still often required for suspected abdominal TB and management of complications, such as infection, perforation, and hemorrhage.

A 6-month course of anti-TB therapy for luminal TB is recommended in treatment guidelines [18, 19]. Two previous prospective, randomized studies confirmed a high cure rate of > 90% after both 6 and 9 months of standard anti-TB therapy [6, 16]. In addition, some retrospective studies have shown that anti-TB agents are usually highly effective and associated with low mortality (0–6%) in abdominal TB [7, 8, 13, 20, 21]. However, abdominal TB has a high mortality rate (6–20%), and the majority of patients had acute complications and

Table 5 Treatment outcomes in 139 patients with abdominal tuberculosis

Characteristic	All patients ($n = 139$)	Luminal TB ($n = 69$)	Peritoneal TB ($n = 28$)	Nodal TB ($n = 7$)	Visceral TB ($n = 23$)	Mixed TB ($n = 12$)
Duration of treatment, days	194.0 (176.0–258.0)	189.0 (175.0–219.0)	200.0 (165.0–258.0)	258.0 (16.0–285.0)	284.0 (178.0–284.0)	245.0 (177.5–349.0)
Side effect	21 (15.2%)	11 (15.9%)	3 (11.1%)	0 (0%)	4 (17.4%)	3 (25.0%)
Drug-induced liver injury	9 (6.5%)	5 (8.7%)	2 (7.1%)	0 (0%)	0 (0%)	1 (8.3%)
Nephrectomy	4 (2.9%)	0 (0%)	0 (0%)	0 (0%)	4 (17.4%) [c, f]	0 (0%)
First-line anti-TB drug	131 (94.2%)	66 (95.7%)	27 (96.4%)	7 (100%)	20 (87.0%)	11 (91.7%)
Second-line anti-TB drug	8 (5.8%)	3 (4.3%)	1 (3.6%)	0 (0%)	3 (13.0%)	1 (8.3%)
Complete response	117 (84.2%)	62 (89.9%)	22 (78.6%)	3 (42.9%) [b, e, h, i]	20 (87.0%)	10 (83.3%)
Partial response	1 (0.7%)	0 (0%)	0 (0%)	1 (14.3%)	0 (0%)	0 (0%)
No response	2 (1.4%)	1 (1.4%)	0 (0%)	0 (0%)	1 (4.3%)	0 (0%)
Lost to follow up	12 (8.6%)	4 (5.8%)	5 (17.9%)	0 (0%)	1 (4.3%)	2 (16.7%)
Recurrence	3 (2.2%)	1 (1.4%)	1 (3.6%)	1 (14.3%)	0 (0%)	0 (0%)
Transfer out	3 (2.2%)	1 (1.4%)	0 (0%)	2 (28.6%)	0 (0%)	0 (0%)
Death	2 (1.4%)	1 (1.4%)	0 (0%)	0 (0%)	1 (4.3%)	0 (0%)

Data are presented as the median (interquartile range) for continuous data and percentages for categorical data
[a]: $P < 0.05$ Luminal TB vs. Peritoneal TB, [b]: $P < 0.05$ Luminal TB vs. Nodal TB, [c]: $P < 0.05$ Luminal TB vs. Visceral TB, [d]: $P < 0.05$ Luminal TB vs. Mixed TB, [e]: $P < 0.05$ Peritoneal TB vs. Nodal TB, [f]: $P < 0.05$ Peritoneal TB vs. Visceral TB, [g]: $P < 0.05$ Peritoneal TB vs. Mixed TB, [h]: $P < 0.05$ Nodal TB vs. Visceral TB, [i]: $P < 0.05$ Nodal TB vs. Mixed TB, [j]: $P < 0.05$ Visceral TB vs. Mixed TB

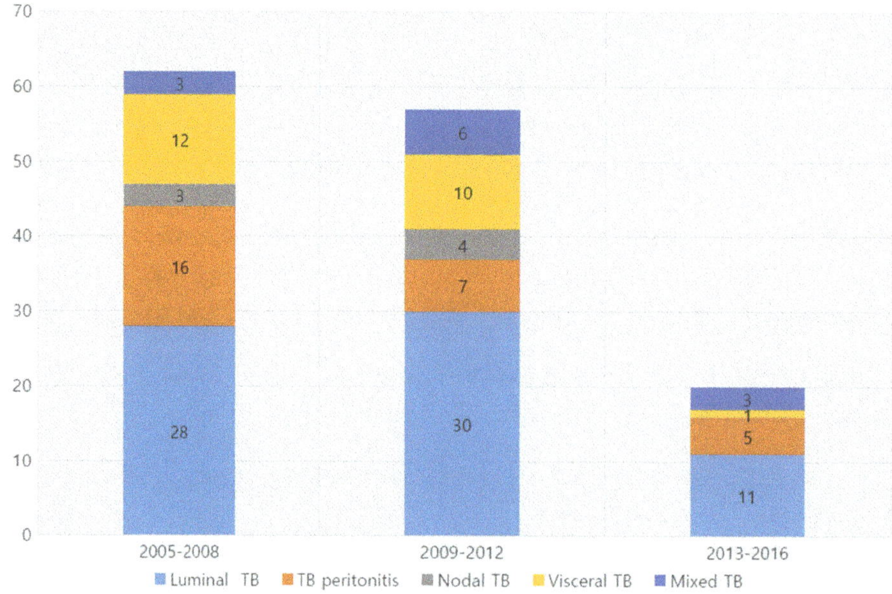

Fig. 2 Cases of abdominal tuberculosis (TB), 2005–2008, 2009–2012, and 2013–2016, respectively. In 2010, incidence of abdominal TB tended to decrease

required emergency exploratory laparotomy in several other studies [22–25]. In our study population, most patients with abdominal TB showed a good response to anti-TB agents and had a good prognosis. Moreover, only 3 cases relapsed and required additional treatment, and the mortality rate was only 1.4%, suggesting that if diagnosed early, abdominal TB can be treated successfully with anti-TB agents, unlike high-mortality study groups. However, nodal TB is difficult to treat based on the low rate of complete response (42.9%), and surgery is often still required for suspected diagnosis.

Drug-induced liver injury during anti-TB treatment is the most common reason leading to discontinuation of therapy [26]. In addition, hepatitis B and C virus are major risk factors for liver injury [27, 28]. We noted drug-induced liver injury in 9 patients (6.5%), including 2 with hepatitis B and 1 with hepatitis C. In 8 patients, all drugs were stopped and a step-wise rechallenge was initiated after complete resolution of hepatotoxicity; 1 patient died due to intestinal obstruction.

The limitations of this study include its single-center, retrospective nature, relatively small sample size, especially in the nodal TB group, and incomplete diagnostic confirmation in all patients. In addition, precise information on alcohol consumption, underlying disease, and drug compliance were unavailable from medical record review. Our study has a low frequency of mixed TB compared to previous studies [14]. Because of the retrospective nature of this study, computed tomography was not performed in all patients with ascites. This is the major limitation of this study. Thus, further prospective studies on abdominal TB including more patients are required.

Conclusion

Abdominal TB can be of various forms, including luminal, peritoneal, nodal, and visceral. A high index of clinical suspicion is required to make a diagnosis of abdominal TB due to the nonspecific clinical symptoms and radiologic features. Early diagnosis with prompt treatment is essential for a promising prognosis. Most cases respond well to medical therapy, and surgery is required in only a minority of cases.

Abbreviations

AFB: acid-fast bacilli; TB: tuberculosis

Acknowledgments

None.

Funding

There was no financial support for this study.

Authors' contributions

Conception and design: SSL, Data collection: HKP, Young Min CRC, WSK, JJK, JML, HongJK, CYH, HyunJK, THK, WTJ, and OJL, Data analysis and interpretation: JKC, YMC and SSL, Manuscript writing: JKC and SSL; Final approval of manuscript: All authors.

Consent for publication

Not applicable.

Competing interests

The authors declare that they have no competing interests.

Author details
[1]Department of Surgery, Gyeongsang National University Hospital, 15, Jinju-daero 816 beon-gil, Jinju-si 52727, Gyeongnam, Republic of Korea. [2]Department of Internal Medicine, Gyeongsang National University School of Medicine and Gyeongsang National University Hospital, 15, Jinju-daero 816 beon-gil, Jinju-si, Gyeongnam 52727, Republic of Korea. [3]Institute of Health Sciences, Gyeongsang National University, Jinju, Republic of Korea. [4]Department of Internal Medicine, Gyeongsang National University Changwon Hospital, Changwon, Republic of Korea.

References

1. Sheer TA, Coyle WJ. Gastrointestinal tuberculosis. Curr Gastroenterol Rep. 2003;5(4):273–8.
2. Farer LS, Lowell AM, Meador MP. Extrapulmonary tuberculosis in the United States. Am J Epidemiol. 1979;109(2):205–17.
3. Donoghue HD, Holton J. Intestinal tuberculosis. Curr Opin Infect Dis. 2009; 22(5):490–6.
4. Lingenfelser T, Zak J, Marks IN, Steyn E, Halkett J, Price SK. Abdominal tuberculosis: still a potentially lethal disease. Am J Gastroenterol. 1993; 88(5):744–50.
5. Marshall JB. Tuberculosis of the gastrointestinal tract and peritoneum. Am J Gastroenterol. 1993;88(7):989–99.
6. Park SH, Yang SK, Yang DH, Kim KJ, Yoon SM, Choe JW, et al. Prospective randomized trial of six-month versus nine-month therapy for intestinal tuberculosis. Antimicrob Agents Chemother. 2009;53(10):4167–71.
7. Ramesh J, Banait GS, Ormerod LP. Abdominal tuberculosis in a district general hospital: a retrospective review of 86 cases. QJM. 2008;101(3):189–95.
8. Mamo JP, Brij SO, Enoch DA. Abdominal tuberculosis: a retrospective review of cases presenting to a UK district hospital. QJM. 2013;106(4):347–54.
9. Lee CM, Lee SS, Lee JM, Cho HC, Kim WS, Kim HJ, et al. Early monitoring for detection of antituberculous drug-induced hepatotoxicity. Korean J Intern Med. 2016;31(1):65–72.
10. Debi U, Ravisankar V, Prasad KK, Sinha SK, Sharma AK. Abdominal tuberculosis of the gastrointestinal tract: revisited. World J Gastroenterol. 2014;20(40):14831–40.
11. Bolukbas C, Bolukbas FF, Kendir T, Dalay RA, Akbayir N, Sokmen MH, et al. Clinical presentation of abdominal tuberculosis in HIV seronegative adults. BMC Gastroenterol. 2005;5:21.
12. Lazarus AA, Thilagar B. Abdominal tuberculosis. Dis Mon. 2007;53(1):32–8.
13. Khan R, Abid S, Jafri W, Abbas Z, Hameed K, Ahmad Z. Diagnostic dilemma of abdominal tuberculosis in non-HIV patients: an ongoing challenge for physicians. World J Gastroenterol. 2006;12(39):6371–5.
14. Sharma V, Mandavdhare HS, Lamoria S, Singh H, Kumar A. Serial C-reactive protein measurements in patients treated for suspected abdominal tuberculosis. Dig Liver Dis. 2018;50(6):559–62.
15. da Rocha EL, Pedrassa BC, Bormann RL, Kierszenbaum ML, Torres LR, D'Ippolito G. Abdominal tuberculosis: a radiological review with emphasis on computed tomography and magnetic resonance imaging findings. Radiol Bras. 2015;48(3):181–91.
16. Makharia GK, Ghoshal UC, Ramakrishna BS, Agnihotri A, Ahuja V, Chowdhury SD, et al. Intermittent directly observed therapy for abdominal tuberculosis: a multicenter randomized controlled trial comparing 6 months versus 9 months of therapy. Clin Infect Dis. 2015;61(5):750–7.
17. Dwivedi M, Misra SP, Misra V, Kumar R. Value of adenosine deaminase estimation in the diagnosis of tuberculous ascites. Am J Gastroenterol. 1990; 85(9):1123–5.
18. Small PM, Fujiwara PI. Management of tuberculosis in the United States. N Engl J Med. 2001;345(3):189–200.
19. Sharma SK, Ryan H, Khaparde S, Sachdeva KS, Singh AD, Mohan A, et al. Index-TB guidelines: guidelines on extrapulmonary tuberculosis for India. Indian J Med Res. 2017;145(4):448–63.
20. Awasthi S, Saxena M, Ahmad F, Kumar A, Dutta S. Abdominal Tuberculosis: A Diagnostic Dilemma. J Clin Diagn Res. 2015;9(5):EC01–3.
21. Singhal A, Gulati A, Frizell R, Manning AP. Abdominal tuberculosis in Bradford, UK: 1992-2002. Eur J Gastroenterol Hepatol. 2005;17(9):967–71.
22. Chalya PL, McHembe MD, Mshana SE, Rambau PF, Jaka H, Mabula JB. Clinicopathological profile and surgical treatment of abdominal tuberculosis: a single Centre experience in northwestern Tanzania. BMC Infect Dis. 2013;13:270.
23. Chou CH, Ho MW, Ho CM, Lin PC, Weng CY, Chen TC, Chi CY, Wang JH. Abdominal tuberculosis in adult: 10-year experience in a teaching hospital in Central Taiwan. J Microbiol Immunol Infect. 2010;43(5):395–400.
24. Chen HL, Wu MS, Chang WH, Shih SC, Chi H, Bair MJ. Abdominal tuberculosis in southeastern Taiwan: 20 years of experience. J Formos Med Assoc. 2009;108(3):195–201.
25. Tan KK, Chen K, Sim R. The spectrum of abdominal tuberculosis in a developed country: a single institution's experience over 7 years. J Gastrointest Surg. 2009;13(1):142–7.
26. Rathi P, Gambhire P. Abdominal Tuberculosis. J Assoc Physicians India. 2016; 64(2):38–47.
27. Kim WS, Lee SS, Lee CM, Kim HJ, Ha CY, Kim HJ, et al. Hepatitis C and not hepatitis B virus is a risk factor for anti-tuberculosis drug induced liver injury. BMC Infect Dis. 2016;16:50.
28. Lee SS, Lee CM, Kim TH, Kim JJ, Lee JM, Kim HJ, et al. Frequency and risk factors of drug-induced liver injury during treatment of multidrug-resistant tuberculosis. Int J Tuberc Lung Dis. 2016;20(6):800–5.

A retrospective study of factors associated with treatment decision for nontuberculous mycobacterial lung disease in adults without altered systemic immunity

Judith Provoost[1], Florent Valour[2,3,4], Delphine Gamondes[5], Sandrine Roux[2], Nathalie Freymond[1], Emilie Perrot[1], Pierre-Jean Souquet[1,4], Lize Kiakouama-Maleka[1], Christian Chidiac[2,4], Gérard Lina[3,4,6], Oana Dumitrescu[3,4,6], Agathe Sénéchal[1] and Florence Ader[2,3,4*]

Abstract

Background: Nontuberculous mycobacteria (NTM) lung diseases are increasingly recognized as chronic opportunistic infections, occurring in individuals with a wide variety of underlying conditions. In the absence of systemic immunodeficiency, decision of NTM lung disease treatment must relies on a careful risk/benefit assessment, given the requirement of long-term administration of multidrug therapies supported by limited evidence. The primary objective was to identify the factors associated with anti-NTM treatment initiation. Clinical and radiological outcome upon treatment were studied.

Methods: This retrospective, single center study (2013–2016, 45 months) addressed the criteria supporting treatment decision among adults with NTM lung disease without systemic immunodeficiency at our institution, with the assigned goal to harmonize the practice. All patients matched the current international definitions of NTM lung disease according to the American Thoracic Society criteria. Factors associated with anti-NTM treatment were investigated by conditional logistic regression. Clinical and radiological outcomes of treated and untreated NTM-disease cases were examined. Mortality rate was assessed. An expert radiologist conducted a blinded computed tomography (CT)-scan review of the treated and untreated patients.

(Continued on next page)

* Correspondence: florence.ader@chu-lyon.fr
[2]Département des Maladies infectieuses et tropicales, Hôpital de la Croix-Rousse, Hospices Civils de Lyon, 103, Grande-Rue de la Croix-Rousse, 69317, cedex 04 Lyon, France
[3]CIRI-Centre International de Recherche en Infectiologie, Inserm, U1111, Université Claude Bernard Lyon 1, CNRS, UMR5308, Ecole Normale Supérieure de Lyon, Univ Lyon, F-69007 Lyon, France
Full list of author information is available at the end of the article

(Continued from previous page)

Results: Among 51 cases of NTM lung diseases, 25 (49%) received anti-NTM treatment. In univariate analysis, a body mass index (BMI) < 18 kg/m^2 (odds ratio (OR), 4.2 [95% confidence interval (CI) 1.2–15.2]; $p = 0.042$), hemoptysis (OR, 11.8 [95% CI 1.35–12.9]; $p = 0.026$), excavation(s) (OR, 4.8 [95% CI 1.4–16.4], $p = 0.012$), prior anti-NTM treatment (OR, 5.65 [95% CI 1.06–29.9]; $p = 0.042$), *Aspergillus* spp. co-infection (OR, 6.3 [95% CI 1.8–22.2]; $p = 0.004$) were associated with treatment initiation. In multivariate analysis, *Aspergillus* spp. co-infection was the only independent determinant of treatment initiation (OR, 5.3 [95% CI 1.1–25.4]; $p = 0.036$). Twenty-one (81%) patients received ≥3 anti-NTM drugs. Median treatment duration and follow-up were 36.3 (interquartile range [IQR], 13.1–64.4) weeks and 17.1 (IQR, 8.7–27.1) months, respectively. Regarding radiological outcome, 85 CT-scans were reviewed, showing similar rates of regression or stabilization in treated and untreated patients. Overall mortality rate was not different in treated and untreated patients.

Conclusion: The most relevant variable associated with anti-NTM treatment initiation was *Aspergillus* spp. co-infection. Radiological regression or stabilization of pulmonary lesions was not different between the treated and untreated patients.

Keywords: *Aspergillus* spp., Bronchiectasis, Chronic obstructive pulmonary disease, Hemoptysis, Mycobacteria, *Mycobacterium avium complex*, Nontuberculous mycobacteria

Background

Nontuberculous mycobacteria (NTM) are ubiquitous bacteria of environmental origin including a widely diverse number of species (> 160), some of which cause disease in humans [1–3]. Prevalence of NTM lung diseases is unexpectedly increasing in industrialized countries, as consistently uncovered by recent studies [3, 4]. The key issue remains to determine whether NTM are the true and single promoter of an evolving lung disease or chronic airway colonizers, among others. To standardize the diagnosis of NTM lung disease, the guidelines for NTM diagnosis of the American Thoracic Society (ATS)/Infectious Disease Society of America (IDSA) and the British Thoracic Society (BTS) require isolation and growth of the same NTM strain on at least two separate samples from the patient [5, 6].

Human host and pathogenic NTM relationship is still poorly understood, as NTM virulence is highly variable from one species to another. NTM lung disease is strongly associated with pre-existing pulmonary conditions such as chronic obstructive pulmonary disease (COPD), cystic fibrosis, idiopathic bronchiectasis, prior active tuberculosis or pneumoconiosis [6]. It is also frequently associated with genetic or acquired systemic immune deficiency such as defects in the pathways of inflammatory cytokines interleukin (IL)-12, tumor necrosis factor (TNF)-α or interferon (IFN)-γ, immunosuppressive treatments (including anti-TNF-α therapy or corticosteroids), solid-organ transplantation, or acquired immune deficiency syndrome (AIDS)/human immunodeficiency virus (HIV) infection [1–7]. However, it may also occur in individuals without recognized severe immune local or systemic deficiency. In the absence of patent predisposition, NTM diseases are overrepresented among the specific morphotype of slender women with a low body fat [8].

Treatment decision for NTM lung disease is challenging. There is debate as to which patients should benefit the most from treatment according to medical background, comorbidities, clinical status, radiologic features and causal NTM strain. Assessment of clinical, microbiologic, and radiologic response to treatment is not standardized as well. We focused on NTM lung diseases in adults without systemic immunodeficiency that met the ATS criteria guidelines. Based on the comparison of a group of treated and untreated patients, the primary objective was to identify the factors associated with physician decision of initiating anti-NTM treatment. Secondary objectives were to study the outcome upon treatment and to propose a standardized evaluation for the diagnosis and decision making to treatment of NTM lung diseases in adults without systemic immunodeficiency.

Methods

Study design and patient population

We conducted a retrospective, observational, single-center study between January 2013 and February 2016 (45 months) among adults (≥ 18 year-old) without systemic immunosuppression presenting NTM lung disease. Exclusion criteria were HIV infection, cystic fibrosis, primary ciliary dyskinesia, active malignant disease, solid-organ transplantation or ongoing immunosuppressant treatments such as TNF inhibitor or high-dose corticosteroid (≥ 1 mg/kg more than 21 days). Case identification was based on cross-referencing the databases of the mycobacteria laboratory and the departments of infectious and pulmonary diseases. Patients eligible for inclusion in the NTM lung disease cohort were those who matched the criteria previously defined by the ATS/IDSA and the BTS guidelines with the minimum requirement of clinical and microbiologic following criteria: *(i)* pulmonary symptoms associated with multifocal bronchiectasis with multiple small nodules on computed tomography (CT)-scan; *(ii)* proper exclusion of other diagnoses; *(iii)* NTM-positive culture results from at least two separate expectorated sputum samples or a NTM-positive culture result from at least one bronchial wash or lavage [5, 6]. Patients' characteristics at diagnosis were collected in order to perform analysis on 146 selected variables: demographics; history of predisposing factors; underlying pulmonary diseases; comorbidities; pulmonary function testing; respiratory bacterial or mycological co-infection(s), which definition was similar to NTM criteria, namely positive culture isolation of the same species from at least two separate expectorated sputum samples or a positive culture result from at least one bronchial wash or lavage; immunologic status; nutritional status; clinical features; microbiologic assessment through identification of NTM species on positive NTM cultures and sample culture conversions; radiologic features on high-resolution CT-scans (fibrocavitary disease or nodular/bronchiectasis disease); prior treatment for NTM lung disease, treatment combination and duration; outcome. Because of the retrospective observational nature of the study and the lack of any modification in patients' management, the need for informed consent was waived with the authorization of the Ethics Committee of Lyon University Hospital (Comité d'Ethique, Hospices Civils de Lyon), which approved the study under the number 17–207.

Radiologic assessment

An independent expert chest radiologist, blinded to the patient information, retrospectively reviewed the CT-scans performed without injection of intravenous contrast media, assigned in random order at diagnosis and six to 24 months after treatment or during the follow up of the untreated patients. The number and size of cavity(ies) and their wall thickness were evaluated in the lung window setting. Nodular opacity(ies) (≥ 10 mm), cluster(s) of small nodules (≤ 5 mm), the tree-in-bud pattern, the presence of bronchiectasis in any of the lobes or multifocal bronchiectasis were evaluated. Based on the number and size of the lesions, the expert classified the lesions as improved, stable or worsening.

Endpoints

The primary endpoint was to identify the factors significantly involved in the decision of initiating anti-NTM treatment by patient referent physician. Secondary endpoints were the assessment of clinical and radiological outcomes upon anti-NTM treatment in comparison with no treatment. Based on these findings, a standardized appraisal was proposed to assist diagnosis management and treatment decision for NTM lung diseases in adults without altered systemic immunity.

Statistical analysis

Descriptive data were used to estimate the frequencies of the study variables. There were expressed as count (percentage, %) for dichotomous variables and as medians (interquartile range [IQR]) for continuous values. The number of missing values was excluded from the denominator. Non-parametric statistical methods Fisher exact test, $\chi2$ test and Mann-Whitney U test were used to compare groups, where appropriate. The probability of treatment initiation over time was evaluated by Kaplan-Meier survival curve analysis, with group comparison using the log-rank (Mantel-Cox) test. Stepwise binary logistic regression analysis was used to assess the determinants for treatment initiation, expressed as odd ratios (OR) with 95% confidence intervals (95% CI). After checking the variables for interactions, variables with medical meaning and with p-values obtained in the univariate analysis of < 0.15 were included in the final multivariate model. A value of $p < 0.05$ was considered significant. All analyses were performed using SPSS software version 24.0 (SPSS. Chicago. IL).

Results

Out of 149 patients eligible to ATS/IDSA NTM lung disease criteria, 51 patients were included in the study, of who 25 (49%) received and 26 (51%) did not receive anti-NTM treatment (Fig. 1). The median age was 68 (interquartile range [IQR], 59–75) year-old with a male/female ratio of 0.76. Etiologic NTM agents were *Mycobacterium avium* (n = 17, 33.3%), *M. chimaerae* (n = 14, 27.5%), *M. xenopii* (n = 9, 17.6%), *M. intracellulare* (n = 9, 17.6%), *M. simiae* (n = 3, 5.9%), *M. kansasii* (n = 1, 2%), and *M. abscessus* (n = 1, 2%), with three patients having ≥2 concomitant NTM lung diseases. Importantly, the evidence of NTM lung disease has led to diagnose six underlying chronic lung diseases, of which a genetically documented cystic fibrosis in a 61 year-old women. On descriptive analysis, patient's characteristics did not significantly differ, to the exception of a lower BMI (p = 0.023) and a higher number of previously known NTM lung disease (p = 0.038) in treated versus untreated patients (Table 1). Notable percentages of missing data at diagnosis have to be acknowledged for active tobacco smoking (64.7%, n = 33), respiratory functional testing (23.5%, n = 12) with a very few patients having a 6-min walk test, baseline arterial blood oxygenation levels (58.8%, n = 30), CT-scan follow up within 24 months after diagnosis in untreated patients (46%, n = 12).

Factors leading the patient referent physician to initiate anti-NTM treatment were assessed using bivariate analysis.

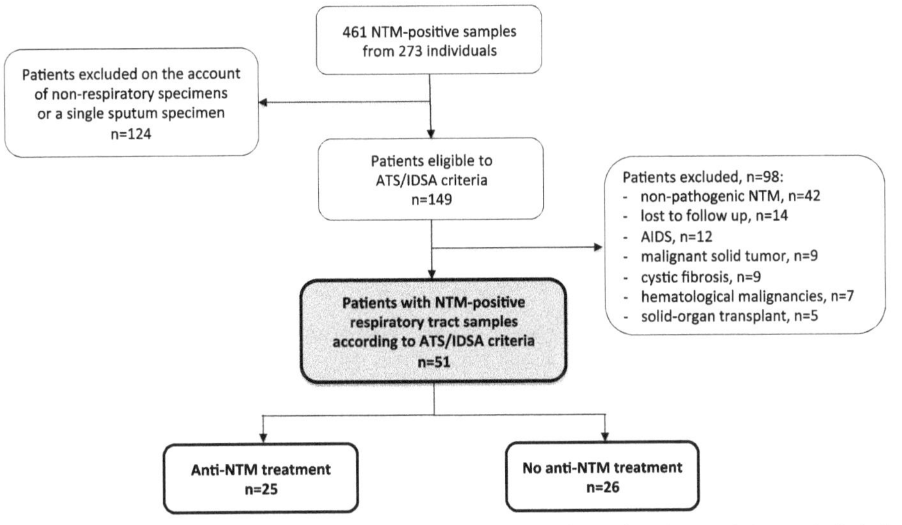

Fig. 1 Flow chart of adult patients with nontuberculous mycobacterial lung disease without altered systemic immunity included in the study. Nontuberculous mycobacterial lung disease defined according to the American Thoracic Society/Infectious Diseases Society of America and the British Thoracic Society [4, 5]

Table 1 Patients' demographic and baseline descriptive characteristics

	Treated patients (*n*=25)	Untreated patients (*n*=26)	*P*-value
Age, median (IQR) years	65 (54-74)	70 (60.8-76)	0.227
Gender (male)	9 (36)	13 (50)	0.4
Active smokers	6 (24)	6 (23)	1
Cumulative tobacco smoking (IQR) pack/year	32.5 (28.8-52.5)	40 (21.3-60)	0.79
BMI (IQR) kg/m^2	17.9 (16.8-19.9)	19.9 (18.3-23.8)	***0.023***
History of tuberculosis	6 (24)	5 (19.2)	0.74
History of NTM lung disease	8 (32)	2 (7.7)	***0.038***
History of croup during infancy	1	1	1
Gastroesophageal reflux disease	4 (16)	2 (7.7)	0.42
History of cured malignant solid tumor	1 (4)	5 (19.2)	0.19
Diabetes mellitus	0	2 (7.7)	0.49
Chronic heart failure	0	4 (16)	0.11
Asthma or atopic disease	6 (24)	2 (7.7)	0.14
Chronic obstructive pulmonary disease	4 (16)	9 (34.6)	0.19
Bronchiectasis	14 (56)	14 (53.8)	1
Chronic interstitial lung disease	2 (8)	5 (19.2)	0.42
Chronic rheumatic disease	6 (24)	2 (7.7)	0.14
Autoimmune disease	3 (12)	4 (15.4)	1
History of thoracic surgery	5 (20)	3 (11.5)	0.46
Corticosteroid inhaled therapy	6 (24)	7 (27)	1

NOTE Data are No. (%) of patients, unless otherwise indicated. Variables were compared using Mann–Whitney U test, $\chi 2$ test or the Fisher exact test, where appropriate
Abbreviations: IQR, interquartile range

Among the factors significantly associated with treatment were the BMI < 18 kg/m^2 (odds ratio (OR), 4.2 [95% confidence interval (CI) 1.2–15.2]; p = 0.042), prior anti-NTM treatment (OR, 5.65 [95% CI 1.06–29.9]; p = 0.042), hemoptysis (OR = 11.8 [95% CI 1.35–102.9]; p = 0.026), the presence of excavation(s) on lung CT-scan (OR, 4.8 [95% CI 1.4–16.4], p = 0.012), *Aspergillus* spp. co-infection (OR, 6.3 [95% CI 1.8–22.2]; p = 0.004) (Table 2). In multivariate analysis, *Aspergillus* spp. co-infection was the single independent factor associated with anti-NTM treatment (OR, 5.3 [95% CI 1.1–25.4]; p = 0.036) (Table 3).

The probability of treatment initiation over time according to the presence or not of targeted variables was investigated. The probability was significantly higher in case of BMI < 18 vs. > 18 kg/m^2 (p = 0.006), of hemoptysis vs. no hemoptysis (p = 0.009), of *Aspergillus* spp. co-infection vs. no co-infection (p = 0.029), of pulmonary excavation(s) vs.

Table 2 Bivariate analysis of the factors associated with treatment initiation in adult patients with nontuberculous mycobacterial lung disease without systemic immunodeficiency

Tested variables	Treated patients (n=25)	Untreated patients (n=26)	*P-value*	OR [95% CI]
Clinical criteria				
BMI < 18 (kg/m^2)	13/24 (54.2)	5/23 (21.7)	***0.026***	4.25 [1.18-15.2]
Weight loss > 5%	17 (68)	10 (38.5)	***0.05***	3.4 [1.07-10.77]
fatigue	13 (52)	7 (27)	0.071	2.94 [0.9-9.46]
chronic cough	16 (64)	14 (54)	0.572	1.52 [0.49-4.69]
night sweats	5 (20)	3 (11.5)	0.465	1.92 [0.41-9.05]
hemoptysis	8 (32)	1 (3.8)	***0.026***	11.8 [1.3-102.8]
Microbiological criteria				
AFB-positive sputum sample on direct examination	13 (52)	8 (30.8)	0.160	2.44 [0.77-7.65]
NTM-positive culture NTM on lower respiratory tract sample	2 (1-2.3)	1 (1-1.8)	***0.044***	**1.79 [1-3.2]**
Functional criteria				
FEV1 (L)	1.6 (1.2-2.2)	1.9 (1.2-2.5)	0.554	0.72 [0.34-1.51]
Immunological and nutritional status				
total lymphocyte count (G/L)	1.3 (1.2-1.7)	1.4 (1.1-2.1)	0.388	0.95 [0.86-1.04]
CD4+ lymphocyte count (%)	54 (4.5-61.5)	40 (37.8-44.3)	***0.031***	**1.07 [0.95-1.21]**
serum albumin (mg/L)	39.5 (36-43)	39 (33-42.5)	0.481	1.05 [0.97-1.14]
serum pre-albumin (mg/L)	0.21 (0.15-0.24)	0.22 (0.15-0.25)	0.974	1.25 [0-1.48]
vitamin D deficiency	6/10 (60)	6/7 (86)	0.338	0.25 [0.02-2.95]
Co-infection(s)				
Mycobacterium tuberculosis	1 (4)	1 (4)	0.35	1.04 [0.06-17.6]
Pseudomonas spp.	2 (8)	3 (11.5)	1	0.68 [0.1-4.4]
Aspergillus spp.	15 (60)	5 (19.2)	***0.004***	**6.3 [1.8-22.2]**
Radiologic features at diagnosis				
nodule(s) (≥ 10mm)	12 (48)	7/23 (30)	0.25	2.11 [0.65-6.9]
cluster(s) of micronodules (< 5mm)	16 (64)	10/23 (44)	0.246	2.31 [0.72-7.4]
cavitation(s)	18 (72)	8/23 (35)	***0.019***	**4.82 [1.42-16.4]**
bronchiectasis	14 (56)	11/23 (48)	0.773	1.39 [0.45-4.3]
emphysema	9 (36)	11/23 (48)	0.559	0.61 [0.19-1.95]
Radiologic review				
regression	8/23 (35)	4/13 (31)	1	1.2 [0.28-5.15]
stabilization	9/23 (39)	6/13 (46)	0.736	0.75 [0.19-2.97]
worsening	6/23 (26)	3/13 (23)	1	1.18 [0.24-5.8]

NOTE Data are No. (%) of patients, unless otherwise indicated. Denominators have been stipulated for variables with missing data. Odds ratios (OR) were determined by conditional logistic regression with 95% confidence interval (95% CI)

Abbreviations: AFB, acid-fast bacilli; BMI, body mass index; CI, confidence interval; FEV1, forced expiratory volume in 1 second; NTM, nontuberculous mycobacteria; OR, odds ratio

Table 3 Multivariate analysis of factors associated with the initiation of anti-nontuberculous mycobacteria treatment

Independent variables	OR [95% CI]	*P*-value
Aspergillus spp.	***5.33 [1.1-25.5]***	***0.036***
weight loss > 5%	2.44 [0.6-10.2]	0.22
hemoptysis	3.2 [0.28-36.3]	0.35
excavation(s)	3.54 [0.83-15.1]	0.087

Abbreviations: CI, confidence interval; OR, odds ratio

no excavation ($p = 0.005$) (Fig. 2a, b, c and d, respectively). In the treated group, 21 (84%) received ≥3 anti-NTM drugs, among whom 23 (92%) received a macrolide as part of a first-line regimen. Median anti-NTM treatment duration was 36.3 (IQR, 13.1–64.4) weeks. Thirteen (52%) of the treated patients developed at least one antimicrobial-related adverse event, among which gastrointestinal disorders ($n = 6$), impaired blood cell count ($n = 5$) and cholestatic and/or cytolytic hepatitis ($n = 4$). According to physician judgment, clinical stabilization and improvement was obtained for 8 (34.8%) and 12 (52.2%) of treated patients, respectively. Patient's median follow-up from diagnosis assessment was 17.1 (IQR, 8.7–27.1) months. Eighty-five CT-scans were reviewed for comparative assessment after treatment or over the course of follow-up in the untreated subset. The median interval between the initiation of NTM treatment and the date of the assessed images was 56.7 (IQR, 43.3–97.7) weeks. Although 34.8% ($n = 8$) and 39.1% ($n = 9$) experienced regression or stabilization of their pulmonary lesions in the treated patients, these rates did not differ from the untreated patients with 30.8% ($n = 4$) and 46.2% ($n = 6$) of regression and stabilization over the course of their follow-up, respectively (Table 2). Finally, all-cause mortality was not different between treated and untreated groups, although lost to follow-up was high in the untreated group ($n = 10$, 38.5%). Regarding the four patients that deceased ($n = 3$ in the treated group and $n = 1$ in the untreated group), the cause of mortality was linked to the underlying diseases rather than NTM-related mortality.

Discussion

In the present study, treated patients were characterized by BMI < 18 kg/m^2, presence of hemoptysis and excavation(s), *Aspergillus* spp. co-infection, and prior anti-NTM treatment. *Aspergillus* spp. co-infection was the only independent factor associated with treatment initiation. A single study from five English centers has recently addressed the factors that influence anti-NTM treatment initiation using similar retrospective design of treated and untreated cohort comparison (2010–2014), to the exception of different

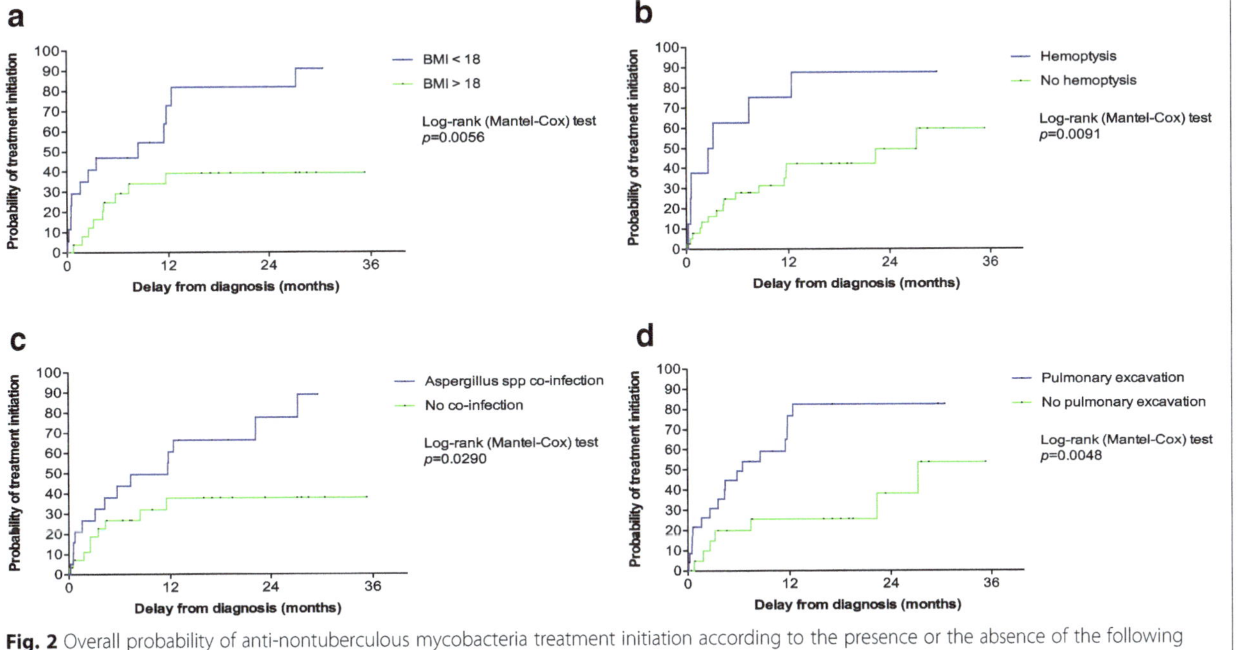

Fig. 2 Overall probability of anti-nontuberculous mycobacteria treatment initiation according to the presence or the absence of the following variables: **a** body mass index < 18 kg/m^2; **b** hemoptysis; **c** *Aspergillus* spp. co-infection; **d** lung excavation(s). Overall survival probabilities were determined by the Kaplan-Meier method and were compared by the log-rank test

Table 4 Standardized appraisal for patients with nontuberculous mycobacterial lung diseases without systemic immunodeficiency referred at our institution

	Comments
Exhaustive history record	
infant respiratory diseases	croup, Influenza, measle
gastro-oesophageal reflux disease	
atopic dermatitis	
eating disorders	anorexia, bulimia
family history of respiratory disease	
prior tuberculosis	
prior anti-NTM treatment	
Environmental exposure	
passive tobacco exposure	
active tobacco smocking	Packs-per-year
other toxic/drug exposure	
chronic alcoholism	micro-inhalations
habitat characteristics	domestic water system, allergens
Blood tests	
serum albumin	nutritional status
serum pre-albumin	
vitamin D (25-OH D3)	
HIV serology	cellular immune defect
T CD4+ and CD8+ lymphocyte counts	
total IgG serum level	hypogammaglobulinemia
total eosinophil count	*Aspergillus*-related allergic lung diseases
total IgE serum level	
Aspergillus-specific IgE	
Aspergillus serology	
galactomannan antigenemia	invasive aspergillosis
Interferon-γ reactive assay	latent tuberculosis infection
Lung function testing	
spirometry including FEV1	lung volumes
plethysmography	
pulse oxymetry	oxygen level
arterial blood gas tests	
6-minutes walk test	stress test
Imagery	
chest X-ray	
lung HRCT scan	Micronodules (≤ 5mm), nodules (≥ 10 mm), pulmonary consolidations, bronchiectasis, tree-in-bud images, cavity(ies)
Cytology and microbiologic tests on respiratory samples	
BALF cytological composition	
sputum/BALF direct examination	
sputum/BALF collection for bacterial culture	Non-fermenting gram-negative bacilli (*Pseudomonas aeruginosa*)
sputum/BALF collection for mycological culture	filamentous fungi
nasal swab/BALF collection for respiratory virus PCR screening	human Respiratory syncytial virus, parainfluenza virus, metapneumovirus, rhinovirus, and coronavirus
Specific tests depending on the setting	
α-1 antitrypsin level	lung emphysema
sweat test	cystic fibrosis
CFTR gene screening	
airway cilia sample	primary ciliary dyskinesia
IFN-γ and IL-12 plasma levels	host predisposition to NTM diseases
blood anti-IFN-γ autoantibodies	
IFN-γ or IL-12 gene screening	

Abbreviations: BALF, bronchoalveolar lavage fluid; CFTR, cystic fibrosis transmembrane conductance regulator, FEV1, forced expiratory volume in 1 second; HRCT, high-resolution computed tomography; IFN-γ, interferon gamma; Ig, immunoglobulins; IL, interleukin

inclusion criteria which allowed non-AIDS/HIV immunosuppressed patients (36 and 33% in the treated and untreated subsets, respectively) to be evaluated. In the multivariate analysis, patients had increased odds of anti-NTM treatment in case of cavitation on CT imaging, night sweats and weight loss [9].

Here, three out of four criteria are part of guideline criteria leading to decision of anti-NTM treatment. They all reflect a degree of severity of NTM lung disease linked with progression of an impaired respiratory condition. The current problematic of NTM lung diseases shifts from distinguishing colonization from infection toward differentiating stable, poorly active vs. progressive active NTM disease, the latter being responsible for further structural lung damage(s). The risk/benefit analysis includes prescribing recommended long-term multidrug regimens with concerns over suboptimal cure rates and frequently reported drug-related side effects. To support these arguments, others have already shown that physician ATS/IDSA guideline adherence is moderate confirming such a trend of intuitive clinical behavior mostly based on evidence of severity and/or patent progression of the disease. A multicenter study has reported a sample of 349 US physicians treating 915 patients with *M. avium* complex (MAC) lung disease. Overall, 55% (n = 411) of patients with MAC lung disease received some type of anti-NTM treatment from their physician and 13% prescribed antibiotic regimens were consistent with ATS/IDSA guidelines [10]. Another study conducted in France has shown that among a cohort of 31 NTM lung diseases, only 12 (38.7%) received appropriate treatment matching ATS/IDSA guidelines [11]. Inappropriate prescriptions were mostly related to shorter treatment duration (6 months or less) and/or off-recommendation regimen, particularly those excluding macrolide from the combination or those using a single-drug macrolide regimen [10, 11]. It has to be acknowledged that guidelines specify that treatment for MAC-associated lung disease in HIV-negative individuals can be a three-times-weekly drug regimen upon culture conversion while on therapy for 1 year, which may favor treatment compliance [5, 12, 13].

Patients with bronchiectasis and NTM lung disease have a higher prevalence of being sensitized to *Aspergillus* than patients with NTM-free bronchiectasis [12]. Allergic airway manifestations in response to *Aspergillus* are termed *Aspergillus*-related lung diseases with a spectrum going from *Aspergillus*-induced hypersensitivity to the severe allergic bronchopulmonary aspergillosis (ABPA) [14]. By itself, the coexistence of NTM and *Aspergillus* in lung airway justifies the need for testing *Aspergillus* serology, total serum immunoglobulin (Ig)E and *Aspergillus*-specific IgE levels as well as mycological direct examination and culture of sputum or bronchial aspirates for presence of filamentous fungi in the diagnosis algorithm of patients with NTM lung diseases. Active co-infections with NTM and *Aspergillus* spp. have also been described, in which patients with NTM lung disease develop chronic forms of pulmonary aspergillosis which definitions and management have been revisited in recent updated guidelines [14–17].

Radiographic improvement may be hampered by concomitant lung disease and the limited potential for resolution of consolidated radiologic abnormalities. A previous study has investigated radiologic response to treatment showing consistent results with those found in the present study. Although anti-NTM treatment led to an improvement or stabilization of lesions for a majority of patients, these modifications were not significantly different from the untreated group who went through CT-scan follow up indicating that anti-NTM treatment did not lead to radiological abnormalities reversion [9]. The present study has strengths and limitations. The strength is the study of the largest cohort so far of NTM lung diseases in patients without systemic immunodeficiency with exhaustive data collection and blinded radiological assessment. We acknowledge the biases that contribute to mitigate conclusions from the study such as being conducted in a single center, the important differences in physician's management resulting in lack of consistency in treatment decision making, the number of missing data. In addition, the CT-scans were not performed at fixed intervals, particularly in the untreated subset of patients. Finally, treatment duration and outcome criteria were not standardized, which prevent to properly assess treatment efficacy. Useful consensus definitions for key outcome parameters to be used in the treatment of NTM lung diseases have been released very recently, which should harmonize data collection regarding NTM treatment [18].

Future researches are necessary to better define criteria associated with progressive active NTM disease in the immunocompetent setting. Concretely, this preliminary study has led to implement in our institution a standardized appraisal for the diagnosis of NTM lung diseases in this particular setting (Table 4). The aim is to provide a future basis for the development of a diagnosis scoring system supporting anti-NTM treatment decision. Future studies should focus as well on the most relevant CT imaging variables associated with response to treatment over time that may be applied in future clinical trials to assess treatment outcome.

Conclusions

In summary, the main factors supporting anti-NTM treatment decision in immunocompetent were low BMI, hemoptysis, lung excavation(s), prior anti-NTM treatment and *Aspergillus* pp. co-infection, the latter being the only independent factor. Anti-NTM treatment did not achieve radiological abnormalities reversion, as pulmonary lesions assessment showed no difference between the treated and the untreated patients. A diagnosis of NTM lung disease in an immunocompetent patient requires investigating the presence of a chronic pulmonary underlying disease.

Abbreviations

AIDS: Acquired immune deficiency syndrome; ATS: American thoracic society; BTS: British thoracic society; COPD: Chronic obstructive pulmonary disease; CT: Computed tomography; HIV: Human immunodeficiency virus; IDSA: Infectious disease society of America; IFN: Interferon; IL: Interleukin; NTM: Non tuberculous mycobacteria; TNF: Tumor necrosis factor

Acknowledgements

The authors gratefully acknowledge Pr Gilles Devouassoux for helpful insights.

Funding

No external funding was received for this study.

Authors' contributions
JP contributed to conception and design of the study, acquisition of the data, interpretation of the data, drafted the manuscript and approved the final version; FV carried out the statistical analysis, participated in revision of the paper for important intellectual content, and approved the final version; DG carried out the blinded review of 85 CT-scans with the examination of each imagery, she participated in revision of the paper for important intellectual content, and approved the final version; GL and OD are in charge of the Mycobacteria laboratory and have provided NTM strain identification and drug susceptibility tests. They participated in revision of the paper for important intellectual content, and approved the final version; SR, NF, EP, PJS, LKM, and CC contributed to acquisition of the data, revision of the paper for important intellectual content, and approved the final version; FA and AS are the project initiators, contributed to conception and design of the study, drafted the manuscript and approved the final version. FA coordinated the project until the submission of the article. All authors read and approved the final manuscript.

Consent for publication
Not applicable.

Competing interests
The authors have no relevant affiliations or financial involvement with any organization or entity with a financial interest in or financial conflict with the subject matter or materials discussed in the manuscript. No writing assistance was utilized in the production of this manuscript.

Author details
[1]Département de Pneumologie, Hospices Civils de Lyon, Lyon, France. [2]Département des Maladies infectieuses et tropicales, Hôpital de la Croix-Rousse, Hospices Civils de Lyon, 103, Grande-Rue de la Croix-Rousse, 69317, cedex 04 Lyon, France. [3]CIRI-Centre International de Recherche en Infectiologie, Inserm, U1111, Université Claude Bernard Lyon 1, CNRS, UMR5308, Ecole Normale Supérieure de Lyon, Univ Lyon, F-69007 Lyon, France. [4]Université Claude Bernard Lyon 1, Lyon, France. [5]Département de Radiologie, Hospices Civils de Lyon, Lyon, France. [6]Institut des Agents Infectieux, Hospices Civils de Lyon, Lyon, France.

References
1. Wassilew N, Hoffmann H, Andrejak C, Lange C. Pulmonary disease caused by non-tuberculous mycobacteria. Respiration. 2016;91:386–402.
2. Aksamit TR, Philley JV, Griffith DE. Nontuberculous mycobacterial lung disease: the top ten essentials. Respir Med. 2014;108:417–25.
3. Raju RM, Raju SM, Zhao Y, Rubin EJ. Leveraging advances in tuberculosis diagnosis and treatment to address nontuberculous mycobacterial disease. Emerg Infect Dis. 2016;22:365–9.
4. Winthrop KL, McNelley E, Kendall B, et al. Pulmonary nontuberculous mycobacterial disease prevalence and clinical features: an emerging public health disease. Am J Respir Crit Care Med. 2010;182:977–82.
5. Griffith DE, Aksamit T, Brown-Elliott BA, Catanzaro A, Daley C, Gordin F, et al. An official ATS/IDSA statement: diagnosis, treatment, and prevention of nontuberculous mycobacterial diseases. Am J Respir Crit Care Med. 2007;175:367–416.
6. Haworth CS, Banks J, Capstick T, et al. British Thoracic Society guidelines for the management of non-tuberculous mycobacterial pulmonary disease (NTM-PD). Thorax. 2017;72:ii1–ii64.
7. Larsson LO, Polverino E, Hoefsloot W, Codecasa LR, Diel R, Jenkins SG, Loebinger MR. Pulmonary disease by nontuberculous mycobacteria-clinical management, unmet needs and future perspectives. Exp Rev Respir Med. 2017;11:977–89.
8. Kartalija M, Ovrutsky AR, Bryan CL, et al. Patients with nontuberculous mycobacterial lung disease exhibit unique body and immune phenotypes. Am J Respir Crit Care Med. 2013;187:197–205.
9. Rawson TM, Abbara A, Kranzer K, et al. Factors which influence treatment initiation for pulmonary non-tuberculous mycobacterium infection in HIV negative patients; a multicentre observational study. Respir Med. 2016;120:101–8.
10. Adjemian J, Prevots DR, Gallagher J, Heap K, Gupta R, Griffith D. Lack of adherence to evidence-based treatment guidelines for nontuberculous mycobacterial lung disease. Ann Am Thorac Soc. 2014;11:9–16.
11. El-Zeenni A, Chanoine S, Recule S, Stahl JP, Maurin M, Camara B. Are guidelines on the management of non-tuberculous mycobacteria lung infections respected and what are the consequences for patients? A French retrospective study from 2007 to 2014. Eur J Clin Microbiol Infect Dis. 2018;37:233–40.
12. Griffith DE, Brown BA, Cegielski P, Murphy DT, Wallace RJ Jr. Early results (at 6 months) with intermittent clarithromycin including regimens for lung disease due to *Mycobacterium avium* complex. Clin Infect Dis. 2000;30:288–92.
13. Jeong BH, Jeon K, Park HY, et al. Intermittent antibiotic therapy for nodular bronchiectatic Mycobacterium avium complex lung disease. Am J Respir Crit Care Med. 2015;191:96–103.
14. Kunst J, Wickremasinghe M, Wells A, Wilson R. Nontuberculous mycobacterial disease and *Aspergillus*-related lung disease in bronchiectasis. Eur Respir J. 2006;28:352–7.
15. Hafeez I, Muers MF, Murphy SA, Evans EG, Barton RC, McWhinney P. Non-tuberculous mycobacterial lung infection complicated by chronic necrotising pulmonary aspergillosis. Thorax. 2000;55:717–9.
16. Kobashi Y, Fukuda M, Yoshida K, Miyashita N, Niki Y, Oka M. Chronic necrotizing pulmonary aspergillosis as a complication of pulmonary *Mycobacterium avium* complex disease. Respirology. 2006;11:809–13.
17. Denning DW, Cadranel J, Beigelman-Aubry C, Ader F, Chakrabarti A, Blot S, Ullman A, Dimopoulos G, Lange C. Chronic pulmonary aspergillosis-rationale and clinical guidelines for diagnosis and management. Eur Resp J. 2016;47(1):45–68.
18. van Ingen J, Aksamit T, Andrejak C, et al. Treatment outcome definitions in nontuberculous mycobacterial pulmonary disease: an NTM-NET consensus statement. Eur Respir J. 2018;51:1800170.

Permissions

All chapters in this book were first published in ID, by BioMed Central; hereby published with permission under the Creative Commons Attribution License or equivalent. Every chapter published in this book has been scrutinized by our experts. Their significance has been extensively debated. The topics covered herein carry significant findings which will fuel the growth of the discipline. They may even be implemented as practical applications or may be referred to as a beginning point for another development.

The contributors of this book come from diverse backgrounds, making this book a truly international effort. This book will bring forth new frontiers with its revolutionizing research information and detailed analysis of the nascent developments around the world.

We would like to thank all the contributing authors for lending their expertise to make the book truly unique. They have played a crucial role in the development of this book. Without their invaluable contributions this book wouldn't have been possible. They have made vital efforts to compile up to date information on the varied aspects of this subject to make this book a valuable addition to the collection of many professionals and students.

This book was conceptualized with the vision of imparting up-to-date information and advanced data in this field. To ensure the same, a matchless editorial board was set up. Every individual on the board went through rigorous rounds of assessment to prove their worth. After which they invested a large part of their time researching and compiling the most relevant data for our readers.

The editorial board has been involved in producing this book since its inception. They have spent rigorous hours researching and exploring the diverse topics which have resulted in the successful publishing of this book. They have passed on their knowledge of decades through this book. To expedite this challenging task, the publisher supported the team at every step. A small team of assistant editors was also appointed to further simplify the editing procedure and attain best results for the readers.

Apart from the editorial board, the designing team has also invested a significant amount of their time in understanding the subject and creating the most relevant covers. They scrutinized every image to scout for the most suitable representation of the subject and create an appropriate cover for the book.

The publishing team has been an ardent support to the editorial, designing and production team. Their endless efforts to recruit the best for this project, has resulted in the accomplishment of this book. They are a veteran in the field of academics and their pool of knowledge is as vast as their experience in printing. Their expertise and guidance has proved useful at every step. Their uncompromising quality standards have made this book an exceptional effort. Their encouragement from time to time has been an inspiration for everyone.

The publisher and the editorial board hope that this book will prove to be a valuable piece of knowledge for researchers, students, practitioners and scholars across the globe.

List of Contributors

Emine Qehaja-Buçaj
Clinic of Infectious Diseases, University Clinical Center of Kosovo, Prishtinë, Kosovo

Diellëza Namani
Smart Center, Prishtinë, Kosov

Sadie Namani
Clinic of Infectious Diseases, University Clinical Center of Kosovo, Prishtinë, Kosovo
Medical Faculty, University of Prishtina, Kongresi i Manastirit 3A, Prishtinë, Kosovo

K. A. T. M. Ehsanul Huq, Michiko Moriyama and Md Moshiur Rahman
Graduate School of Biomedical & Health Sciences, Hiroshima University, Kasumi 1-2-3 Minami-ku, Hiroshima 734-8553, Japan

Khalequ Zaman, Mohammod Jobayer Chisti, Shahed Hossain, Habiba Shirin and Mohammad Jyoti Raihan
International Centre for Diarrhoeal Disease Research, Dhaka, Bangladesh

Julie Long
University of Colorado, Denver, USA

Akramul Islam
Health Programme, BRAC, Dhaka, Bangladesh

Sajeda Chowdhury
Institute of Biomedical & Health Sciences, Hiroshima University, Hiroshima, Japan

D. Vallois and C. Rioux
APHP, Hôpital Bichat Claude Bernard, Service des Maladies Infectieuses et Tropicales, Paris Diderot University, Paris, France

S. Jaureguiberry, H. Guillot, M. Jaspard and E. Caumes
APHP, Hôpitaux Universitaires Pitié Salpêtrière-Charles Foix, Service des Maladies Infectieuses et Tropicales, Paris, France

N. Houhou
Virology Department, APHP-Bichat-Claude Bernard Hospital, Paris, France

D. Boutolleau
AP-HP, Hôpitaux Universitaires Pitié Salpêtrière-Charles Foix, Service de Virologie, et Sorbonne Universités, UPMC Univ Paris 06, CR7, CIMI, INSERM U1135, Paris, France

J. C. Lucet
APHP, Infection control unit, Bichat Claude Bernard hospital, Paris Diderot University, Paris, France
INSERM, IAME, UMR 1137, Paris, France
Univ Paris Diderot, IAME, UMR 1137, Sorbonne Paris Cité, Paris, France

A. Bleibtreu
APHP, Hôpital Bichat Claude Bernard, Service des Maladies Infectieuses et Tropicales, Paris Diderot University, Paris, France
APHP, Hôpitaux Universitaires Pitié Salpêtrière-Charles Foix, Service des Maladies Infectieuses et Tropicales, Paris, France
INSERM, IAME, UMR 1137, Paris, France
Univ Paris Diderot, IAME, UMR 1137, Sorbonne Paris Cité, Paris, France

F. X. Lescure and Y. Yazdanapanah
APHP, Hôpital Bichat Claude Bernard, Service des Maladies Infectieuses et Tropicales, Paris Diderot University, Paris, France
INSERM, IAME, UMR 1137, Paris, France
Univ Paris Diderot, IAME, UMR 1137, Sorbonne Paris Cité, Paris, France

J. Robert
AP-HP, Hôpitaux Universitaires Pitié Salpêtrière-Charles Foix, Bactériologie-Hygiène Hospitalière, Paris, France
Faculté de Médecine P. & M. Curie Paris-6 - Site Pitié, Centre d'Immunologie et des Maladies Infectieuses (CIMI) - E13, Paris, France

B. Mourvillier
INSERM, IAME, UMR 1137, Paris, France
Univ Paris Diderot, IAME, UMR 1137, Sorbonne Paris Cité, Paris, France
APHP- Hôpital Bichat Claude Bernard, Service de Réanimation médicale et Infectieuse, Paris, France

J. Delemazure
Service de pneumologie et réanimation Département R3S, AP-HP, Hôpitaux Universitaires Pitié Salpêtrière-Charles Foix, unité de Soin de Réadaptation Post Réanimation (SRPR), Paris, France

Dao Nguyen Vinh and Nguyen Thi Hanh
Wellcome Trust Major Overseas Programme, Hospital for Tropical Diseases, Oxford University Clinical Research Unit, 764 Vo Van Kiet Street, District 5, Ho Chi Minh City, Vietnam

Dang Thi Minh Ha
Wellcome Trust Major Overseas Programme, Hospital for Tropical Diseases, Oxford University Clinical Research Unit, 764 Vo Van Kiet Street, District 5, Ho Chi Minh City, Vietnam
Pham Ngoc Thach Hospital, Ho Chi Minh City, Vietnam

Guy Thwaites, Hannah E. Clapham and Nguyen Thuy Thuong Thuong
Wellcome Trust Major Overseas Programme, Hospital for Tropical Diseases, Oxford University Clinical Research Unit, 764 Vo Van Kiet Street, District 5, Ho Chi Minh City, Vietnam
Centre for Tropical Medicine and Global Health, Nuffield Department of Medicine, University of Oxford, Oxford, UK

Maciej F. Boni
Centre for Tropical Medicine and Global Health, Nuffield Department of Medicine, University of Oxford, Oxford, UK
Center for Infectious Disease Dynamics, Department of Biology, Pennsylvania State University, Pennsylvania, USA

Setegn Eshetie
Department of Medical Microbiology, School of Biomedical and Laboratory Sciences, College of Medicine and Health Sciences, University of Gondar, Gondar, Ethiopia

Animut Alebel and Fasil Wagnew
Department of Clinical Nursing, College of Health Sciences, Debre Markos University, Debre Marqos, Ethiopia

Demeke Geremew
Department of Immunology and Molecular Biology, College of Medicine and Health Sciences, University of Gondar, Gondar, Ethiopia

Alebachew Fasil
Department of Clinical Chemistry, College of Medicine and Health Sciences, University of Gondar, Gondar, Ethiopia

Ulrich Sack
Institute of Clinical Immunology, Medical Faculty, University of Leipzig, Leipzig, Germany

Qing Yu, Peng Jia, Li Su and Chengli Que
Department of Respiratory and Critical Care Medicine, Peking University First Hospital, Beijing 100034, China

Hong Zhao
Department of Infectious Disease, Peking University First Hospital, Beijing 100034, China

Rhiannon Ions and Gary Stiefel
Children's Hospital, University Hospitals of Leicester, NHS Trust, Leicester, UK

Manjith Narayanan and Erol A. Gaillard
Children's Hospital, University Hospitals of Leicester, NHS Trust, Leicester, UK
Infection, Immunity and Inflammation, University of Leicester, Leicester, UK

Michael Browning
Immunology, University Hospitals of Leicester, NHS Trust, Leicester, UK

Julian W. Tang
Infection, Immunity and Inflammation, University of Leicester, Leicester, UK
Clinical Microbiology and Virology, University Hospitals of Leicester NHS Trust, Level 5 Sandringham Building, Leicester Royal Infirmary, Infirmary Square, Leicester LE1 5WW, UK

Diya Surie and Eleanor S. Click
Division of Global HIV and TB, Centers for Disease Control and Prevention, Atlanta, GA, USA

Martien W. Borgdorff
Center for Global Health, Office of the Director, Centers for Disease Control and Prevention, Kisumu, Kenya

Kevin P. Cain
Division of Global HIV and TB, Centers for Disease Control and Prevention, Kisumu, Kenya

Kevin M. DeCock
Division of Global HIV and TB, Centers for Disease Control and Prevention, Nairobi, Kenya

Courtney M. Yuen
Division of Global Health Equity, Brigham and Women's Hospital, Boston, MA, USA
Department of Global Health and Social Medicine, Harvard Medical School, Boston, MA, USA

Asfaw Ayalew, Zewdu Gashu, Tadesse Anteneh, Nebiyu Hiruy, Dereje Habte, Degu Jerene and Muluken Melese
Management Sciences for Health, Help Ethiopia Address the Low Performance of Tuberculosis (HEAL TB) Project, Bole Sub City, Kebele 02, House Number 708, Code 1250 Addis Ababa, Ethiopia

Genetu Alem
Amhara Regional Health Bureau, Bahir Dar, Ethiopia

Ilili Jemal
Oromia Regional Health Bureau, Addis Ababa, Ethiopia

Pedro G. Suarez
Management Sciences for Health, Health Programs Group, 4301 North Fairfax Drive, Suite 400, Arlington, VA 22203, USA

Vittoria Offeddu
Saw Swee Hock School of Public Health, National University of Singapore and National University Health System, Singapore 117549, Singapore

Clarence C. Tam
Saw Swee Hock School of Public Health, National University of Singapore and National University Health System, Singapore 117549, Singapore
London School of Hygiene & Tropical Medicine, WC1E7HT, London, UK

Kathryn B. Anderson
University of Minnesota, Minneapolis 55455, USA
Armed Forces Research Institute of Medical Sciences, Bangkok 10400, Thailand

Alden L. Weg, Louis R. Macareo, Damon W. Ellison and Stefan Fernandez
Armed Forces Research Institute of Medical Sciences, Bangkok 10400, Thailand

Ram Rangsin
Phramongkutklao College of Medicine, Bangkok 10400, Thailand

Robert V. Gibbons
University of Texas at San Antonio, San Antonio 78249, USA

In-Kyu Yoon
International Vaccine Institute, Seoul 08826, South Korea

Sriluck Simasathien
Phramongkutklao Hospital, Bangkok 10400, Thailand

Jonathan Underwood
Division of Infectious Diseases, Imperial College London, London, UK

Fiona Cresswell
Lawson Unit, Brighton and Sussex University Hospitals NHS Trust, Brighton, UK

Alex P Salam
King's College London, London, UK

Alex J Keeley
Department of Medicine, Western Sussex Hospitals Trust, Worthing, UK

Charles Cleland
Royal Free Hospital, London, UK

Laurence John and Robert N Davidson
Department of Infectious Diseases, Northwick Park Hospital, Northwest London Teaching Hospitals NHS Trust, London, UK

Kent J. Koster and Lishi Qian
University of Hawaii at Manoa, Honolulu, HI, USA

James T. Douglas
University of Hawaii at Manoa, Honolulu, HI, USA
Pathogen and Microbiome Institute, Northern Arizona University, Flagstaff, AZ, USA

Angela Largen
Hawaii State Department of Health, Honolulu, HI, USA

Kevin P. Drees
University of New Hampshire, Durham, NH, USA

Ed Desmond
California Department of Public Health, Richmond, CA, USA

Xuehua Wan and Shaobin Hou
Advanced Studies in Genomics, Proteomics and Bioinformatics, Honolulu, HI, USA

Jeffrey T. Foster
University of New Hampshire, Durham, NH, USA
Pathogen and Microbiome Institute, Northern Arizona University, Flagstaff, AZ, USA

Roger C. Tine, Léon A. Ndiaye and Oumar Gaye
Service de Parasitologie, Faculté de Médecine, Université Cheikh Anta Diop de Dakar (UCAD), BP5005 Dakar-Fann, Senegal

Mbayame N. Niang, Davy E. Kiori and Ndongo Dia
Laboratoire des Virus respiratoires, Institut Pasteur de Dakar, Dakar, Senegal

Hélène Broutin
Service de Parasitologie, Faculté de Médecine, Université Cheikh Anta Diop de Dakar (UCAD), BP5005 Dakar-Fann, Senegal
MIVEGEC, UMR CNRS -IRD -University of Montpellier - 911, Avenue Agropolis BP 64501, Cédex 5 34394 Montpellier, France

Manlio Monti, Angelo Delmonte, Valentina Fausti, Paola Cravero, Giulia Marcantognini and Giovanni Luca Frassineti
Department of Medical Oncology, Istituto Scientifico Romagnolo per lo Studio e la Cura dei Tumori (IRST) IRCCS, Meldola, Italy

Danila Diano
Radiology Unit, Istituto Scientifico Romagnolo per lo Studio e la Cura dei Tumori (IRST) IRCCS, Meldola, Italy

Francesco Allegrini
Department of Infectious Diseases, Morgagni-Pierantoni Hospital, Forlì, Italy

Jin Li, Mingyu Tang, Bailu Du and Qing Cao
Department of Infectious Diseases, Shanghai Children's Medical Center, Shanghai Jiaotong University School of Medicine, Shanghai, China

Yue Tao and Xi Mo
The Laboratory of Pediatric Infectious Diseases, Pediatric Translational Medicine Institute, Shanghai Children's Medical Center, Shanghai Jiaotong University School of Medicine, Shanghai, China

Yijun Xia
Medical Affairs, Great China | bioMérieux (Shanghai) Company, Limited, Shanghai, China

Denise Andrews, Yumela Chetty and Philip A. Kelly
Division of Acute Medicine, King's College Hospital NHS Foundation Trust, London SE5 9RS, UK

Ben S. Cooper
Mahidol-Oxford Tropical Medicine Research Unit, Faculty of Tropical Medicine, Mahidol University, Bangkok 10400, Thailand
Centre for Tropical Medicine and Global Health, Nuffield Department of Clinical Medicine, University of Oxford, Oxford, UK

Manjinder Virk and Malur Sudhanva
South London Specialist Virology Centre, King's College Hospital NHS Foundation Trust, London SE5 9RS, UK

Stephen K Glass and Dakshika Jeyaratnam
Department of Medical Microbiology, Cheyne Wing, King's College Hospital NHS Foundation Trust, Denmark Hill, London SE5 9RS, UK

Andrew Letters
Infection, Prevention and Control Team, King's College Hospital NHS Foundation Trust, London SE5 9RS, UK

Tao Shi
Department of Orthopedics, The Third Affiliated Hospital of Chongqing Medical University (Gener Hospital), No. 1, Shuanghu Branch Road, Yubei District, Chongqing 401120, China

Tongxin Li, Jungang Li and Jing Wang
Department of Clinical Laboratory, Public Health Medical Center, No. 109, Baoyu Road, Shapingba District, Chongqing 400036, China

Zehua Zhang
Department of Orthopedics, Southwest Hospital, Third Military Medical University, No. 30, Gaotanyan Main Street, Shapingba District, Chongqing 400038, China

Mebrahtu Teweldemedhin
Department of Medical Laboratory Sciences, College of Health Sciences, Aksum University, Aksum, Tigray, Ethiopia

Negasi Asres and Hailay Gebreyesus
Department of Public Health, College of Health Sciences, Aksum University, Aksum, Tigray, Ethiopia

Solomon Weldegebreal Asgedom
School of Pharmacy, College of Health Sciences, Mekelle University, Mekelle, Tigray, Ethiopia

Lili Xu, Chunyan Liu, Yali Duan, Yun Zhu and Zhengde Xie
Beijing Key Laboratory of Pediatric Respiratory Infection Diseases, Key Laboratory of Major Diseases in Children, Ministry of Education, National Clinical Research Center for Respiratory Diseases, National Key Discipline of Pediatrics (Capital Medical University), Beijing Pediatric Research Institute, Beijing Children's Hospital, Capital Medical University, National Center for Children's Health, Beijing, China

Jun Liu and Baoping Xu
National Clinical Research Center for Respiratory Diseases, Resiratory Department, Beijing Children's Hospital, Capital Medical University, National Center for Children's Health, Beijing, China

Alessandro Bidossi, Roberta De Grandi, Marta Bottagisio and Elena De Vecchi
Laboratory of Clinical Chemistry and Microbiology, IRCCS Orthopedic Institute Galeazzi, Milan, Italy

Lorenzo Drago
Laboratory of Clinical Chemistry and Microbiology, IRCCS Orthopedic Institute Galeazzi, Milan, Italy
Department of Biomedical Sciences for Health, Laboratory of Clinical Microbiology, University of Milan, Milan, Italy

Marco Toscano
Department of Biomedical Sciences for Health, Laboratory of Clinical Microbiology, University of Milan, Milan, Italy

Matteo Gelardi
Department of Basic Medical Science, Otolaryngology Unit, Neuroscience and Sensory Organs, University of Bari Aldo Moro, Bari, Italy

Kyaw Ko Ko Htet
Department of Medical Research (Pyin Oo Lwin Branch), Pyin Oo Lwin 100201, Myanmar

Tippawan Liabsuetrakul, Edward B. McNeil and Virasakdi Chongsuvivatwong
Epidemiology Unit, Faculty of Medicine, Prince of Songkla University, Hat Yai, Songkhla 90110, Thailand

Saw Thein
Ministry of Health and Sports, National Tuberculosis Programme, Mandalay 100107, Myanmar

V. Q. Hoa
Vietnam National Lung Hospital, National Tuberculosis Programme Vietnam, 463 Hoang Hoa Tham street, Badinh District, Hanoi, Vietnam

N. B. Hoa
Vietnam National Lung Hospital, National Tuberculosis Programme Vietnam, 463 Hoang Hoa Tham street, Badinh District, Hanoi, Vietnam
Centre for Operational Research, International Union Against Tuberculosis and Lung Disease, Paris, France

P. D. Phuc and N. T. Hien
Center for Public Health and Ecosystem Research, Hanoi University of Public Health, Hanoi, Vietnam
Institute of Environmental Health and Sustainable Development, Hanoi, Vietnam

P. H. Thuong and P. T. Anh
Hanoi Lung Hospital, Hanoi, Vietnam

N. V. Nhung
Vietnam National Lung Hospital, National Tuberculosis Programme Vietnam, 463 Hoang Hoa Tham street, Badinh District, Hanoi, Vietnam
Vietnam Association for Tuberculosis and Lung Disease, Hanoi, Vietnam

Giuseppe Lapadula
Division of Infectious Diseases, "San Gerardo" Hospital, Via GB Pergolesi 33, Monza, Italy

Anna Maria Peri
Division of Infectious Diseases, "San Gerardo" Hospital, Via GB Pergolesi 33, Monza, Italy
Infectious Diseases Unit, Fondazione IRCCS Ca' Granda, Ospedale Maggiore Policlinico, University of Milan, Milan, Italy

Andrea Gori
Infectious Diseases Unit, Fondazione IRCCS Ca' Granda, Ospedale Maggiore Policlinico, University of Milan, Milan, Italy

Davide Paolo Bernasconi
Centre of Biostatistics for Clinical Epidemiology, School of Medicine and Surgery, University of Milano-Bicocca, Milan, Italy

Nadia Galizzi
"San Raffaele" Hospital, "Vita-Salute" University, Milan, Italy

Alberto Matteelli
Department of Infectious and Tropical Diseases, WHO Collaborating Centre for TB/HIV and TB elimination, University of Brescia, Brescia, Italy

Luigi Codecasa
Regional TB Reference Centre, "Villa Marelli" Institute, Niguarda Hospital, Milan, Italy

Vincenza Giorgio
"L. Fallacara" Hospital, Triggiano, BA, Italy

Antonio Di Biagio
Infectious Diseases Department, IRCCS AOU San Martino-IST, Genova, Italy

Fabio Franzetti
"L. Sacco" Hospital, University of Milan, Milan, Italy

Antonella Cingolani
Policlinico "Gemelli", "Sacro Cuore" Catholic University, Rome, Italy

Yi Liu, Xuxia Zhang, Yuqing Zhang, Yong Sun, Cong Yao, Wei Wang and Chuanyou Li
Department of Bacteriology and Immunology, Beijing Key Laboratory on Drug-Resistant Tuberculosis Research, Beijing Tuberculosis and Thoracic Tumor Research Institute/Beijing Chest Hospital, Capital Medical University, Beijing 101149, China

Jin-Kyu Cho
Department of Surgery, Gyeongsang National University Hospital, 15, Jinju-daero 816 beon-gil, Jinju-si 52727, Gyeongnam, Republic of Korea

Young Min Choi
Department of Internal Medicine, Gyeongsang National University School of Medicine and Gyeongsang National University Hospital, 15, Jinju-daero 816 beon-gil, Jinju-si, Gyeongnam 52727, Republic of Korea

Ra Ri Cha, Wan Soo Kim and Jin Joo Kim
Department of Internal Medicine, Gyeongsang National University School of Medicine and Gyeongsang National University Hospital, 15, Jinju-daero 816 beon-gil, Jinju-si, Gyeongnam 52727, Republic of Korea
Department of Internal Medicine, Gyeongsang National University Changwon Hospital, Changwon, Republic of Korea

Sang Soo Lee, Jae Min Lee and Hyun Jin Kim
Department of Internal Medicine, Gyeongsang National University School of Medicine and Gyeongsang National University Hospital, 15, Jinju-daero 816 beon-gil, Jinju-si, Gyeongnam 52727, Republic of Korea
Institute of Health Sciences, Gyeongsang National University, Jinju, Republic of Korea
Department of Internal Medicine, Gyeongsang National University Changwon Hospital, Changwon, Republic of Korea

Hong Jun Kim, Chang Yoon Ha, Tae Hyo Kim, Woon Tae Jung and Ok Jae Lee
Department of Internal Medicine, Gyeongsang National University Changwon Hospital, Changwon, Republic of Korea
Institute of Health Sciences, Gyeongsang National University, Jinju, Republic of Korea

Hye Kyong Park
Department of Internal Medicine, Gyeongsang National University Changwon Hospital, Changwon, Republic of Korea

Judith Provoost, Nathalie Freymond, Emilie Perrot, Lize Kiakouama-Maleka and Agathe Sénéchal
Département de Pneumologie, Hospices Civils de Lyon, Lyon, France

Sandrine Roux
Département des Maladies infectieuses et tropicales, Hôpital de la Croix-Rousse, Hospices Civils de Lyon, 103, Grande-Rue de la Croix-Rousse, 69317, cedex 04 Lyon, France

Christian Chidiac
Département des Maladies infectieuses et tropicales, Hôpital de la Croix-Rousse, Hospices Civils de Lyon, 103, Grande-Rue de la Croix-Rousse, 69317, cedex 04 Lyon, France
Université Claude Bernard Lyon 1, Lyon, France

Florent Valour and Florence Ader
Département des Maladies infectieuses et tropicales, Hôpital de la Croix-Rousse, Hospices Civils de Lyon, 103, Grande-Rue de la Croix-Rousse, 69317, cedex 04 Lyon, France
CIRI-Centre International de Recherche en Infectiologie, Inserm, U1111, Université Claude Bernard Lyon 1, CNRS, UMR5308, Ecole Normale Supérieure de Lyon, Univ Lyon, F-69007 Lyon, France
Université Claude Bernard Lyon 1, Lyon, France

Pierre-Jean Souquet
Département de Pneumologie, Hospices Civils de Lyon, Lyon, France
Université Claude Bernard Lyon 1, Lyon, France

Delphine Gamondes
Département de Radiologie, Hospices Civils de Lyon, Lyon, France

Gérard Lina and Oana Dumitrescu
CIRI-Centre International de Recherche en Infectiologie, Inserm, U1111, Université Claude Bernard Lyon 1, CNRS, UMR5308, Ecole Normale Supérieure de Lyon, Univ Lyon, F-69007 Lyon, France
Université Claude Bernard Lyon 1, Lyon, France
Institut des Agents Infectieux, Hospices Civils de Lyon, Lyon, France

Index

CPSIA information can be obtained
at www.ICGtesting.com
Printed in the USA
LVHW060855030122
707669LV00002B/180

9 781639 274673